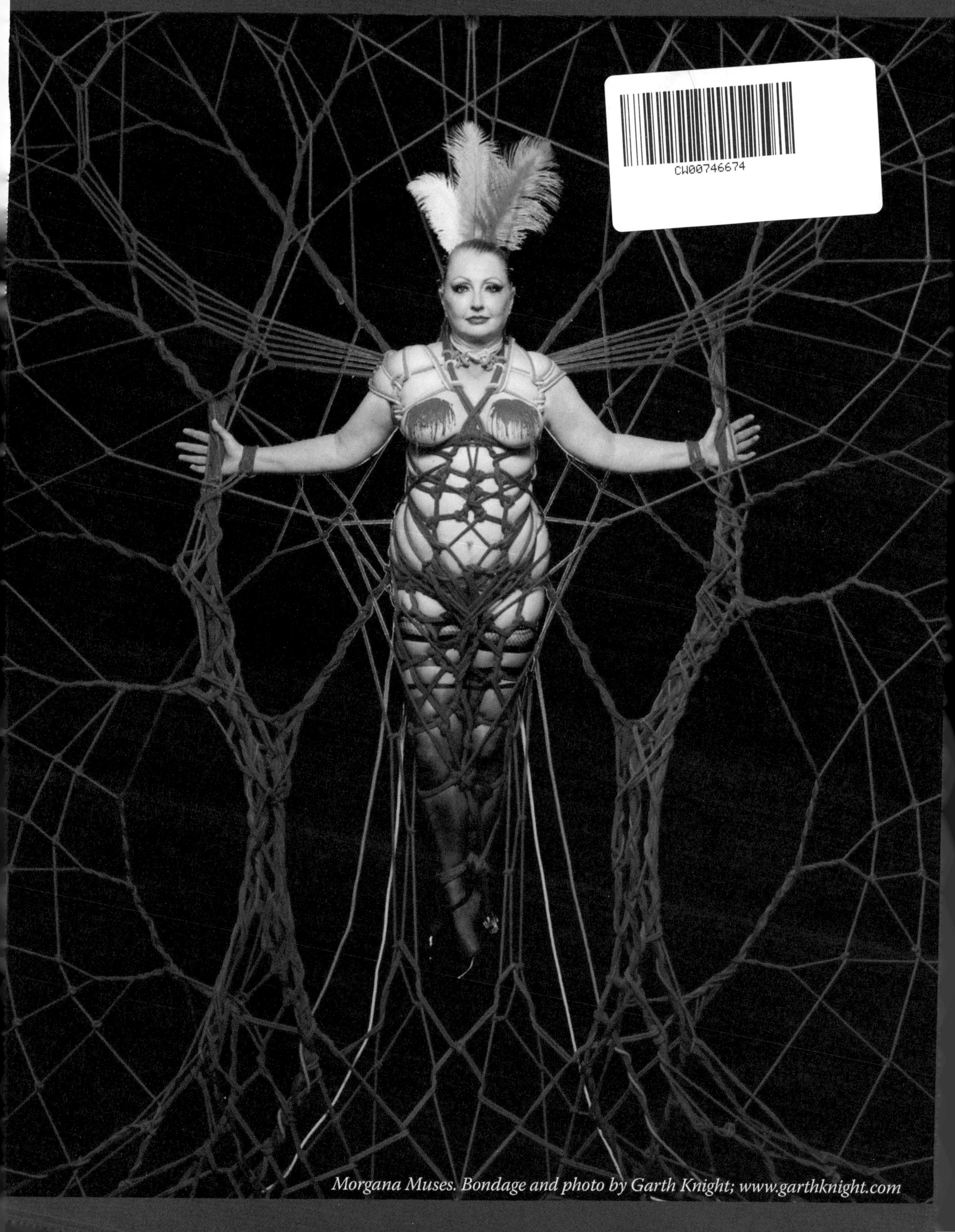

Morgana Muses. Bondage and photo by Garth Knight; www.garthknight.com

For my angel, Lily.
May the world be even more accepting
by the time you grow up.

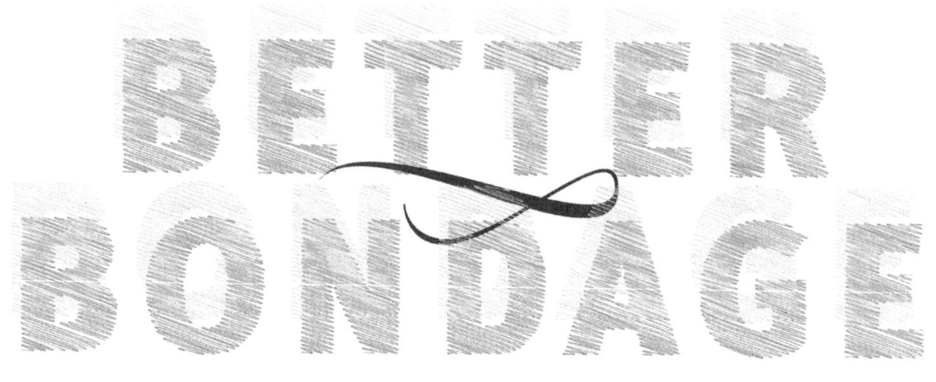

for EVERY BODY

Evie Vane

Wanton Press
San Francisco

© 2017 by Evelyn Vane. All rights reserved. All photos are © their original owners and are used with permission.

No part of this publication may be reproduced, stored, or introduced into a retrieval system, or transmitted, in any form or by any means (electronic, mechanical, photocopying, recording, or otherwise), without the prior written permission of the author or, for photos, of the original copyright holder.

The scanning, uploading, and distribution of this book via the Internet or via any other means without the permission of the author is illegal and punishable by law.

For permission requests, write to the publisher, addressed "Attention: Permissions Coordinator," at the address below.

Wanton Press

P.O. Box 210739

San Francisco, CA 94121

www.RopeBottoming.com

ISBN 978-1533152114

This book contains explicit material and is intended for mature audiences. All photos depict consensual scenes.

Cover design by David Delp

Cover photo by The Silence; location courtesy of _impysh_

Book design by MJ Maxam

Photo credits for back cover (top to bottom):

Terri F. Bondage by Demonsix and Zetsu Nawa. Photo by Retrotie. Hair and makeup by Anastasia Panagiotidis

Luis Miguel Jiménez Villalba. Bondage by BrAxTeR. Photo by Tentesion

Ashley Lane and Kel Bowie. Bondage by Kel Bowie. Photo by The_Silence

Cat. Bondage by -EM-. Photo by iambic9

Bradley Cuttlefish and FredRx. Bondage by FredRx. Photo by Cam Damage

Also by Evie Vane: *The Little Guide to Getting Tied Up*

Introduction

Has it been two and a half years already since *The Little Guide to Getting Tied Up* was published? Time flies when you're in rope! That book got an outpouring of support that makes my heart all melty. And although it was focused on rope bottoming, rope tops got into it too, saying it helped them understand their partners better—which I hadn't even thought of but which now seems obvious.

I've learned a lot more since then too! Some things were "duuuuuh" moments, some are tips and tricks gleaned from other rope lovers, and some are lessons from that greatest of teachers: making mistakes.

Rope bottoming as a "thing" has really taken off in the past few years. You'll now find a slew of resources on my FetLife profile (and at the end of this book), and some of those links even take you to other slews of links. Education for rope bottoms has grown exponentially, and even many instructors on the top side are now including components for bottoms in their teachings. Writings on being in rope have reached FetLife's Kinky & Popular page, and are appearing on more personal profile pages and blogs than ever before. There are even videos besides the pornographic kind, and some are even free.

The days of "using up" bondage models, of uncommunicative rope scenes in which the bottom's needs and safety aren't considered, seem to have greatly diminished. Maybe one day they will be completely a thing of the past.

This book builds on *The Little Guide to Getting Tied Up*—and if you haven't cracked that one yet, please consider it. It covers a lot of safety stuff, which is important because rope can be highly dangerous. **Do not attempt what you see in the photos here without the proper training.** You could experience injuries from rope that last from hours to years. You could die from rope bondage, especially if it's combined with breath play. Know what you're getting yourself into.

Minimizing risk was the biggest goal of the previous book. The focus of this one is more on ways to deepen the enjoyment of being in rope and on understanding the experience better. And there's quite a bit for tops too! Most of all, it's a celebration of community and of all of us in rope. Because let's get something straight: The majority of us are *not* the models flooding the pages of Facebook's secret rope groups, FetLife's Kinky & Popular page, and most fetish magazines. I hope this book has a ripple effect leading to more exposure and celebration of ropesters in all their diverse beauty. It's about time, don't you think?

As for community, this book was an "it takes a village" effort if ever there was one! Experts and ropesters at large from around the world generously contributed their time and effort to write, consult, answer survey questions, provide photos, and speak with me in person. Many also sent heartfelt messages of support that kept my motivation strong while holed up alone working on this day after day. I want to hug everyone who helped out until my arms ache! This book shows that we really *are* a community, despite all of our different styles, preferences, and opinions.

Bliss and photo by Marcuslikesit; www.marcuslikesit.com

All names, quoted material, and photos are used with permission; most of the names are FetLife handles or scene names to protect privacy. The photos are a mix of professional and amateur shots. There are no doubt countless more stunning photos that never hit my radar, so please consider the ones here a small sampling and not by any means a "best of" collection.

No single book can be a one-stop shop for those who love being in rope. I recommend being proactive about exploring for yourself and discovering complementary practices. And please know that you alone are ultimately responsible for your safety in rope. By reading this book, you absolve me and all contributors of any and all liability should you experience a rope-related injury. Use what you find herein at your own risk.

As noted in *The Little Guide*, I'm not a medical or fitness pro. I'm just a rope bottom on a journey, like you are. So if anything here doesn't resonate with you, toss it out the window and come up with something that does—and then maybe consider writing about that so the rest of us can benefit too. Learning about what works for you and how to make it happen is key to enjoying your time in rope. Rope bottoming is a practice of self-exploration, and in the end only you can figure out how to get to where you want to be.

I hope this book helps you on your journey, and wish you the best of luck on it!

Love and hugs,

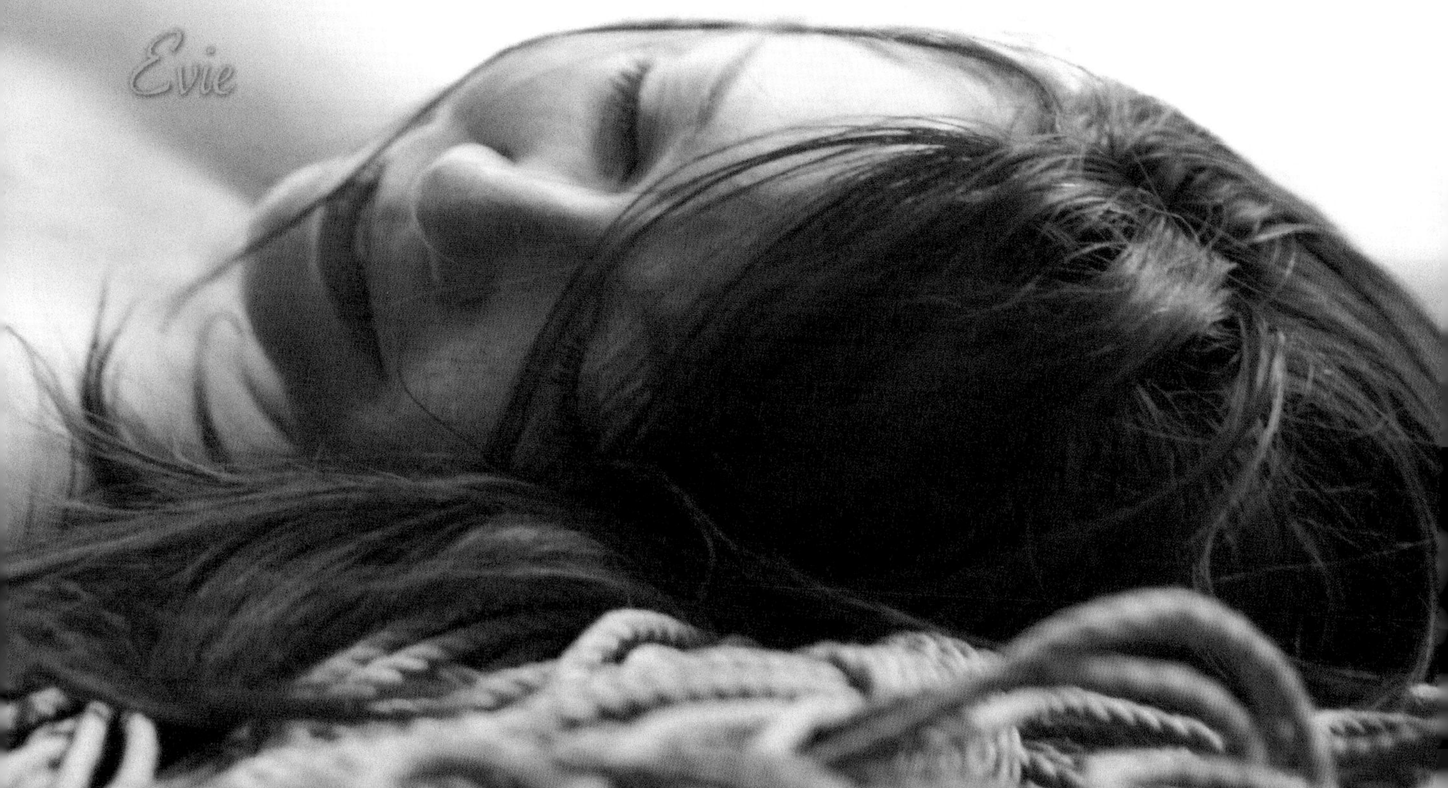

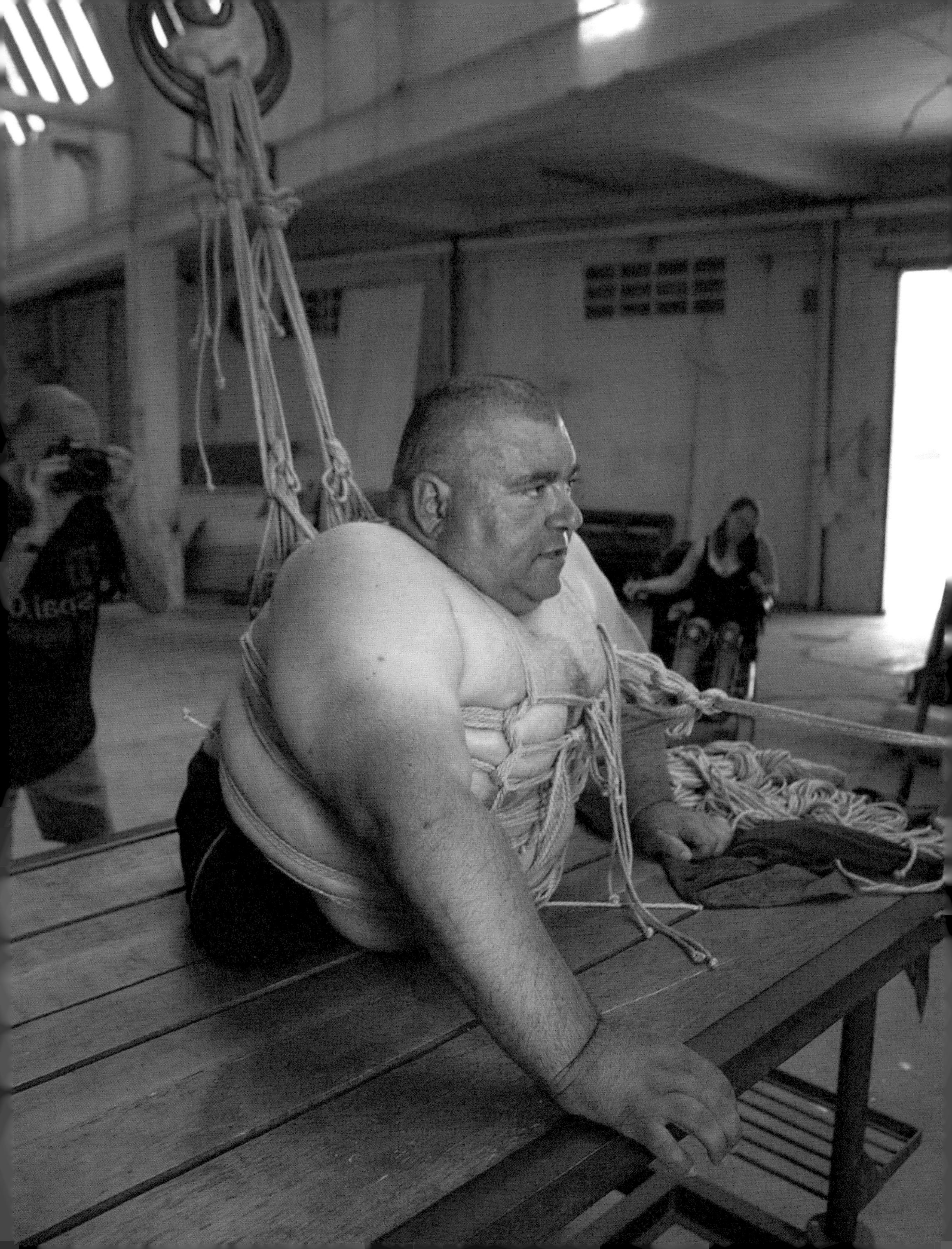

Chapter 1
Inspiration

Whether you're having trouble finding the courage to try bondage, certain issues are making your rope journey a challenge, or you're comparing yourself to others and feeling bad about it, these three blog posts might help. I actually return to these myself whenever I'm struggling with something about my rope bottoming!

A Motto for Rope Bottoms Facing Challenges

So you can't touch your toes or fit into size-0 pants, or ibuprofen is your constant companion. Is rope bondage destined to just be forever a dream?

Not likely. While you should always consult a medical professional before trying bondage if you have concerns, and should research all the risks (nerve damage, for instance)[1] along with consent and negotiation,[2] so many kinds of rope bondage exist that there could easily be one that suits you. It may just take a little figuring out.

You may benefit from modified ties or positions. You may need to find a partner who can work with your issues. You may find changing your own assumptions, perceptions, or mindset beneficial. And you may find my own motto, which I came up with to help me deal with being an older (47-year-old) rope bottom, helpful too:

Patience. Persistence. Resilience

1. Patience. An older body may take longer to warm up and heal. A male body, a curvy one, or one with physical issues may take longer for a rope top to learn how to tie. A gender-nonconforming body may be going through stages of changes over a long period of time. Instead of seeing this time needed as a negative, we can see it as a gift that allows us to more deeply experience our bodies than someone who takes the body for granted because things come more easily.

In my 20s I was so impatient and restless that I couldn't really enjoy anything in the moment—I was always wondering what was next, how the situation could be improved, was there something better/more fun/more worthwhile somewhere else? Two decades later as I slowly and carefully stretch before a rope scene or see marks that linger for months, I savor the joy of just being and offer gratitude for my body that it has taken me so far and done so much, and gratitude for life that over many years has given me the gift of more patience.

Patience applies to our minds when we compare ourselves to others and when self-doubt arises too. I've started thinking in terms of meditation: how when we meditate, we treat those random thoughts that wander in as clouds floating by—we notice them and move on, without judgment or self-criticism. When I find myself looking at photos of younger, bendier rope bottoms in amazing poses and comparing myself in a negative way, I notice the thought and then let it float past. I'm patient with my thoughts instead of lamenting them. Those photos have nothing to do with the beauty and magic of my own rope scenes. And amazing poses are certainly not required for an amazing scene anyway!

Jaume and Iris. Bondage by NoShibari and Glü Wür. Photo by Xavier Basiana Vers

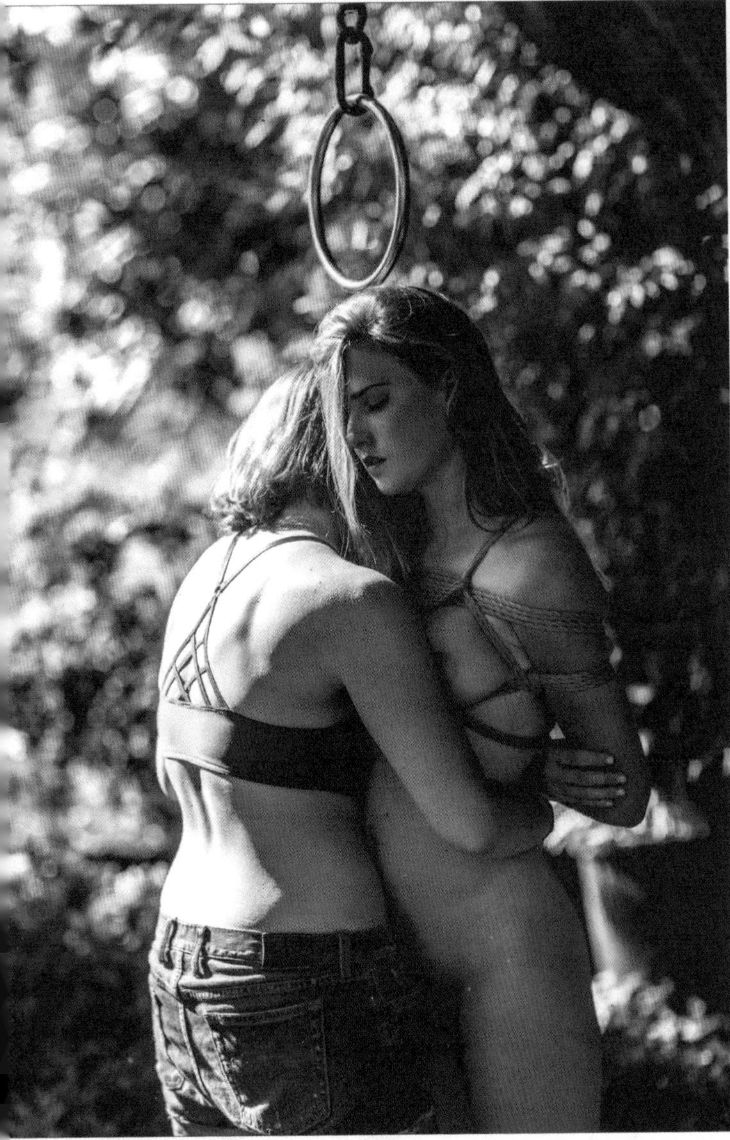

Kel Bowie and Ashley Lane. Bondage by Kel Bowie. Photo by The Silence

2. *Persistence.* "Find 12 ways around the word 'no,'" recommends TMZ founder Harvey Levin in an interview in an in-flight magazine. Sage advice for a rope bottom facing challenges, and it applies to ourselves and our bodies as well as to things like finding partners.

Persistence might be needed for working around physical issues, whether from age or size or shape or things like chronic pain or limited mobility. Some rope bottoms have found ways around the body's saying no that will make your heart sing.

Persistence might be needed for finding partners, because rope bottoms facing challenges may have to work harder at this. Finding ways around no doesn't mean hounding someone until they give in to playing with us, by the way. It means honoring one person's no and moving on to someone who may say yes. We may have to do this way more times than someone else, but think of it like being an actor who gets rejected over and over before landing a big part. Oscar nominee Naomi Watts made her film debut in 1986 but didn't hit it big until *15 years* later, with *Mulholland Drive* (2001).[3] She sometimes thought, "I can't handle it. I'm giving up"[4] during all those years of low-profile or no roles, but did she give up? Nope, and now she's a celebrity. That's persistence.

3. *Resilience.* Rope bottoms facing challenges may have to deal with more frustrations, setbacks, and rejections than other rope bottoms. Not internalizing those things—learning how to deal with them without letting them define us, rising above them—is key to getting the most out of our rope journeys. We can't experience the heights of rope joy if we're stuck in the muck of feeling regret, self-pity, bitterness, or any other feeling that doesn't serve us.

My resilience as an older rope bottom comes from reminding myself that my body has done amazing things, like given birth to a child, climbed a mountain in Switzerland, held the hand of a loved one as she passed from this earth. Other people's resilience might come from remembering that they've changed even one person's stereotypical perception, or had the courage to be true to themselves when no one else

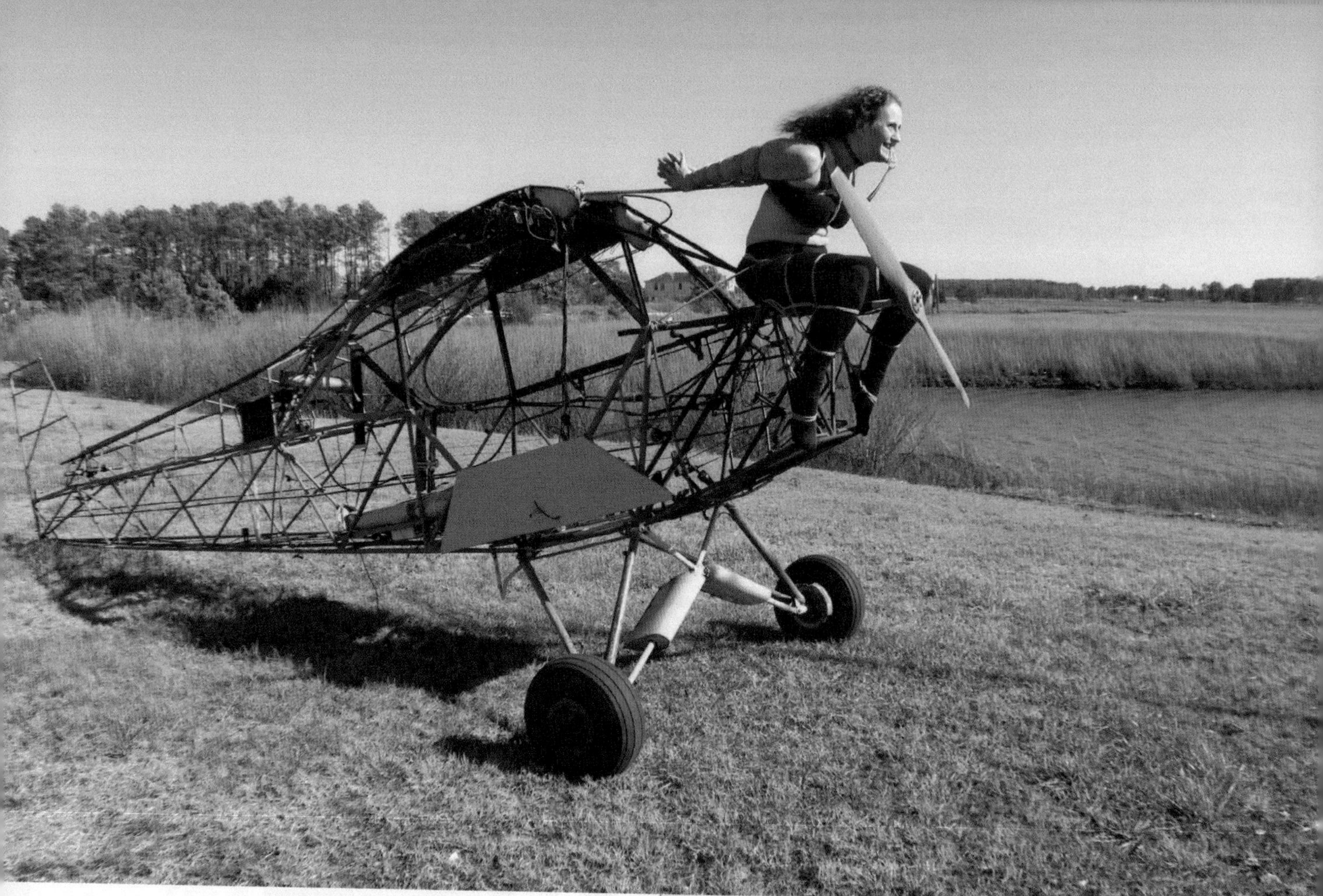

Anne-X. Bondage and photo by KnotRod

they knew was like them, or did a challenging rope scene after they were told it wasn't possible. Whatever renews and reaffirms our confidence and sense of self-worth in the face of challenges can help our resilience.

And resilience may be helped by reminding ourselves that the more we've been through, the more we've grown and deepened. All of our experiences, whether we consider them positive or negative, are our teachers. They teach us compassion; they give us a greater understanding of ourselves and the world. They make our lives richer and more meaningful. They allow us to live our lives more fully.

With patience, persistence, and resilience, we can all celebrate what makes us uniquely us, and how we make the rope community as a whole richer, deeper, and more vibrant. A single musical note doesn't make a song, let alone a symphony.

All of us, with every unique note we contribute, make the rope community a symphony. And that's something to celebrate.

• • •

The "Not Good Enough" Rope Bottoming Mentality

After the bliss of a rope scene fades, maybe in an hour or two, maybe in a day or two, thoughts of all my shortcomings start rearing their ugly heads. I curse my lower back's inflexibility, feel ashamed about asking for adjustments, wish I had been able to stay in the rope longer, wish I had been more graceful or more attractive...just more. Better.

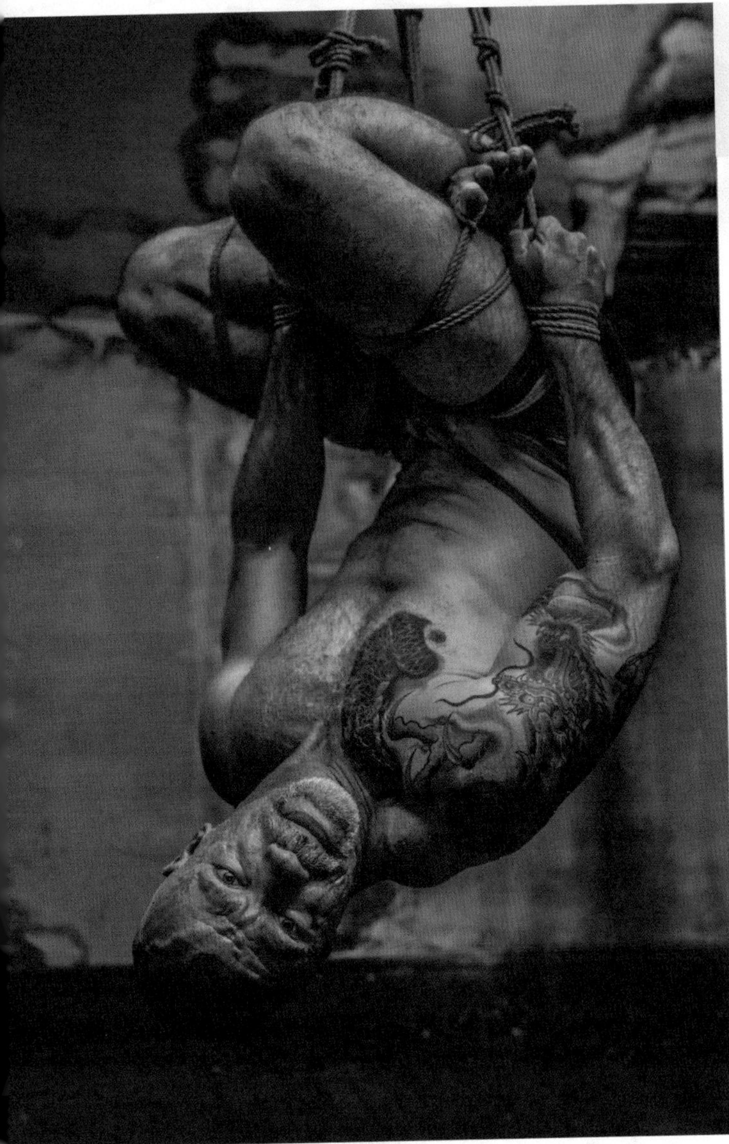

Bill Dudley. Bondage by Aeolis Est. Photo by Tyler Neuroth Photography; www.NeurothPhotography.com

Maybe it's the rope drop talking. What goes up must come down, and maybe the self-doubt is on the other side of bliss on the pendulum's swing. Or maybe it's just my perfectionistic personality. Whatever the reason, I know my perception is warped. But warped or not, there it is, that dark cloud of self-doubt hovering relentlessly.

Surely other rope bottoms have felt this at some point. The question is, What can we do about it?

We could try to eliminate all the things we have the self-doubt about. For example, I could finally buy that darn contortionist DVD and seriously strive for more flexibility. I could lose those extra pounds and get more fit. I could find someone to do more rope bottoming "lab time" with to work on improving.

But something tells me I'd still feel not good enough. Because there's always room for improvement. If you eradicate those particular issues, others will just slide in to take their place. Because beating back self-doubt doesn't happen by letting it control you.

Of course, improvement can be a worthy idea, as long as our self-esteem isn't tied to the results—as long as we aren't attached to the outcome, which is a Zen concept and which is much easier said than done, for me anyway.

If "fixing" the issues won't make the self-doubt go away, what will?

Talking with the partner in the rope play seems like a good idea. But I'm loath to unleash all of my insecurities on someone I'm hoping will find me desirable enough to want to tie with again. Telling a rope top all the ways you think you fell short as a rope bottom... not so sexy I think. It could also make them think they did something wrong. Besides, I know my perception is warped and that the feelings will ease eventually (ease but not entirely disappear).

Journaling helps a little. So does writing down one positive thought for every negative one, in two columns. For instance, in column A goes "stupid embarrassing inflexible lower back," and in column B goes

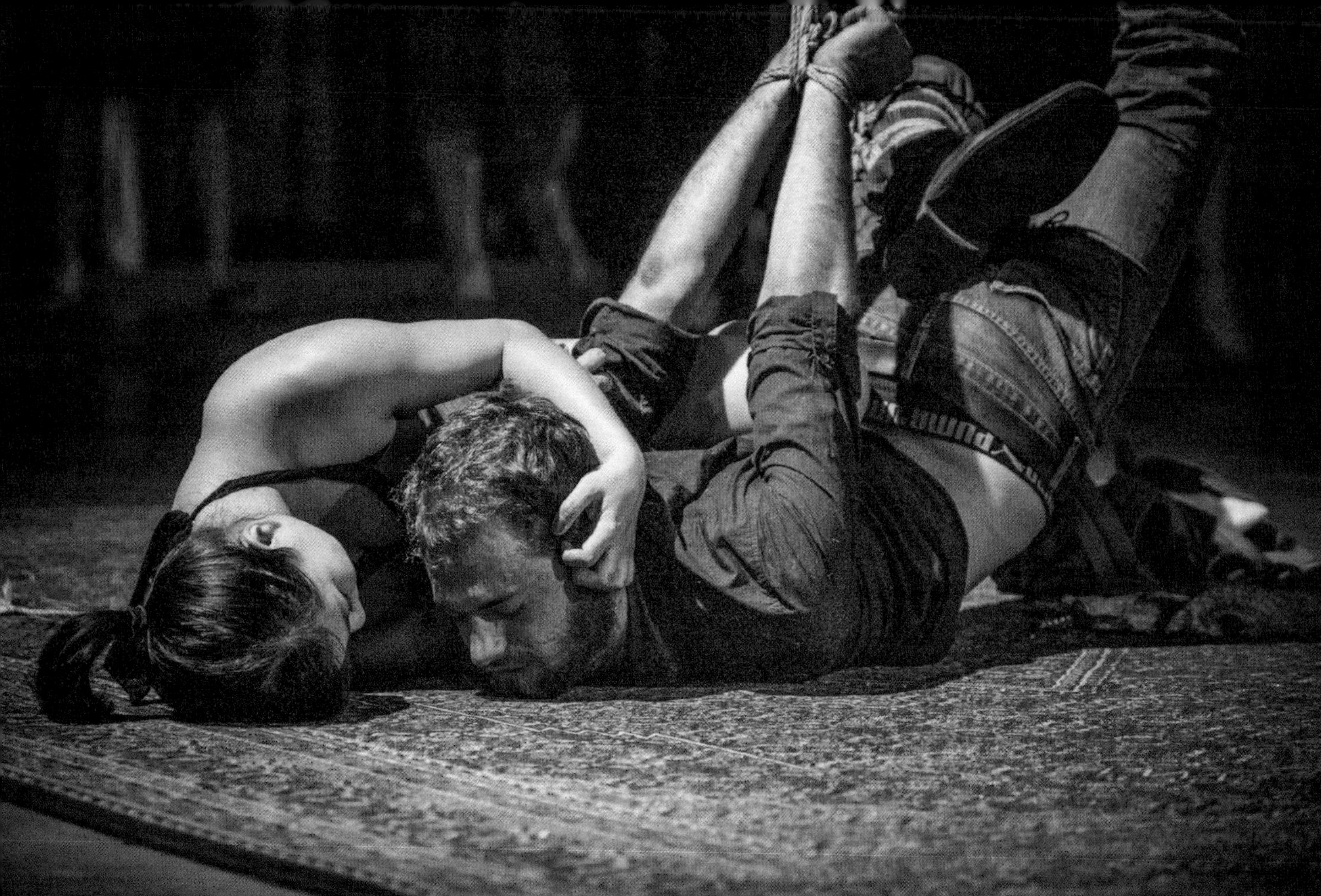

E-mechanic and Kat. Bondage by Kat. Photo by iambic9

"was totally present." But I tend to give more weight to the negative side, so that's not a complete solution.

What seems to help the most is talking with other rope bottoms, in person or online. Every time I've spoken or posted something about my mistakes, thoughts, or feelings, someone if not many someones has been right there saying, "Me too." I think a lot of us feel like our issues and problems and insecurities as rope bottoms (or even just in general) are unique just to us. But I'm also pretty sure that no matter what it is, someone else can identify with it—and often can even offer wisdom or insight that helps.

That's one of the reasons I feel so strongly about the idea of a rope community, and in particular a rope bottoming community. This thing we do, there's no road map for it. You can't study rope bottoming in college or read reams of rope bottoming studies and manuals, because they don't exist. All we have is one another and our collective knowledge and experiences. And the more we can share that knowledge and those experiences, the more we can support one another, the better off we'll all be.

• • •

The One Thing That Will Make You a Super Rope Bottom

You gaze in awe at the gorgeous bondage models, their slender limbs stretched into unbelievable poses by artfully placed rope, their faces enrapt or etched beautifully with suffering. "Well, hell," you might think. "I could never be as good a bondage bottom as they are."

And you would be wrong.

What makes a great rope bottom? This question comes up often in the rope community. You'll hear answers like flexibility, stamina, an ability to surrender...and yes, those things do help expand the range of bondage play possibilities. You may hear about good communication, which is essential, since rope play even with experienced partners can cause nerve damage and other injuries. You may hear about being a petite size, which is utter bullshit (see Shay's article in Chapter 6). What you might never hear is the one thing I consider to be the most important of all:

Be honest.

"That's it?" you might be thinking, shaking your head in disbelief. "How is honesty going to help me touch my toes to my head in a full backbend 10 feet in the air while spinning around blindfolded? How is honesty going to make me 20 pounds thinner so the rope doesn't squeeze my flesh like an overstuffed sausage?"

It's not. But those things aren't what makes a great rope bottom. A great rope bottom—a *super* rope bottom—is simply one who is an active participant in creating a successful scene. And what exactly makes for a successful scene, the kind that lingers long after it's over, causing those sweet little shivers of joy at random moments? It's one where you meet each other in a place beyond everyday mundanities, where you feel raw or intimate or connected or like the whole world is in its place. You see and are seen like never before. And that has zero to do with physical feats of derring-do or supermodel looks.

How does being honest help make a scene successful?

You will choose partners you instinctively and honestly feel good about, as opposed to playing with people because you feel bad about turning them down or for whatever other reason. It's hard to have a beautiful, memorable scene with someone you don't really feel good about (duh, right?).

Being honest about both your desires and limits (physical and mental) will help set the intention, help you relax, and help keep you safe. If you haven't been honest that you'd like a sensuous seduction and you're playing with a hard-core sadist, what are your chances of success? (Hint: not good.) And if you haven't been honest about, say, your troublesome shoulder, a scene featuring many common ties can tank pretty quickly.

When you let your honest self shine through in the rope, the one who is scared or shy or thrilled or passionate, you open the door to that otherworldly place and invite your partner to enter with you. When you drop into the moment with your partner, feeling whatever you're feeling instead of trying to be that film-worthy bondage model, seeing your partner for who they are too, you are summoning the deepest magic you have as a bondage bottom.

When you are honest with yourself about what did and didn't work in a scene, and the things you can do to make future scenes better, you put yourself on the path to improvement. And having the mindset of always looking to improve—while still understanding that you are perfect exactly as you are—you will continually grow and contribute new and wondrous things to your rope scenes and partners.

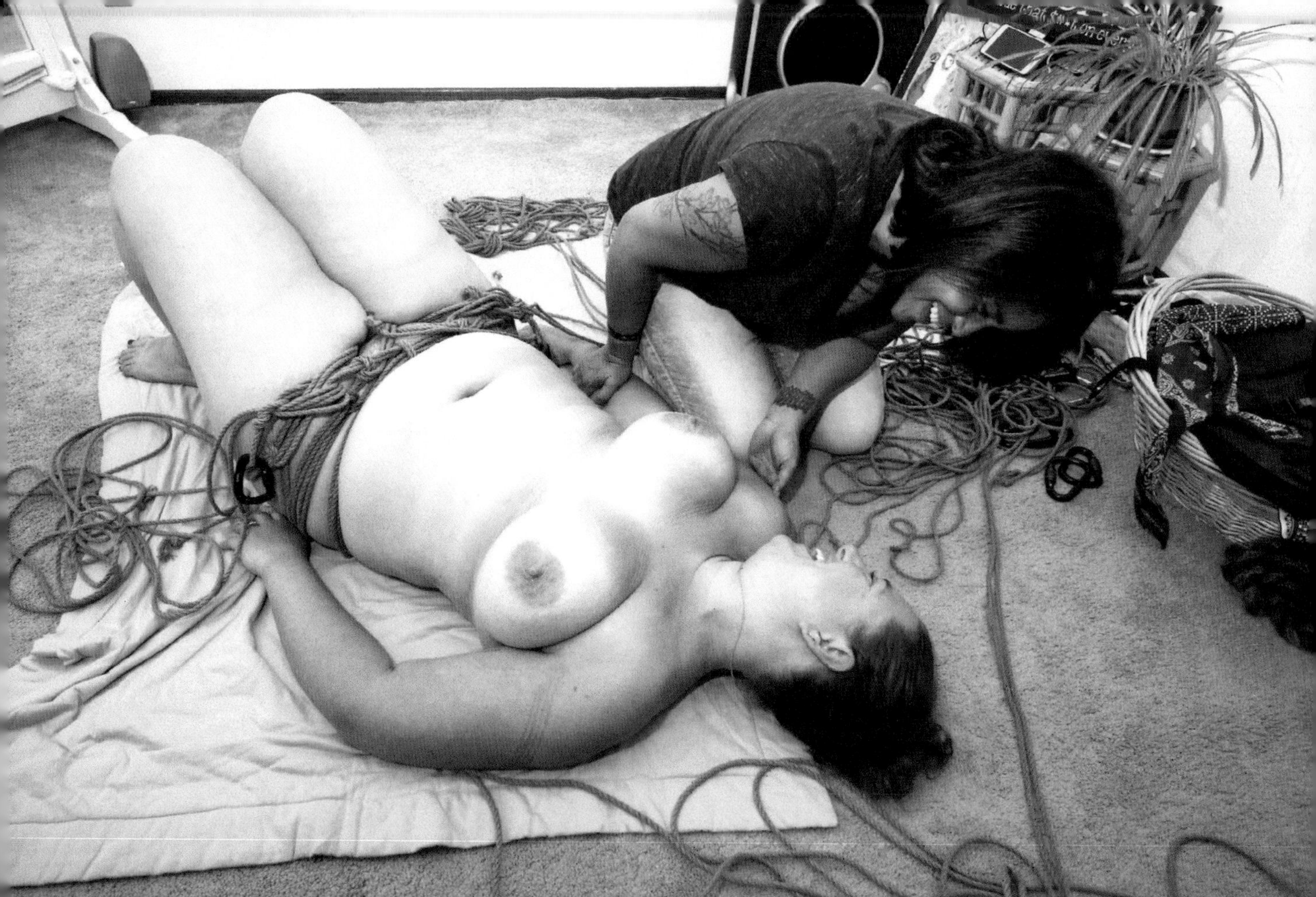

SaucyBelle and ShesANatural. Bondage by ShesANatural. Photo by Conroy

Without honesty, you may as well be a sack of potatoes. With it, you offer your partner the most precious gift of all: your true self. With it, you become an empowered, active contributor to a wonderful experience for you both. In my opinion, that makes you the very best kind of rope bottom. (And btw, the bondage models whose photos tend to be so compelling are the ones whose honest, real commitment to their partner and the scene just radiates off the image, don't you think?)

Notes

1. RemedialRopes.com offers articles on nerve damage and other potential issues.
2. Jay Wiseman offers both comprehensive and shorter forms for general BDSM negotiation at http://www.evilmonk.org/a/wiseman10.cfm
3. http://www.lifetimetv.co.uk/biography/biography-naomi-watts
4. http://www.pearlanddean.com/news/naomi-watts-i-was-ready-give

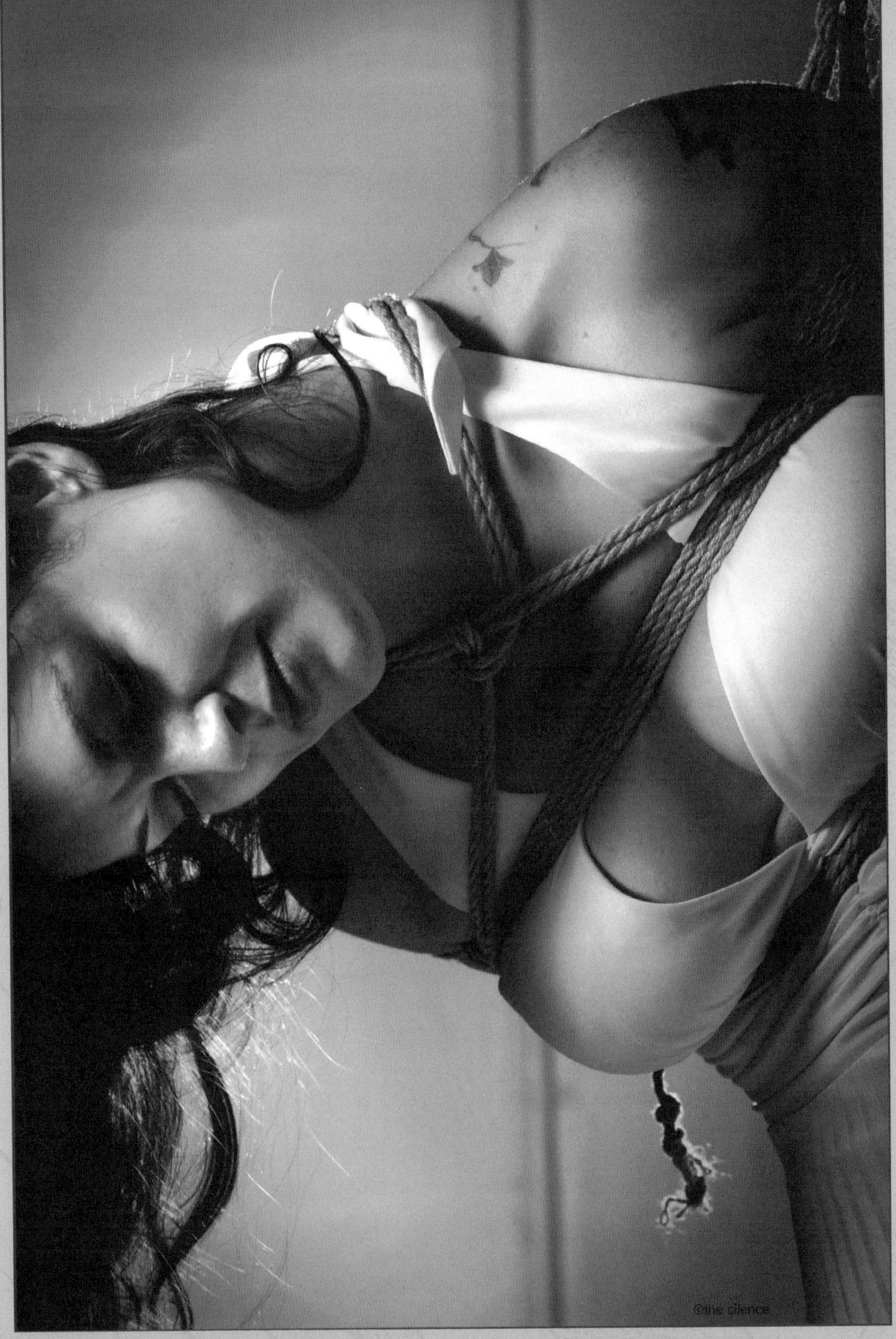

©the silence

Chapter 2
Anatomy for Rope Bondage

by MissDoctor

MissDoctor is a kink-friendly practicing physician who works in primary care with an emphasis on musculoskeletal medicine, endocrinology, and women's health. She has been in private practice for five years and has been involved in the world of bondage for over 18 years.

Key

X = vulnerable area of nerve

—— = area where nerve runs more superficially

- - - - = area where nerve runs more deeply (protected by overlying muscles)

Dotted areas = places where you will feel sensation corresponding to the same color-coded nerves

RADIAL NERVE (red areas)

- Helps extend the wrist
- Provides sensation on side of thumb and back of hand/wrist
- Damage to upper portion of nerve can cause wrist drop; damage to lower portion of nerve affects sensation only

ULNAR NERVE (blue areas)

- Helps ring and pinkie fingers move from side to side and flex
- Provides sensation on ring and pinkie fingers and part of palm
- Damage at wrist limits side-to-side finger movement; damage at elbow also limits flexion of these fingers

MEDIAN NERVE (green areas)

- Helps flex thumb, index finger, and middle finger; helps rotate palm downward
- Provides sensation for most of palm and thumb, index finger, and middle finger
- Damage at wrist limits ability to make a fist

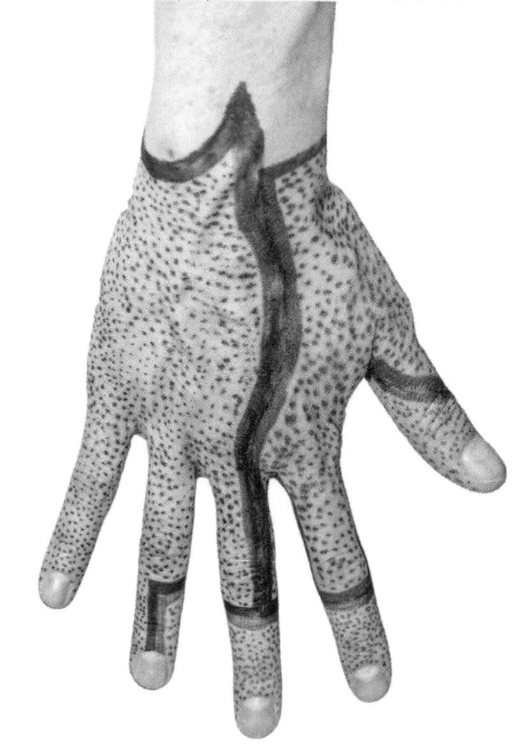

Anatomy photo credits

Model: Greta Poley

Photos by Samir Rengifo

"Rope play is edge play."

This phrase gets thrown around a lot in the world of rope bondage. But what does it mean, and why should you as a rope bottom pay attention?

Rope is a tool that can be used for bondage, just like leather, fabric, metal chains...pretty much anything you can imagine! What makes rope riskier than some of these

MissDoctor. Bondage and photo by The Silence

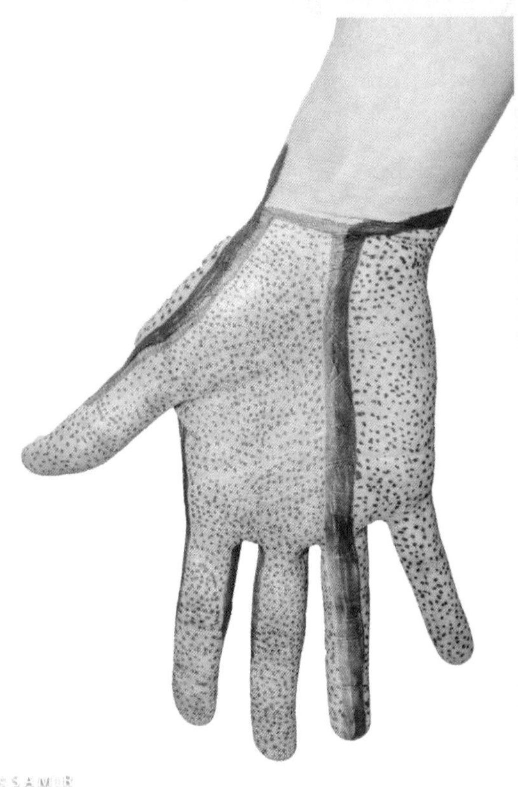

© SAMIR

other materials, however, is how tightly and precisely it can compress and create a shearing force on important parts of your anatomy (more on those concepts below). If rope is improperly placed or tensioned over a nerve, it can cause temporary or even permanent damage to that nerve and the parts of the body connected to it.

The goal of this chapter is to make you much more aware of your own anatomy so that you can communicate better with your rope partner(s) to prevent and mitigate injuries.

Nerves 101

Let's start with some basic information about nerves. Nerves are like long, thin wires connecting your brain to all the different structures in your body—your skin, organs, muscles, joints, etc. Nerves are made up of bundles of microscopic fibers that are each individually wrapped in a protective coating, called myelin. These bundles are then bound together by layers of connective tissue to make up the larger nerve, which can in some cases be seen by the naked eye. One of the things about nerves that is often overlooked is that each large nerve actually contains very small blood vessels. These vessels run the length of the nerve, bringing the fibers oxygen and nutrients and removing toxins. Compression of a nerve can interrupt that blood supply.

Nerves in the arms and legs (the ones that we care the most about in rope bondage) fall into two categories: sensory and motor. Sensory nerves carry information about stimuli like temperature, vibration, pressure, and pain from the periphery to the brain, where it can be interpreted. Yes, there are specific fibers that carry pain signals, and they are some of the most easily damaged components of a nerve! An example of sensory nerve damage is not being able to feel an area on the front of your thigh, although you can still move the entire leg just fine. Motor nerves are involved in movement—they carry instructions from the brain out to muscles in the body, telling them to tense or relax. An example of motor nerve damage is wrist drop, when the wrist cannot move on its own into an extended position—it hangs limply when the arm is parallel to the floor.

Both sensory and motor nerves are very important in our day-to-day lives, and the loss of either sensation or movement in a part of our bodies can be anything from minor to devastating. Imagine your job involves typing on a computer, and for three weeks after a rope session you are unable to feel what is happening in your finger-

RADIAL = red; ULNAR = blue; MEDIAN = green

tips. Or perhaps you cannot lift your dominant hand for three days, and you have an art project due in a week. It is very important in rope bondage (or any bondage for that matter) to understand the risks and decide what level of risk you are comfortable with. If an injury like those described above would be unacceptable to you, you must take extra caution in preventing it!

Preventing Nerve Injury

OK, so nerves are important. How do they actually get injured in rope?

Nerves can be damaged by rope in two ways: **compressive force** (for example, a wrap is too tight or on for too long) and **shearing force** (for example, when a wrap moves across a limb under pressure, such as during transitions in suspension). Think of a nerve like a bundle of uncooked spaghetti strands wrapped in plastic wrap. If you squeeze it hard enough, some of the pieces will break. If you hit it with something, more pieces will likely break. These are both types of compressive forces. Now, consider what would happen if you grip the opposite ends of the bundle with both hands and twist in opposite directions. Most of the pieces will break! This is a shearing force, and it is by far the most damaging thing to a nerve.

When you are in rope, pay attention to the tension of each wrap (its looseness or tightness). If you notice a wrap is uncomfortably tight, consider its position—is it in a dangerous area where a nerve could be damaged? We'll talk more about where those trouble zones are shortly. If you are doing a dynamic suspension or being moved around actively in rope, pay attention to the rope in those trouble zones. Traction or pulling along those wraps may create a risky shearing force, so you need to monitor that limb closely.

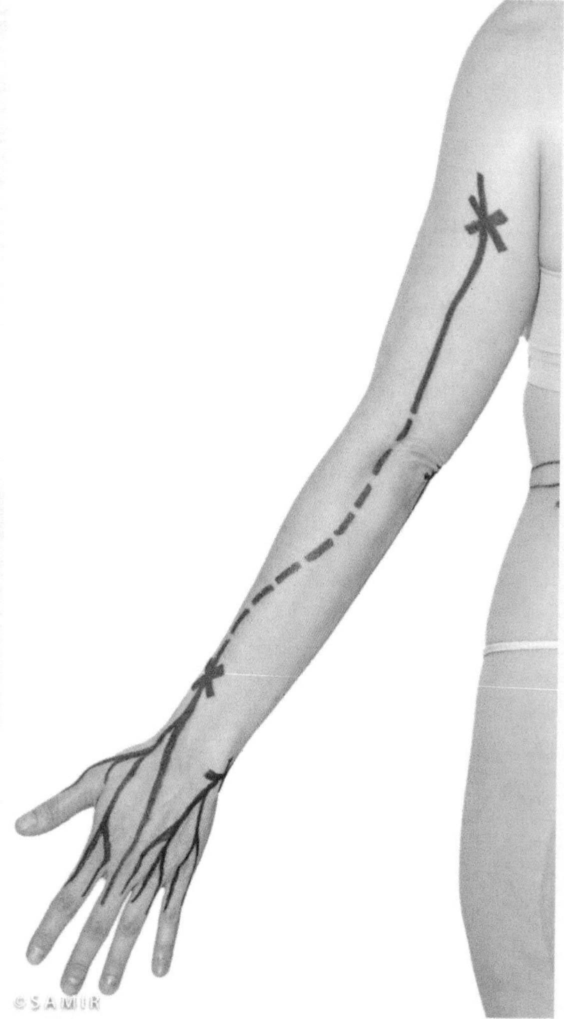

This sounds great in theory, but how do you know if there is a problem?

We will start with sensory nerves. Symptoms of sensory nerve damage usually come in phases. First, most people will notice a tingling or burning sensation in the part of the limb that is affected by the nerve in danger. Sometimes the area will also feel cold. This is typically a very specific feeling in terms of location—a couple of fingers, one side of a leg, etc. Sometimes you will simply lose sensation on an area of the skin without any tingling or burning at all.

X = extra-vulnerable spot; —— = nerve runs more superficially; - - - - = nerve runs more deeply; dotted areas show sensation

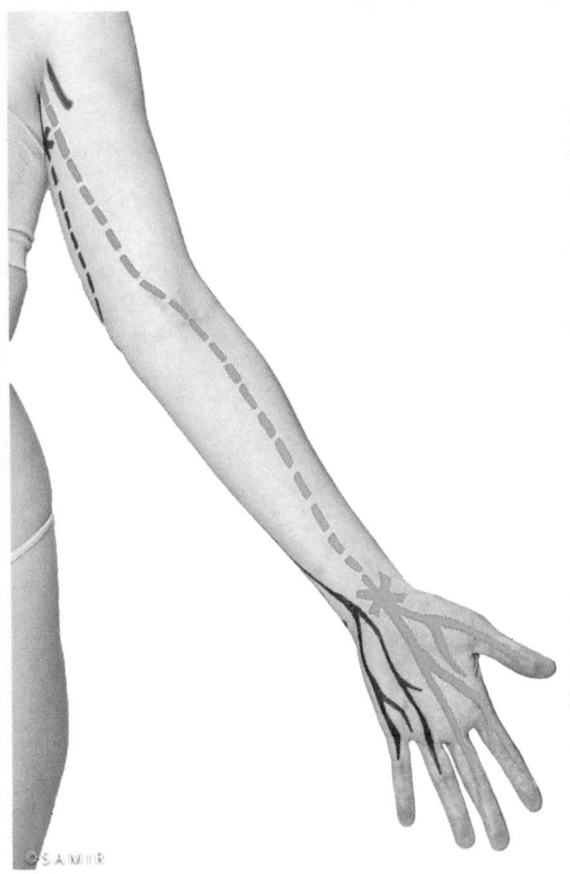

If the wrap causing the issue is not adjusted, this can progress to numbness or complete loss of sensation. Tingling and burning usually improve as soon as the wrap is adjusted, but numbness can take minutes, hours, even days or weeks to improve.

When your arms are bound, it is helpful to run your thumb over the tip of each of your fingers periodically to see if the sensation experience is the same for all fingers. You should also run your index finger along the back side of your thumb. If the sensation varies from one finger to another, this may mean that a nerve is in danger, and you should consider communicating the specific information to your rigger. For example: "I am starting to feel tingling along the back of my right thumb."[1] Your rigger can then look at your wraps and deduce where an adjustment should be made.

Sensory nerve issues are more common and in most cases less debilitating. Quick adjustments by a millimeter or two might be all that is needed, and the scene can progress. They are also usually the first things you will notice. Motor nerve issues are more concerning, however.

Motor nerve fibers are thicker and more resistant to damage, so if you are developing weakness, it was likely preceded by sensation problems along the same large nerve bundle. Weakness typically starts as a sluggish feeling, like you are trying to move a limb through molasses. This will then progress to the inability to move at all. For example, you try to extend a hand at the wrist, but nothing happens.[2] This is something you should communicate with your rigger immediately, and it is a reason to consider stopping the scene to fix the problem. If you are so numb that you cannot tell if your hand(s) or fingers are responding to your brain's commands, ask your rigger to look for you.

Many bottoms and riggers will develop specific systems to check on sensation and motion. One of my favorite examples is a rigger's taking the bottom's hand and giving it a squeeze—if you can feel the squeeze and the rigger's touch equally on all your fingers, then sensation is OK. If you can squeeze back and pull against the rigger's hands by extending yours at the wrist, then the motor function in your hand is OK. It is a good idea to test both wrists at the same time. Extension of the wrist, opening and closing the fingers, and squeezing are the functions that you need to be sure work in your hands while bound. If your hands are bound behind your back,

RADIAL = red; ULNAR = blue; MEDIAN = green

you can extend your wrists so that they press against the small of your back—even if you are a little tingly in the hands, you will feel the pressure of your hands against your back.

Circulation

When people teach about the risks of rope bondage, they tend to focus on nerve damage. But circulation issues can also cause numbness, sluggish movement of a limb, and sometimes even dramatic color changes in the skin. Sometimes it can be hard to tell the difference between a problem with circulation and with nerves. We will review the basics of the peripheral circulatory system to help clarify these issues—it's not actually as hard as it might seem!

Arteries carry blood away from the heart and out to the periphery. There, they spread out into tiny little **capillaries** where the oxygen and other nutrients that the blood is carrying can be delivered to their targets—muscles, skin, organs, etc. After the important contents of the blood have been delivered, waste products from the tissues are then absorbed through the thin walls of the capillaries. Capillaries then feed into larger **veins**, which collect the blood from the periphery and bring it back to the heart.[3]

Arteries have thick muscular walls that make them harder to compress. They also tend to run deeper inside our limbs and be more protected by muscle tissue. This usually protects them during bondage. If an artery is compressed to the point of blocking blood flow, the limb downstream from it will turn white. It will go numb fairly quickly as well. This is a bad sign, as lack of blood flow can cause fairly rapid damage to nerves and muscles. You have a matter of a minute or so to adjust or loosen the wrap on a white limb. Once a wrap is shifted or loosened, you will notice the limb start to get pink again, and sensation will slowly but steadily return. Fortunately, you will almost never see or hear of issues from compressing arteries in rope bondage!

Veins have thin, easily compressible walls, which makes them much more vulnerable. Some veins run deep between layers of muscle, but many are quite superficial. When ties are placed on your arms, you will often notice the veins in your hands start to plump up and become more prominent. Blood in the arteries is still able to get past the rope into your hands, but the pressure from the rope on your veins is just enough to trap it there. This will cause blood to gradually pool in the arm, and the tissue will start

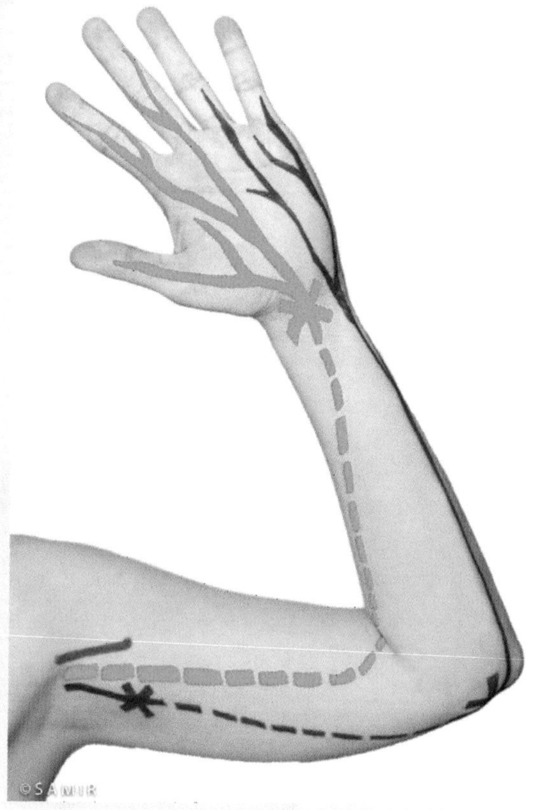

X = extra-vulnerable spot; —— = nerve runs more superficially; - - - - = nerve runs more deeply; dotted areas show sensation

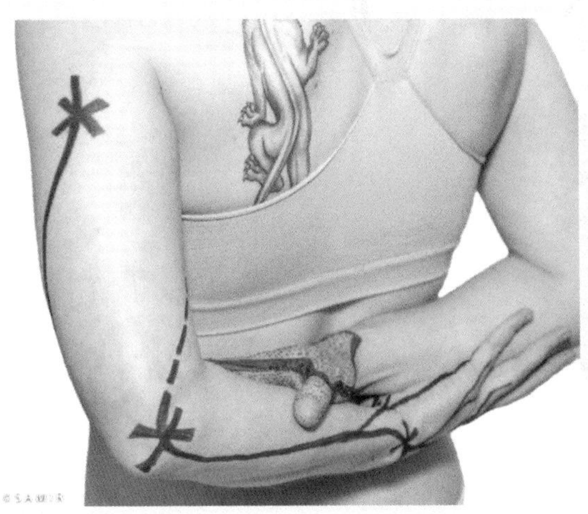

to swell. This process tends to create a wide array of color changes in the skin—**red, blue, and purple** are the most common. If blood is trapped there long enough and there is enough pressure on the limb, it can even cause capillaries to burst and red speckles will form within minutes. The good news, however, is that at least all your tissues are getting the nutrients they need survive, because fresh blood keeps pumping in. **Color change does not necessarily mean there is a problem!**

With veins, you usually have at least 10 to 15 minutes of significant compression and blood-trapping before you need to worry about any damage. There is a caveat, however. When you have significant blood-trapping in a limb, you will tend to go diffusely numb (rather than in specific smaller areas like you do with nerve compression). **If you are completely numb from circulatory issues, you cannot accurately perform sensory checks to be sure your nerves are safe. Additionally, if your movement is sluggish from blood-logging of the muscles, you cannot reliably test your motor function.** These are reasons to consider loosening, adjusting, or removing a tie.

The Nerve Pathways

In the diagrams throughout, you can see each nerve outlined on the body. The nerves are drawn with a solid line where they are more superficial and with a dotted line where they are buried deeply underneath layers of muscle. The most exposed and therefore most vulnerable area of each nerve is marked with an X. Bear in mind, however, that every person is different and there are many possible variations. It is important to explore your own body to see where you are most sensitive. There are also diagrams with dotted zones. These are color coded to match the nerves and show the sensory areas to correspond to each nerve. Damage to the nerve anywhere upstream from the dotted area may cause numbness, tingling, or the sensation of temperature change in that zone.

In this chapter we are focusing on the nerves of the upper extremity, as these are easily irritated and injured in rope bondage. The three most important nerves to consider when binding the upper half of the body are the radial nerve, the ulnar nerve, and the median nerve. All of these nerves carry both motor and sensory fibers above the elbow, but from the wrist and below their functions are primarily sensory. Certain common ties, like the takate-kote (box tie) can place these nerves at risk, but if you learn your body and how these nerves run, you can better avoid or quickly diagnose and correct problems.

Here is an example. Let's say you are bound in a box tie, and after five minutes your left pinkie finger starts to tingle and burn. Where might the problem be? First, you need to figure out what nerve is involved. As you can see on pages 17 and 18, this area is marked blue, corresponding to the ulnar nerve. In

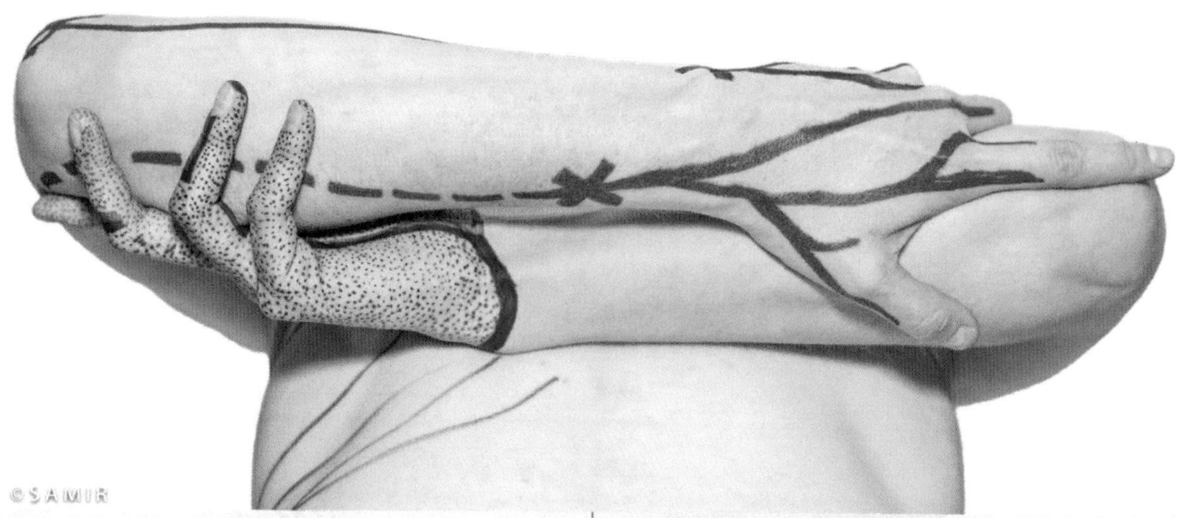

the images on pages 20 to 22, this nerve is vulnerable in the armpit, the elbow, and the pinkie side of the wrist. Now you assess the tie that you are in. Are there upper cinches running through your armpit? If so, is the one on the left causing compression? Is the wrist cuff too tight? Can you adjust your wrist slightly to avoid putting pressure on the nerve? You can ask your rigger to dress your wraps, to adjust the location of the cinch or the wrist cuff, or perhaps even release your wrists if the sensation is worsening. Practice running through scenarios like this with a partner so that you can quickly identify trouble areas. The images on this page and page 22 will help you see where the nerves travel when the arms are in a box tie position.

• • •

Treatment for nerve injuries is constantly evolving and is beyond the scope of this book. If you've been injured, it's highly recommended that you seek the attention of a medical professional. (You could even do your own research to be armed with the latest information to discuss with your doctor.) Also, it's good to have an emotional support system, as getting injured can cause you to blame or doubt yourself and your abilities, or otherwise feel bad about yourself. Having support from your partner, other rope bottoms, friends, or even just online can help alleviate those feelings.

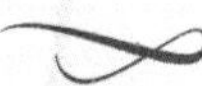

Notes

1. This may be a sign of right radial nerve compression.
2. This may also be a sign of right radial nerve compression. As mentioned above, this is commonly called wrist drop.
3. Please note this is a description of systemic circulation. We will skip pulmonic circulation to avoid confusion.

X = extra-vulnerable spot; —— = nerve runs more superficially; - - - - = nerve runs more deeply; dotted areas show sensation

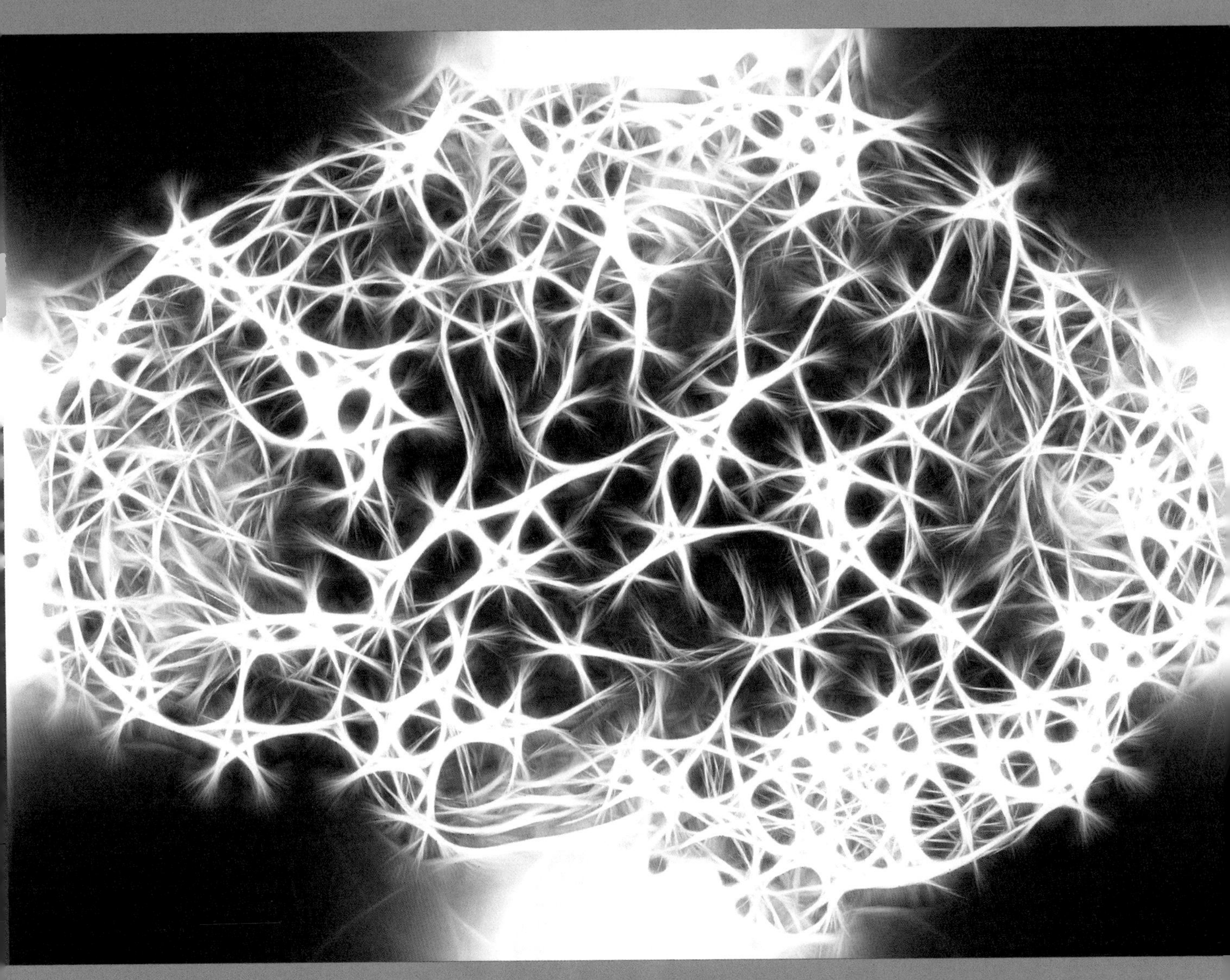

Chapter 3

Neuroscience Meets Rope

by Neuromancer28

Neuromancer28 has been a neuroscientist for 15 years and is a rope switch.

My past four years have been an odyssey of trying to understand why rope bondage affects us so strongly. Here I'll delve into neuroscience and psychophysiology to explore its effects, including providing results from some case studies in which awesome riggers and rope bottoms agreed to have their brains and bodies measured with all sorts of technology during their ties.

A few disclaimers: 1. I've included many references to scientific studies. In general, these studies didn't investigate people in rope. Rather, they focused on physiological reactions to stimuli that might inform our understanding of rope—for instance, how the brain reacts to pain or pleasurable touch. 2. I also reference medical texts, but this is not a medical guide and should not be used to understand or diagnose any medical conditions. Please consult a medical professional if you have any medical questions.

Terms to Know

Neuroscience: The scientific study of the nervous system, which includes the brain, spinal cord, and nerves.

Psychology: The scientific study of mental processes and behavior.

Psychophysiology: The scientific study of the interaction between mind and body.

Neurophysiology: The scientific study of the functioning of the nervous system.

Not Just the Rope

Psychological processes that affect our reactions to rope can begin long before the first strand is placed. Establishing the relationship context with our rope partner, negotiating, composing ourselves, doing our pre-scene rituals like stretching or meditation, and having our first bits of physical contact with our partner help to determine our mindset at the time of the tie. I'll suggest that resulting feelings of trust or mistrust in our partner, relaxation or tenseness, and feeling centered or scatterbrained could all influence how our body will respond in rope later on.

For example, research suggests that how we think of ourselves and our relationships can affect how we react to emotional situations, like being in rope. Increased feelings of self-worth decrease subsequent pain tolerance.[1] And higher levels of perceived support are associated with decreased inflammation and threat-related brain activity,[2, 3] which can yield increased pain tolerance and flexibility.[4] So if your sense of self-worth is on the high side before you're planning to do a very painful scene, you might consider getting extra support from your partner to tolerate it better. Or maybe a bit of humiliation play is in order.

Our daily practices may also be important. People who regularly meditate increase their ability to engage with exciting or threatening experiences for prolonged periods, for instance, while those who don't meditate tend to shut down their threat responses after a while.[5] So if you meditate, you may be increasing your ability to maintain the emotional tone of challenging rope scenes.

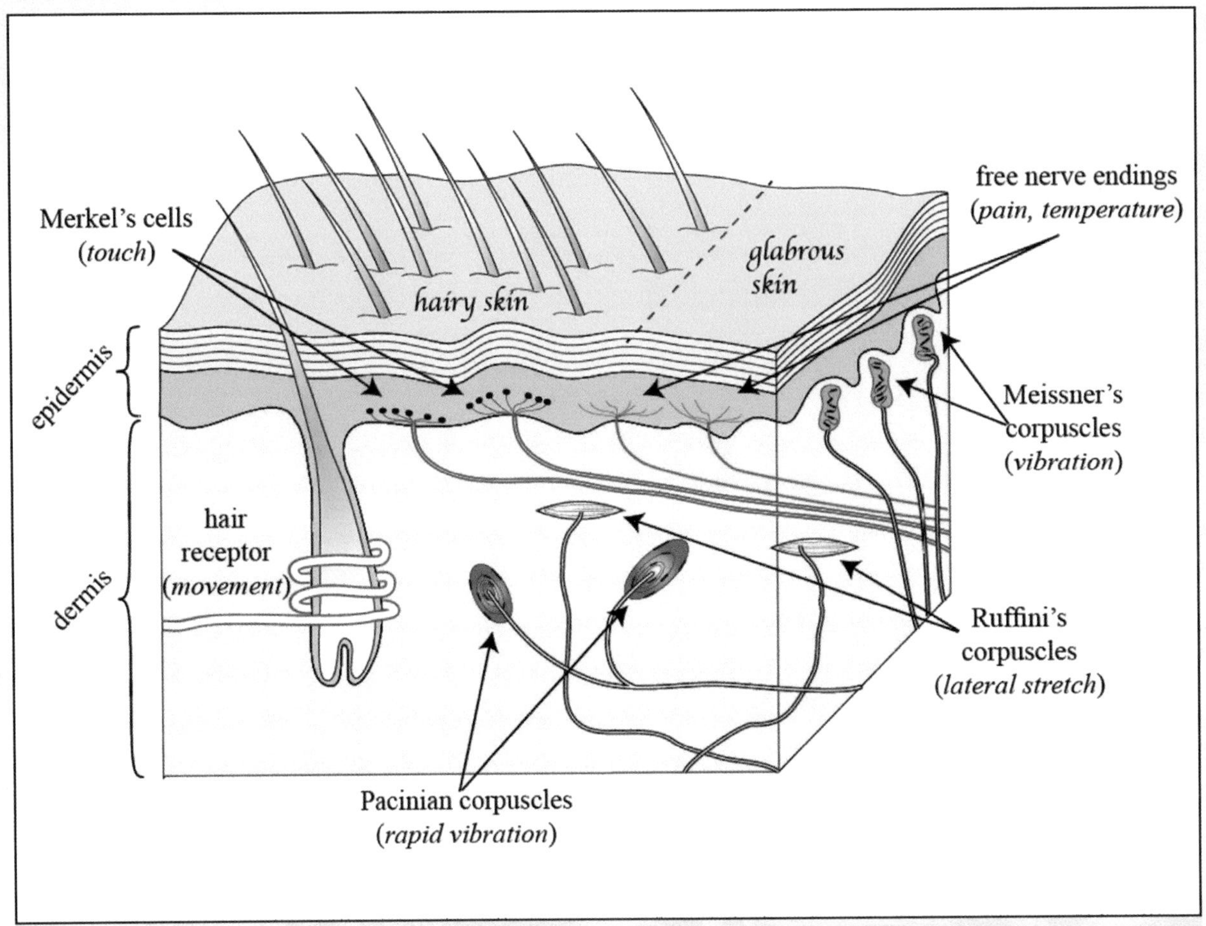

Fig. 1. Skin receptors. Image courtesy of and © neurones.co.uk and HumanPhysiology.academy

Understanding what will go on can also affect our experience. Before any activity, the brain sets up expectations. For example, by hearing you will be doing a relaxing rope scene, you may expect that there will be stroking, pressure, and continuous touch. You may relax and not prepare for possible other reactions. Conflicts with these expectations (e.g., getting threatened unexpectedly) can generate a ton of brain activity associated with avoidance of threat and working to figure out how to respond in the face of conflict with expectations.[6] Uncertainty (e.g., not knowing how play will go) particularly increases the readiness of brain systems that detect and react to conflict, so that we are prepared to react flexibly to what might happen (e.g., being yanked around). So your brain will prepare to have heightened attention, and be ready to respond to challenges.[7] This could mean that if your goal is to have a high-arousal (exciting), high-fear scene, then having your rope top keep you in the dark about what to expect could be good. If you want a trancy, meditative experience, on the other hand, where you are not "on edge," then more negotiation, discussion of the exact ties and sequencing, and focused preparation may be useful.

Bodily Responses to Rope

The Skin: Touching Base

Our primary bodily connection to rope is through our skin, the heaviest organ in our body, so let's get to know it a little better.

The outer layer is called the **epidermis**, and below that is the **dermis**, which contains **mechanoreceptors** (see Fig. 1). Mechanoreceptors process touch and other stimuli, such as pressure and vibration. The ones closer to the surface of the skin (Meissner corpuscles in nonhairy areas and Pacinean corpuscles in hairy areas) tend to be more sensitive to light touch, have smaller receptive fields (sense over a smaller area), and adapt (stop feeling) quickly. The ones buried deeper (Merkel cells, Ruffini's corpuscles) are sensitive to stronger touch, have wider receptive fields, and adapt more slowly (over a few minutes).[8] Rope can affect all of these receptors.

If the rope is not moving and is not tight, only the receptors that quickly habituate (decrease in response over time) are likely to receive the sensory input, so we may stop feeling the rope quickly. Nonhairy areas (fingers, palms, soles of feet, lips, labia minora, and glans penis) are especially sensitive to rope that touches the skin lightly and is moving. After a short time in nonmoving rope, we stop noticing whether it is smooth or rough—for instance, jute and silk shouldn't feel much different at this point. If the rope is not moving but is creating deep pressure, the deeper receptors will still recognize it, and we will still feel it for a bit.

Because surface receptors are sensitive to light touch and have smaller receptive fields than deeper receptors, if two rope strands are dragged near each other lightly, we should be able to distinguish them. But if we are wrapped tightly—engaging the deeper receptors—the receptive fields are large enough that we cannot distinguish between strands of rope next to each other, meaning we wouldn't know if we have on one wrap or two.

Skin receptors are far apart on our calves, thighs, and belly, yielding lower sensitivity—for example, to how many wraps we have on and the distance between them. They are dense in our arms and especially in our fingers, yielding higher sensitivity there.

You may already have figured out that the experience of the same rope interaction may be sensorily very different for tops and bottoms. This sensory difference may be due, in part, to touch receptor function. The fingertips, which are the top's primary contact with the rope, are specialized to give a more complete and integrated perception of a touched stimulus than other places on the body.[9] Thus, the top may have a strong understanding of exactly how the rope is slipping across the bottom's skin as they use their fingertips to move it, while the bottom will sense the rope differently. (Takeaway: Tops and bottoms shouldn't assume they understand each other's sensory experience.)

The Skin: Beyond Touch

Aside from processing touch, the skin has other receptors that process pain, pleasure, and temperature.

Nociceptors are sensory nerve cells that process pain—that is, stimuli that can cause damage. These are fast-acting and bypass the brain's cortex, resulting in an immediate emotional reaction. Their habituation can vary, meaning you may be able to prolong pain more than other kinds of touch with rope. Regardless, the response to pain can be increased by varying the stimulation sites over time,[10] which is why, even when you start to adjust to a futomomo, you may still cringe if a crotch rope is tugged on.

C-tactile (CT) fibers are pleasure receptors. Scientists actually just discovered these recently. Gentle, slow stroking (as when rope is slowly dragged across skin) optimally activates these. People who like touch more than others appear to have more CT fibers[11]—highly enthusiastic rope bottoms may be in this set. It also may suggest that if someone doesn't like rope play, it could be due to a lower number of CT fibers and not just psychological reasons.

Thermoreceptors process temperature. They interact with CT fibers, so a cold stimulus will likely be less pleasant than a body-temperature one.[12] Hint: Don't tell a sadistic rope top this unless you want fresh-from-the-freezer rope in your next scene.

Sight input also comes into play in how we respond to rope. You may have experienced the feeling of time slowing down when you see something that could cause you harm. Through our sense of sight we process looming threats, like hands or rope coming toward the face, which causes time dilation (the feeling that time has sped up or slowed down).[13] The constant processing of looming threats during rope play may explain why you can't remember afterward whether you were in a suspension for 10 minutes or 30.

You may also have gotten "tunnel vision" or experienced other alterations to your vision while in rope. It may be because vision (and touch as well) may be difficult for the brain to integrate when parts of it are otherwise occupied or not functioning—at least, that's what brain damage studies would suggest.[14] Seeing only a partner's hands and the rope in them, and not the rest of the person, is a form of tunnel vision that seems particularly common for rope bottoms, and is consistent with stress-induced changes in visual processing.[15, 16]

Moving On Up: From Skin to Brain

Now that we've discussed how the skin responds to rope, let's consider what happens as the information travels north.

Information gathered by the skin receptors travels via nerves to the spinal cord and then on to the somatosensory cortex in the parietal lobe of the brain, which creates the awareness of sensation in different areas of the body such as the arms or legs. If the pathways to the spinal cord and brain—that is, the nerves—are damaged, then even though the skin receptors will register touch, you may not know you are being touched, because the sensory information won't be reaching the brain. That's why nerve damage causes an area to feel numb. (See Chapter 2 for more on anatomy and nerve damage.)

In the somatosensory cortex, areas of the body are represented to different degrees. The largest area is devoted to the hands. This means our hands are particularly sensitive to touch—rope across palms, between fingers, and so on will be processed in great detail. The area devoted to what is touching us is separate from the one devoted to where we are being touched.[17] So in the throes of ropespace, it would not be weird to be able to identify where you are feeling something but not be able to identify exactly what is touching you, or vice versa.

Methodology

The technique: Primarily electroencephalography (EEG)[20, 21]—electrodes on the scalp measured brain activity. I used a 14-channel Bluetooth wireless EEG™ rig.

The data processing: I processed the data to remove the effects of motion, jaw clenching, etc. and then transformed it to the "frequency" domain, from which four psychologically meaningful types of brain oscillation were extracted, including:

- **Theta oscillations** (4 to 7 times per second), which are associated with meditative and trance-like states

- **Alpha oscillations** (8 to 12 times per second), which are associated with relaxation and a lack of thinking

- **Beta oscillations** (15 to 25 times per second), which are associated with attention, and

- **Gamma oscillations** (30 to 45 times per second—often measured higher), which are associated with arousal (general, not just sexual), cognitive effort (e.g., trying to solve problems), and integrating features (such as putting eyes and nose together to understand one is looking at a face).

In truth, oscillations in these bands are more complicated than that (for instance, expert meditators have lots of gamma band activity), but these basic notions can help guide you in understanding what we saw.

The measurements: Figures will show how much "power," or signal, there was at each of these frequency bands as specific events of interest in the tie unfolded over time (shown from the earliest events at the top to later events at the bottom of each graph). Separate lines are plotted for signals from the front of the head (frontal) and the middle-to-rear area of the head (temporoparietal). In general the lines are parallel, and I comment only when they diverge. Axes labeled "z" show power for some period compared to the rest of the session, in "standard deviation" units, where z = 0 is the average for the session, 68 percent of the session has z between -1 and 1, and 94 percent of the session has z between -2 and 2. So if you see z > 2, that's pretty rare for that person in that session.

Delving Deeper

As rope bottoming is not a simple activity, there are many other brain reactions to consider. I'll break down some of the brain processes associated with rope a bit and use some case studies to illustrate the concepts in action.

Rope touch cues are sent, in parallel, to areas of the brain that are active during physical interactive tasks, particularly strenuous, engaging ones. Involved in this are brain networks associated with **cognitive processes** such as planning, preparation, attention, and conflict recognition (things not working out as we would expect); **motor processes** (keeping balance, moving in space); **social processes** (recognizing another person's mental states and intentions, conveying our own mental state); and networks more involved in **emotional functions**, including recognizing and generating emotion (the amygdala, insula, and striatum, for example), and regulating emotion (the prefrontal cortex, for instance).[18]

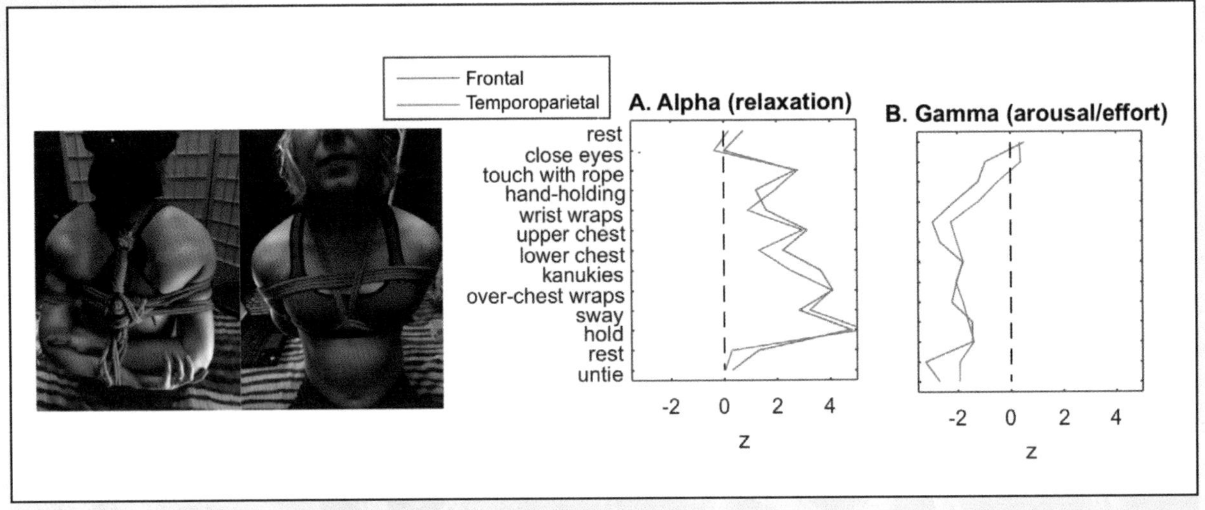

Fig. 2. EEG from two-rope TK. Rope bottom: Vixy_Pixie. Rope top: Neuromancer28.

A. As the tie progressed, alpha activity (relaxation/lack of thinking) increased, up until we said the tie was over. After the TK was in place, my holding Vixy_Pixy and swaying with her raised her alpha above and beyond what the ropes had done alone.

B. Gamma activity (arousal/cognitive processing) decreased from the time she closed her eyes until the wrist wraps were done, and stayed low throughout, consistent with our intent for this tie to be more meditative than arousing.

Emotions can be generated not just from present inputs but from our interpretation of bodily cues[19] based on previous experiences as well. So it is not surprising that rope touching an area that has been touched in other contexts—that is, the area has previously been associated with aches, caresses, or pain—could generate strong feelings even if the present context is different. This may be especially good to be aware of if you have been subject to abuse.

Much of kinky play seems to be about manipulating our ability to regulate emotion—that is, it helps to free us of prefrontal control over emotion generation so we can freely emote: yell, laugh, scream, cry. I believe rope is no exception—it can free the mind from its own shackles, allowing us to fully experience our emotions, unfettered by our own internal protests.

Below I'll share some vignettes that illustrate brain reactions to specific ties. We can all thank the amazing rope bottoms and tops who got tied up literally for science. I've used FetLife names only, and their identities, data, and pictures are used with permission.

Responses to the Takate-Kote

The takate-kote (TK) is a common tie, one many people learn early in their tying "career," and it is the foundation of many types of rope suspensions. Its popularity may stem not just from its structural integrity for suspensions, however—there are psychological and physiological reasons too. The TK progresses from psychologically "safe" areas (the hands) through less safe areas (the shoulders) to a much less safe area (under the chest).[22] And each of the steps appears to create physiological responses that could systematically increase relaxation and intimacy. We can thus use this common type of tie to see how physical, mental, and emotional responses all work together in creating an experience in rope.

Check out Fig. 2 as we move along through the tie; it shows Vixy_Pixy's brain responses to each stage of a two-rope TK, largely in the style of DeGiotto[23] with an additional wrap over the shoulders.

I was the tyer. This tie was done for the book, with little talking or psychological context beyond "Let's do a TK like we have done it before." Thus, there was very little uncertainty—we'd done this tie countless times before and in every case it had gone well, so our psychological states were relaxed and positive.

Initial hand-holding: Following preliminaries like getting situated, a TK often begins in earnest when the rope top moves the bottom's hands behind their back, either toward the elbows or in a "high-hands" position. Holding hands decreases neural activity in brain regions that generate threat responses, even when we are threatened,[24] possibly fostering feelings of safety. It also changes our time perception. In a doctor's office, touch by the doctor upon greeting decreases patients' estimates of the time they spent waiting to see the doctor, and may increase time estimated to be spent with the doctor.[25] If this translates to rope, it could mean that initial touch can help the bottom focus on what is happening during the tie, eliminating their memory of the preliminaries and helping them be more present in the scene.

Tying the forearms creates vibration on the wrists, which increases parasympathetic responses.[26] The parasympathetic nervous system, also sometimes called the "rest and digest" system, conserves energy by slowing heart rate and relaxing muscles in the gastrointestinal tract, among other things—in other words, increasing feelings of relaxation. It also increases how much the time between heartbeats varies with the breath ("respiratory sinus arrhythmia"), which appears to govern our ability to react as we would like to in response to emotional stimuli.[27] With higher respiratory sinus arrhythmia, we may be able to regulate our emotions more effectively if we find ourselves reacting emotionally or if a situation like a tie goes differently than we had expected; it may specifically decrease our rumination and worry.[28, 29] These responses also increase touch sensitivity.[30] Both human and mechanical forearm pressure also increase brain responses to social emotional information,[31] potentially suggesting that forearm ties make us more receptive to emotional aspects of rope.

Wraps over the chest create compression. Such intrathoracic pressure could trigger a baroreceptor reflex response (which lowers blood pressure), again increasing the parasympathetic response of relaxation and increased ability to regulate emotion. Chest wraps may also be processed like mechanical hugging, which reduces the activity of the sympathetic nervous system (the "fight or flight" response, which raises arousal) and decreases anxiety.[32]

Wraps under the chest have a number of potential physiological and psychological effects. They are in an area of notoriously high skin conductance (i.e., low electrical resistance)—such regions are often considered susceptible to acupressure. These wraps could also trigger increased feelings of intimacy through two routes. The first is that if you are relaxed, given increased parasympathetic tone from the previous steps, despite being touched in a conventionally taboo area of the body such as under the breasts, you may, without thinking about it, resolve that "cognitive dissonance"[33, 34] (not wanting to believe you are OK with someone's doing something counter to your basic principles, you create an internal "story" consistent with entering a safe situation), leading to the conclusion that you have a high level of comfort and intimacy with the top, based only on that made-up story.

The second potential route is that being touched on and below the breasts could lead to sexual arousal, which yields both analgesia[35] (decreased sensitivity to pain) and the potential for "misattributed arousal"[36-38]—that is, your brain could associate your arousal and the associated disappearance of pain with being with your top, leading to a narrative about how you must feel close to or have a special connection with them, when in reality the reaction is due only to the chest wraps. I will digress and suggest that as sexual arousal could lower your ability to feel pain, it's a good idea to use caution when mixing sexual stimulation and rope bondage. That lovely vibrator, for instance, could cause you to miss out on signs of impending nerve damage or other injuries.

Kannukis (cinches under the armpits) are part of some TKs. If you are comfortable, given all of the previous steps, with the kannukis, it could lead, through further resolution of cognitive dissonance, to a narrative such as, "If I am comfortable despite their messing around with my armpits, I must have great trust in my top." This could lead to increased comfortability in the rest of the tie. In truth, of course, the reaction may be due, in part, to the tie itself, and not necessarily to a profound relationship with your top.

Some bottoms aren't comfortable with being touched in this area. Even outside rope, many people are particularly uncomfortable being touched under the armpits, as it's a particularly ticklish area. If you perceive touch in this area as uncomfortable and the tie continues anyway, you may generalize and subconsciously invent other reasons for the discomfort—for instance, low intimacy or poor safety. The tendency to overgeneralize negative interpretations appears to involve the insula, a brain area that interprets reactions to touch.[39]

One takeaway is that touch, particularly in traditionally taboo areas, notoriously leads to states of high arousal, which could easily flip to be positive or negative. Pre-tie communication, the relationship you have with your partner, and other interaction during the tie during these types of touch can help dictate how the scene will play out.

Other wraps around the chest. Some TKs include additional wraps, which often go over the shoulders and which interact with the chest wraps. These may or may not provide structural stability, based on the tie. Even when they are not structurally important, they provide an opportunity for the top and bottom to connect with touch in the most intimate parts of the TK, allowing for "caring" fiddling in taboo places, which the top and bottom can use to facilitate the narrative they have created throughout the rest of the tie.

A takeaway lesson from all of the preceding elements is that it may be useful to be aware of how rope affects us so that we can separate the effects of rope from our relationships. This awareness can keep us from making more, or less, of a tie than it is. My editorial take here is that with good communication, rope need not be considered creepy even if it affects our reactions—rather, in the best cases, we are willingly, and with upfront communication, putting ourselves in a rope situation knowing it could lead to an increased feeling of intimacy. It is the responsibility of the rope bottom and top to consider this possibility in advance.

Other common TK elements may be useful to consider. The TK is often tied in a kneeling or seated position with the top behind the bottom. This has a few effects:

1. You're being put in a position of being physically manipulated or controlled by the top. Again, attempts to resolve cognitive dissonance may lead you to conclude that you're therefore submissive to the top, increasing your comfort level in the rope dynamic.

2. You and your partner aren't making eye contact. Seeing the whites of a person's eyes yields increased amygdala reactivity,[40] which is associated with increased arousal. Making eye contact allows a more intense processing of social connection. Some people, especially those who identify on the autism spectrum, have particular uncomfortability looking at a person's eyes, which is attributed specifically to the high level of neural threat response (amygdala reactivity) that occurs from eye contact.[41] For such individuals, the top-behind-bottom positioning of the TK may particularly put the bottom at ease.

In contrast, if increased social connection and arousal are a goal, as you and your partner aren't making eye contact when you're facing the same direction, other factors may be necessary to promote these feelings. Physical contact may be particularly useful in this regard. The common habit of grazing the bottom's neck or ears with fingers, lips, or breath can yield increased arousal, given the potential for light touch to activate the sympathetic nervous system.[42] Sympathetic terminals at the top of the spine may be particularly apt targets in this regard. Touch or heat along terminals of the vagus nerve in the neck and ears could also yield an increased parasympathetic response,[43-46] as can moderate blood pressure more generally.[39] This simultaneous activation of sympathetic and parasympathetic systems may be resolved as a comfortable or safe-feeling aroused state. As a possible bonus, animal data suggests that light touch can inhibit pain responses.[47]

3. Another practice common during TK tying is rocking. Repetitive physical behaviors such as rocking back and forth are often associated with emotion regulation and stress coping.[48] Slow whole-body movements (about 1 rock every 3 to 100 seconds) are specifically associated with feelings of pleasantness and increased parasympathetic response[49, 50]—that is, relaxation.

All of these effects of the TK happen whether or not it ends in a suspension. Being suspended brings its own neurophysiological responses, which we'll discuss later.

Elements of Rope Play in General

Now that we've covered the effects of a specific tie, let's zoom out to the bigger picture and look at some general elements of being tied up.

Restraint-Induced Immobility/Loss of Control

Restraint stress has been studied extensively, but primarily in animals.[51] To the extent that observations of nonconsensually restrained animals can be gener-

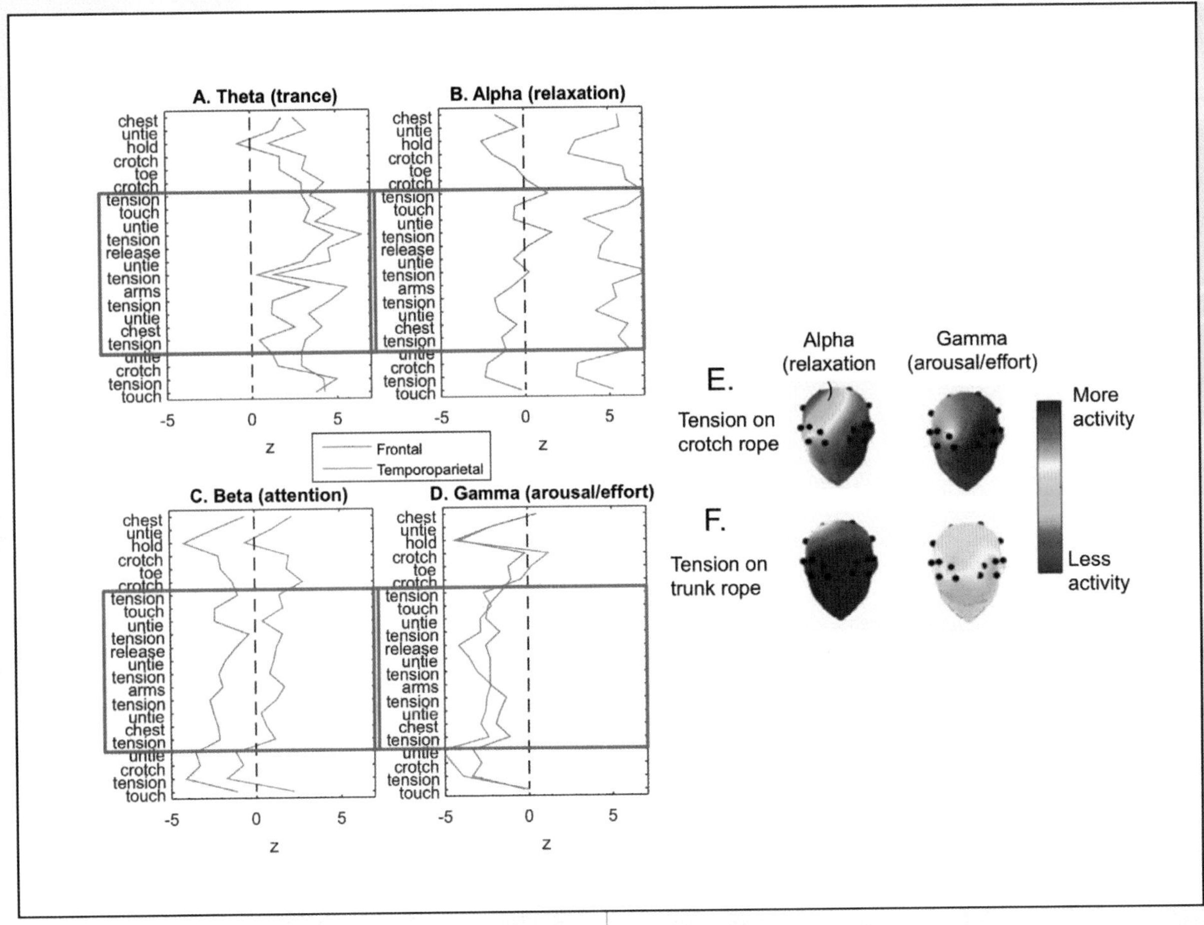

alized to consensually restrained humans, we may infer that phasic (short-term) and chronic restraint are likely to cause profound changes in the brain's neurochemical environment. Effects of phasic restraint appear largely positive, including:

- An increase in the release of dopamine[52] (a neurotransmitter that plays a critical role in motivation and reward).

- An increase in protein kinases, which promote learning in areas such as the hippocampus,[53] which is associated with emotional memory. (That's why you may remember certain restraint scenes particularly well.)

- An increase in indices of activity in brain regions associated with recognizing emotion (for example, the amygdala) and processing stimuli as rewarding or punishing (for example, the nucleus accumbens region).[54] Restraint may thus be perceived as particularly emotional and be processed as particularly rewarding or punishing.

Other effects of phasic restraint:

- It could affect "bratty" behavior one way or the other—animals have been observed to hit each other more[55] and also to stop fighting[51] after being restrained.

Fig. 3. EEG segment from a long session of ichinawa (one rope, kept moving throughout a tie). Rope bottom: tangle_. Rope top: Neuromancer28.

This segment illustrates two things:

1. Tangle_'s style: Her rope journeys with me consistently involve high levels of frontal alpha (B, high blue line, associated with relaxation/lack of thinking), from the time rope is put on her until the time it comes off. The primary variations throughout the tie thus happen in other frequency bands.

2. The session began and ended with tension on a tight crotch rope that was accompanied by high levels of beta (C, attention) and gamma (D, arousal). The middle of the segment involved repeated tension, touching, tying, and untying. It had higher levels of theta (A, trance-like) and lower levels of beta and gamma, possibly consistent with "leaning into" (allowing herself to experience without second-guessing or internally narrating) the tie or her reactions.

E and F show alpha and gamma, throughout the head, for one segment of crotch rope tension and one segment of trunk rope tension (mostly around the upper chest), respectively. Blue is less activity and red is more activity. Whereas alpha was high the entire time, and highest for trunk rope tension, gamma (arousal/cognitive processing) was higher in response to momentary crotch rope tension.

On discussing it with tangle_, I learned that leaning into trunk tension was consistent with her experience. Thus, her rope experience with me was seemingly one of alternately higher and lower arousal and more trance-like periods. Putting tension on the trunk, holding her, and releasing her from tension deepened the trance-like experience. Acute arousal snapped her out of it, but not so far that she couldn't dip back in. The journey was in the transitions.

• It affects the amygdala[56] in ways that might increase relaxation, like increasing amygdala serotonin[57] and changing signaling (for example, via endocannabinoids—as in a runner's high) in the amygdala.[58] This could explain why short-term restraint seems to make animals more docile/easy to handle, and able to accept reward[51] from humans. And the docility seems to continue the next day.[59]

You may or may not find it particularly interesting that following restraint, animals might be more aggressive toward other animals but more docile toward humans. I've found no explanation for this, and will leave any speculations about the potential importance of perceived power dynamics and status differences—for instance, feeling dominated—to you.

In contrast to brief restraint, restraint that is done for long periods, very frequently, or chronically, is associated with poorer outcomes in animal models, including poor memory, ulcers, stress, inflammation, poor appetite, decreased wound healing, and poor coordination. If these results translate to humans, watching how much time you're spending in rope and, if you're feeling at a particular loss for control or experiencing negative effects, considering spending some more time outside rope may be interesting.

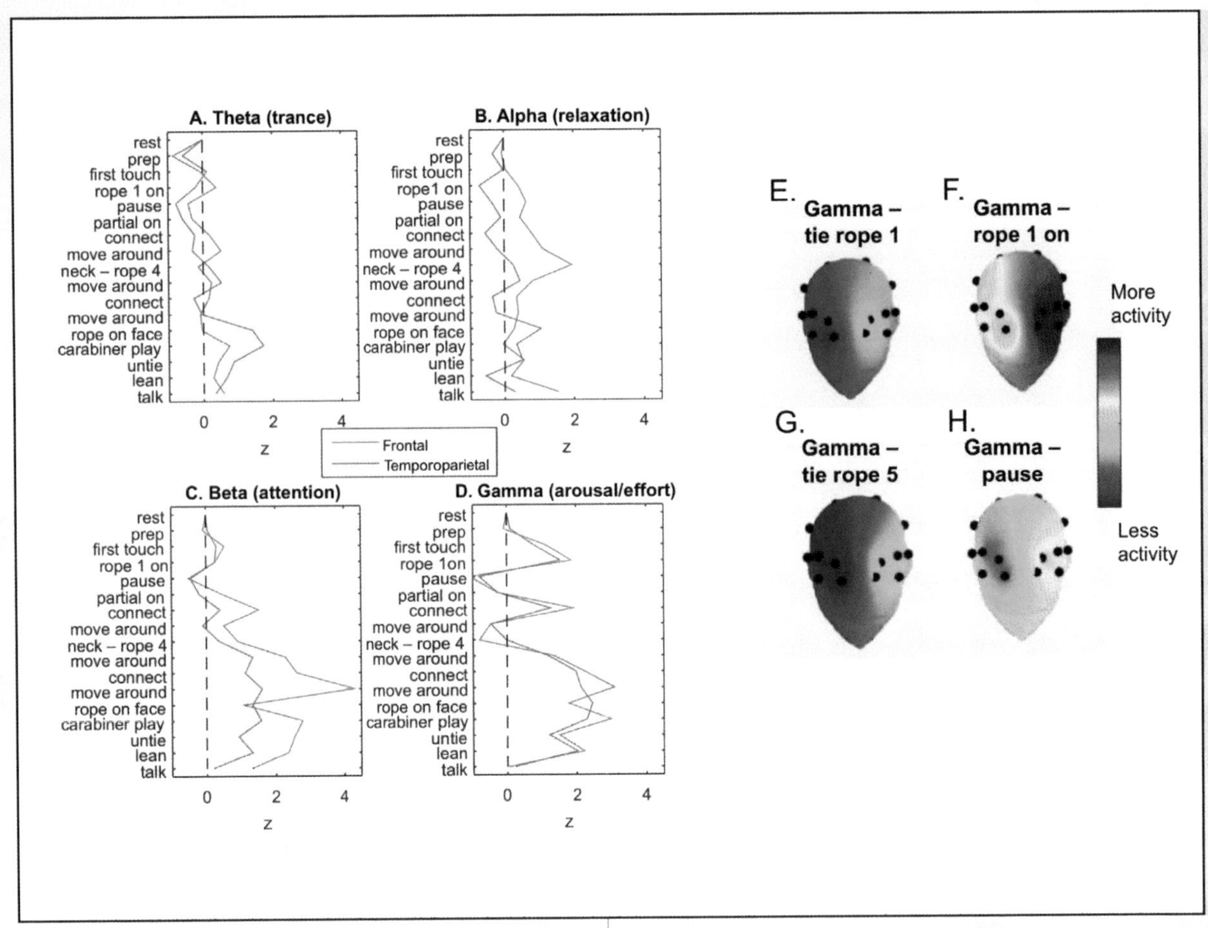

Pain

Pain and pleasure are intimately intertwined in the brain, as pretty much anyone who's ever engaged in any kind of BDSM knows. Playing with both can change a rope experience dramatically. For example, pain systems activate reward circuitry,[60] likely making us more responsive to reward—meaning that caress may feel extra sweet after an intensely painful segment. And laughing increases pain tolerance[61]—which bottoms who crack jokes or tops who make lighthearted comments during a tough tie may intuitively be tapping into. Oxytocin (released during intimate social encounters) appears to dampen pain responses, likely through modulation of the A-delta and C-fiber nociceptive inputs we discussed before.[62] So, increased intimacy—socially, sexually, etc.—between top and bottom could increase pain tolerance.

More generally, higher relationship quality and good social interactions with a close partner predict stronger ability to complete challenges with a low-level threat of pain[63] (though this doesn't hold for challenges with a threat of intense pain). Of course, different people respond very differently to pain. Factors from gender to social network size to conditions such as PTSD are all associated with pain tolerance.[64-66]

Fig. 4. EEG excerpts from a long session that moved from floorwork to partial suspension to full suspension. Rope bottom: True Blue. Rope top: Kanso.

This session highlights the potential of the rope journey in those highly experienced in the art. Kanso and True Blue are performance partners and experienced rope teachers.

Their tie used 8 ropes, each of which yielded what True Blue described as profoundly different headspaces. This subjective journey was mirrored by extraordinary variation in all frequency bands, with the greatest theta (A; trance) occurring in response to rope being put on her face, the greatest alpha (B; relaxation/lack of thinking) happening in response to neck rope, the highest beta (C; attention) occurring when she was fully suspended and being moved through space, and the greatest gamma (D; arousal/cognitive feature integration) occurring for playful elements like having her chest threatened with a snapping carabiner. Thus, True Blue was constantly experiencing variations in mood, headspace, and physical placement. The different elements of the rope scene each took her to an observably different brain state.

One of the most moving elements, for me, was how well Kanso knew True Blue's reactions and worked with them. For example, he would consistently tie a rope and then wait for its effects to "set." Each time, when he deemed the rope had set, there were profound changes in brain activity at that moment. So, E and G show gamma (arousal and cognitive feature integration) during the tying of ropes 1 and 5. F and H show how gamma EEG increased at the very moment he deemed the rope to have set—as if he knew she "got" it and was able to fully process the state she was in. Only then would they move on.

The scientific literature is just starting to iron out how and why different people respond to pain differently. Initial data suggests, particularly, that masochists' pain tolerance is increased and perceived unpleasantness of pain is decreased only in conditions of consensual masochistic interaction.[67] Brain imaging data from that study suggested that in masochistic contexts, masochists' brain areas associated with sensation but not with emotional pain, and areas that sense internal body states (e.g., feeling uncomfortable), become less strongly communicative with other parts of the brain.

Timing and Rhythm

Timing in rope play is hugely important. The rhythm of a tie is often thought of as critical, and indeed, the brain responds strongly to different tempos.[68] Fig. 3 shows how repeated tension and relaxation of rope during the practice of ichinawa (a one-rope technique) was associated with an apparent deepening of trance-like reactions in one rope bottom, whereas just one level of tension and no relaxation did not create that effect.

Also in terms of timing and rhythm, it may be important to consider the time course of a bottom's reaction to a given rope manipulation—like putting on or taking off a wrap. In particular, physiological reactions do not end when the stimulation stops. So, for example, the effects of a single shock last many hours in the brain.[69] For this reason, some tops "wait for the rope to set," as rope bondage instructor Kanso puts it (shown in a tie with longtime partner True Blue, in Fig. 4). Human touch affects us immediately in a perceptual way and later in a cognitive way,[70] though they both happen pretty fast.

Connection

A lot of brain space is devoted to aspects of social connection, with different areas associated with understanding what another person is thinking, empathy, and perceiving connection.[71] Of particular note, many of the same brain areas are active when we perceive another's emotion as when we have our own emotions,[72] suggesting that time spent connecting and perceiving another person's emotional states could increase our own emotions, possibly yielding powerful connective experiences. For example, in Fig. 4, C and D show the increase in EEG indices of beta (attention) and gamma (arousal/effort) power that occurred each time Kanso stopped actively tying, during which he and True Blue made eye contact and connected. During our discussion, they described these moments as some of the most profound of their tie.

Sexual Arousal

Being sexually aroused shuts off a lot of brain function responsible for executive control (doing what our "everyday head" wants us to, and regulating or decreasing emotional reactivity).[73] Sexual arousal also interacts with other pleasure mechanisms,[74] so sexual arousal can be used as a tool for manipulating brain function. For example, during sexual arousal, disgust responses are decreased, as brain regions that process disgust are recruited for other purposes.[75-77] So if you're sexually aroused, you may be more OK with that skanky crotch rope previously used on a hundred people than if it's brought out before you're highly sexually aroused. This may also be considered a point in favor of the argument that renegotiating in the middle of a scene can be unwise.

In women, nipple and vaginocervical stimulation are associated with oxytocin release, which increases pair bonding—meaning it may make you feel closer to your partner; there is conflicting but initially promising evidence for the effect of sexual arousal more generally regarding oxytocin release.[74] Sexual arousal also increases activity in brain regions associated with emotional empathy, potentially increasing the sense of connection between bottom and top in other ways.

Asymmetry

For centuries, symmetry has been recognized as an "efficiency" of the body, in that one action can be used to guide movements of a wide network of muscles on both sides of the body.[78] Skin receptors are distributed similarly, and the information they pick up is fed to the same brain regions from each side of the body.

Asymmetric loads on limbs mess with our ability to perceive our own body,[79] yielding interesting novelties in perception. For example, if you tie a person's arm to be weighted asymmetrically (e.g., pulled at the wrist) and blindfold them, they may misestimate where their arm is pointed, where their hand is in space, and even their arm's length.[79] So, asymmetric ties may be harder to "process"—they require more

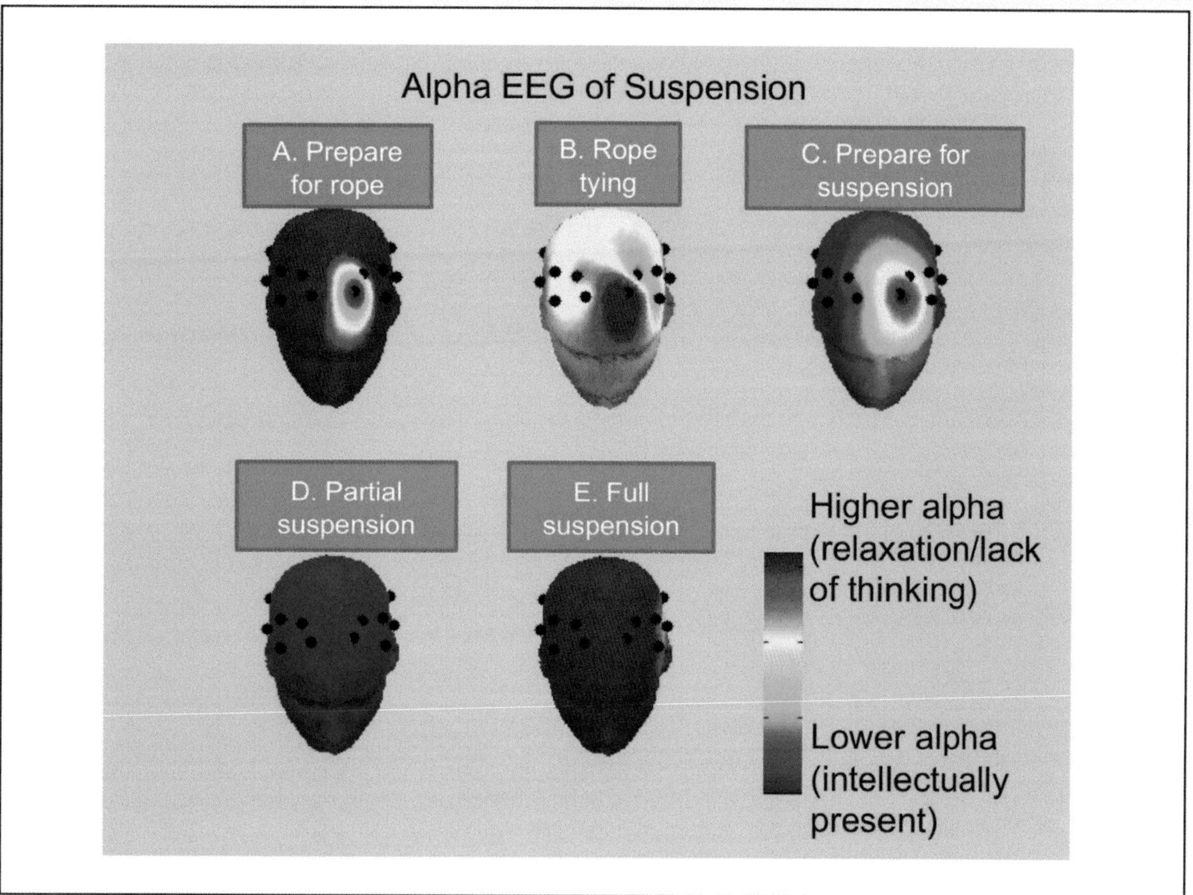

Fig. 5. Alpha EEG leading up to and during a facedown TK-anchored suspension. Rope bottom: FierySubmissive. Rope top: DamienSaint.

This tie shows EEG alpha (relaxation/lack-of-cognition) reactivity associated with a full suspension tie. FierySubmissive's initial state, and that of other bottoms I have measured, involves a meditative state characterized by high levels of alpha EEG (A). This largely remained unchanged with the first wraps (B), in this case wrist wraps. As the tie progressed toward suspension (C), we see a more cognitive process characterized by high levels of "helping" rigger DamienSaint, involving body adjustments and attending to her position, which seemed to increase during partial suspension (D). She describes these two phases as a less meditative experience. Finally, in full suspension, when FierySubmissive had hardly any physical control over her position, we see a stronger return to a more relaxed meditation-like state (E; higher alpha).

work for you to understand where the parts of your body are when you're in them.

Asymmetry can be particularly interesting when you're tied to things, as the perceived weight of something you're holding may be inaccurate if you're tied to it asymmetrically. Tops might therefore use asymmetry to keep their bottoms "off-balance" and challenge them more, instead of tying symmetrically, even if the resulting tie does not look standard or conventionally "pretty." (Pro tip: To play most effectively with perceptual inaccuracy from weighted asymmetric ties, it's useful for the bottom to be blindfolded or to have their limbs tied where they can't see them—sight can make up for some of the perceptual misinformation caused by asymmetric limb restriction.)

Limb Movement, Squeezing, and Touch

We have different brain mechanisms for moving our limbs and the perception of having our limbs moved.[80] For example, studies with monkeys suggest that 75 percent of motor neurons that perceive leg and arm movements respond only to being moved, and not to voluntary movement.[81] Similarly, pain from a ring being squeezed around your hand by someone else is perceived as more intense than the pain that would come from squeezing that same ring yourself. When someone else squeezes the ring, sensory, pain, and conflict-perception circuits in the brain are more strongly activated than when you squeeze the ring.[82] So, voluntary movement and squeezing actions inhibit sensory systems. That doesn't happen for being moved or squeezed. Having our body moved around, squeezed, etc. during tying is a given.

There are a few possible takeaways here. One is that just because you can tolerate a tie when you do it on yourself, e.g., in a self-suspension, this doesn't necessarily translate to when someone else does it to you. And you probably know intuitively that being moved and tied "like a package" doesn't feel as good as being moved and tied with intention. (Note that being objectified and tied up as an actual piece of luggage may still be fun when it's intentional.)

So, the way we are touched and moved strongly affects our brain responses, and thus, our experience. For example, as we have noted, interactions in which more oxytocin is released (e.g., more intimate interactions) are more likely to increase pain tolerance.[62] This could mean that if the way someone is touching and moving you doesn't feel good, you may have a negative overall experience with them in rope even if you like the way the tie looks when it's finished.

Responses to Suspension

Being suspended in rope is often described as more intense, physically and mentally, than doing rope play on the floor. When the ropes are bearing the body's weight in a full or partial suspension, the pain response can be high due to increased pressure; fear can be increased, which can actually lead to greater intimacy by misattributing the arousal to the relationship rather than the actual risk; and a sense of disorientation may result, because the usual cues we rely on for balance when we're firmly on the ground aren't present—or are present in a distorted form.

Of course, some partial and full suspensions can be incredibly comfortable, and some floor scenes can be incredibly intense, so there is no hard and fast rule as to what responses will occur. That said, in this section we'll explore some responses that are more distinct to suspensions.

Psychological Elements

Because of the added risk due to having the ropes support the body's weight, suspension often involves more preparation and more considerations than floor tying for both the top and bottom. This includes the top's concentration on details that are not just about the bottom's psychological experience: "Are all my carabiners in reach?" "Where should I attach the upline?" "How can I make the transition as smooth as possible here?" Suspensions can also involve extended periods of anticipation moreso than floor tying—for example, it may take a while for your top to get that three-rope TK just right. The psychological context for suspension is thus often different than for floor tying.

Fig. 5 shows brain reactivity leading up to and during a facedown TK-anchored suspension. If we extrapolate the results to suspensions in general, we can surmise that the experience goes something like this:

1. A bottom begins in a somewhat meditative state as the first wraps are put on.

2. During the time a top is working on an upline, their attention toward the bottom may be decreased, yielding a break in connection—this can manifest in the bottom's moving away from a meditative state toward a higher level of attention.

3. As the tie progresses into a partial suspension, some bottoms "help" their top by adjusting their position, maintaining balance, etc. This can lead to a further intellectual presence and even less of a meditative state.

4. In full suspension, when movement is highly restricted or difficult, the bottom experiences the most trance-like state—cognitive abandon—showing neural activity characteristic of a deeply meditative state (e.g., high theta EEG).

Throughout a suspension, there are moments of awkwardness, high anticipation, and abrupt movements that further affect the bottom's cognitive state. Together, all of these elements create a physical and mental journey that is highly variable—which can make it significantly different from the experience of a floor tie.

Physical Elements

The body's position during suspension also affects brain activity.

In face-up suspensions, the bottom is often in a V-position in which their upper torso is at a 45- to 60-degree angle to the floor, which is one of the Fowler's positions (doctors place patients in these when they're in respiratory distress). This position maximizes respiratory sinus arrhythmia (how much the heart varies with breathing),[83] which increases the parasympathetic (calming) response, and thus promotes relaxation and emotion regulation. Also, characteristic of face-up suspensions, the supine position (on the back) reduces neural responses to aggression.[84]

Inverted positions (feet toward the ceiling and head toward the ground) change how our brains process common visual stimuli—for instance, we stop processing inverted faces quickly[85] and process them more like objects than faces.[86] We are less likely to remember bodies seen upside down too.[87] So after an inversion, you may remember the visual details of what went on less well than in a noninverted suspension.

Things that are moving generate more amygdala reactivity (associated with more emotion) than things that are not moving.[88-91] It hasn't been researched yet whether moving a person (as in lifting them from the ground into a suspension, or moving them through transitions) induces these effects, as self-motion and other kinds of motion have different perceptual mechanisms. But I think it would apply.

Responses to Untying

Considering only the responses to tying and to being in the air would leave out one of the most profound parts of the rope experience—untying. Untying is important for many reasons. Many rope bottoms find that thoughtless untying (getting ropes off without the connection, intimacy, and attention to timing present in the rest of the session) can reduce the blissful and intimate feelings they experienced while in rope.

Untying affords the opportunity not just for prolonging the emotional connection but for prolonging the physical connection through touch and providing sensation. For instance, slowly dragging the rope across the skin can maximize pleasurable touch responses.[11] The reduction in uncertainty and in anticipation of stress or pain, along with the expectation of friendly, supportive contact, can all lead to a reduction in arousal system activity.[24] This reduction in arousal system activity is one reason why you may suddenly feel cold after all the ropes are off. (See the next section for more reasons.)

Because the top is no longer concentrating on tying, they can "let go" a bit—decreased engagement of the prefrontal cortex (the area of the brain that carries out the executive function) allows them to be more emotional, likely yielding stronger emotional responses in the bottom via emotional contagion[92] (emotional convergence) and perception of emotion.[72]

Responses After the Rope Is Off

Immediately after the rope comes off, the body and brain go through a number of changes. You may be chilly and start yawning, for instance. High levels of energy expenditure, as are present in a challenging tie, involve oxygen's being directed to muscle cells to fuel their metabolism. After 35 to 45 minutes, your body will need to begin to dissipate the associated rise in heat. If you are expending energy, as in a challenging tie, you won't feel the heat dissipation, because you are continuing to generate heat. But after the tying session is done—that is, when you're no longer expending energy—dissipation continues through sweat and you can become cold or get the chills.

This is a natural process that is thought to be helpful, for example, in reducing muscle soreness. Actions like walking after rope (instead of collapsing), wearing a blanket, hydrating, and having reasonable carbohydrate intake before rope (to prevent hypoglycemia afterward) can all help to mediate the chills. Just as sweat cools the body, yawning is thought to cool the body and brain[93, 94] and is thus often observed after strenuous activities like rope play.

In addition, the brain immediately encodes (remembers) lots of information directly after stressors and emotional situations. This means that intense, soul-searing, uplifting, or strenuous rope could be deeply encoded. This "plasticity" is likely high because the brain wants to know how to approach or avoid such experiences again later. For this reason, it may be useful to plan for an explicitly positive aftercare experience: one that includes warmth, chocolate, human contact, kind words or whatever makes you feel good.

Memories are encoded with the place in which the

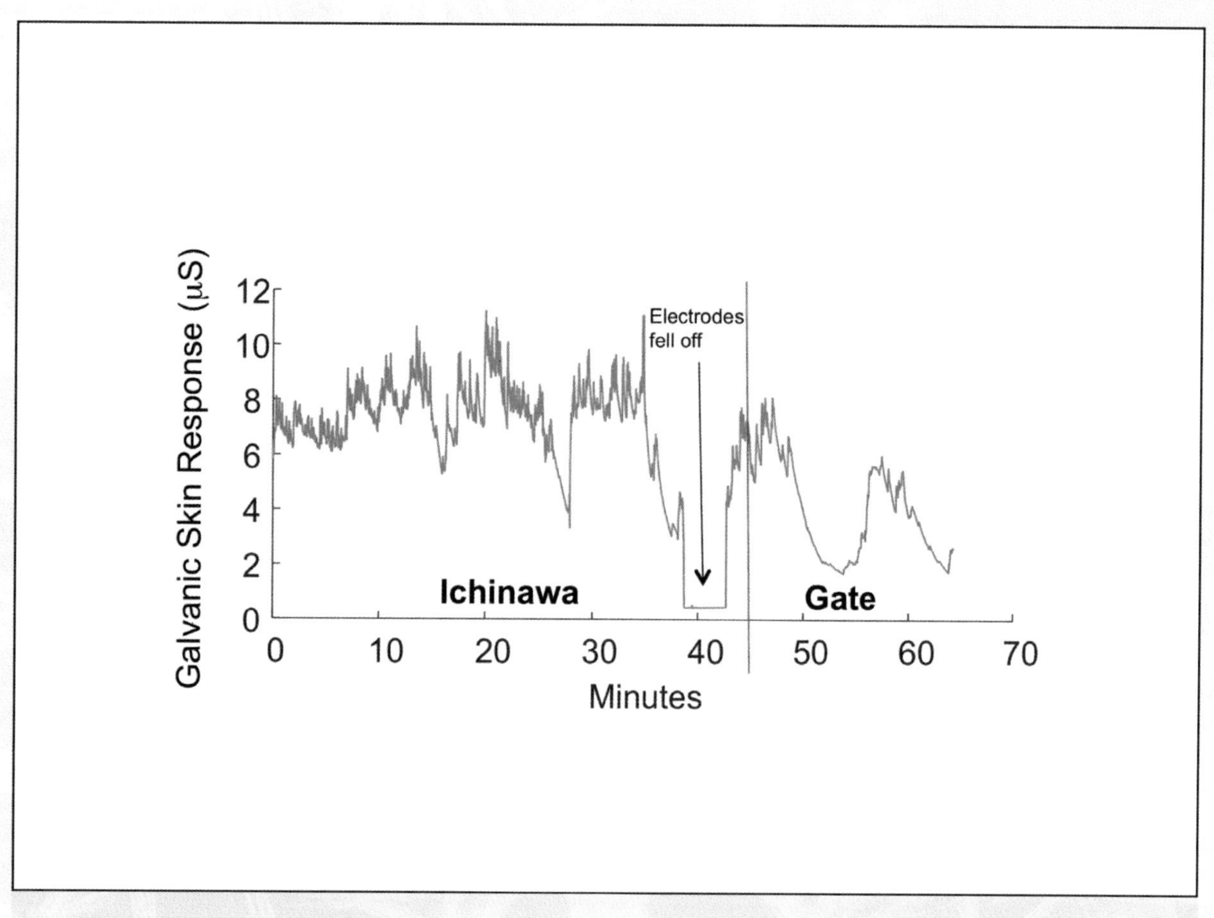

Fig. 6. Galvanic skin responses to ichinawa. Rope bottom: Evie Vane. Rope top: Neuromancer28.

experience happened. So doing the aftercare in the same place as the rope scene—as close to where the scene occurred as possible, could be useful in pairing the caring with the experience to avoid later memories of mostly pain or stress.

Despite all of this memory-making, remember also that you may have experienced time dilation, and the way your sight and touch inputs were perceived may have been altered from the way they are normally perceived, so you may struggle to remember certain parts of the rope play while remembering others in great detail.

The Following Days

Rope drop, which many bottoms experience from minutes to days after rope play, is a notoriously vulnerable time often characterized by feeling low or being in a bad mood, difficulty concentrating, and a host of other features that represent a startlingly accurate one- to three-day facsimile of a clinical depression. Much has been written about drop in general. Here I'll recap some related brain regions we have already discussed, and point out how they may be involved in drop.

As we have noted, the amygdala recognizes emotion. It also helps us decide that information is good or bad, whether we're facing a threat or whether we're safe. It's highly reciprocally connected to much of the rest of the brain—in particular, structures like the hippocampus, which is associated with retrieving memories. So when we feel something intense, memories may bubble up that reactivate the amygdala in a loop. And when the amygdala turns on, it tends to shut off much of the brain's more cognitive processing.

So, after an intense rope experience, any little trigger in the following days—the brush of clothes against a nipple, sitting on a sore spot, or smelling the rope used, for instance—could bring on a rush of memories and feelings that leaves you effectively zoned out for a while. This suggests that as part of aftercare, both you and your top might figure out a way together to integrate a scene with the rest of your lives days after the scene is over, so you don't have an isolated powerful memory that sucks you away.

Similarly, as we have noted, the insula processes body cues, can be triggered by the amygdala, and is associated with time dilation (feeling like time has sped up or slowed down).[13] So, if the amygdala is active, or you have a bodily sensation that takes you back to the scene, you can easily be back in a land without time.

One brain system that helps to regulate the amygdala begins with the prefrontal cortex. Ideally it helps us think about what we want to do (like a job) rather than what we are automatically programmed to react to. But if what's recently happened is exactly the type of thing we want to think about, we can be conflicted about shutting off these processes—and we get lost in reverie. This suggests that as part of aftercare days later, it could be helpful for the top and bottom to remind each other to perform "executive control" activities, like eating or exercising.

Finally, the nucleus accumbens processes information as rewarding or punishing. There's a current theory that reward perception is calibrated to the most intense recent rewarding stimulus. So if the best thing that's recently happened in your life is that you found a quarter, that quarter might be amazing. But if you've had an epic rope scene, finding a quarter might barely register. A takeway for rope is that after a scene, it may be hard to find everyday life interesting. But you can remember that by living your everyday dull life for a while, ideally with gusto, it will get back to being more interesting as the rope scene fades from view.

Putting It All Together: Physiology Case Study

To put this chapter in context, let's walk through a specific tie from the first time I met Evie (who put together this book you're reading). At that point I knew very little about her aside from her rope bottoming reputation and what we discussed in our short conversation beforehand. In that chat, Evie said she likes to be "blissed out" but also likes to connect with and learn about her partner. Our goal was to see if psychophysiology could add anything to her understanding of rope bottoming, and also to see how accurately it could "read" her as a rope bottom.

We decided on ichinawa for the rope play, as it is a fairly simple and safe style: One rope is repeatedly wrapped around, tensioned, and loosened to allow continual unfolding of experience. Our measurement was simply and only galvanic (electrical) skin response, or electrodermal activity. Electrodes on two of her fingers measured, effectively, how much they sweat, with the response measured in microsiemens. This is a (messy) proxy for sympathetic nervous system activity, which roughly signifies general (not just sexual) arousal. An iPad gave us a dynamic readout of her physiology. Fig. 6 plots the result, unfolding in time (minutes) over the course of about an hour.

Timing and Rhythm

Just touching Evie with a coil of rope provoked an immediate increase in galvanic skin response. But as soon as the rope went away, her skin response shot back down—meaning it seemed like she took no time savoring or otherwise riffing on that first sensation. With even a moment of respite, she came back immediately to a quiescent, perhaps contemplative state.

This would become a theme for the evening. Each time I put rope on her, when it was tensioned in a new way, or if the rope were tied in a way we had not yet tried, her skin response would rise for about three to five seconds and then immediately fall. Given what she had told me earlier, I asked if she was using those respite times to think and learn about me, to which she coyly admitted yes, but assured me that was OK.

Psychological Context

Evie's physiology changed over time as we were increasingly able to predict and understand each other's reactions. Increasingly, I had to be more and more dramatic, or novel, or sadistic to get a physiological reaction (rise) out of her. Doing anything Evie could expect or predict—and the field of what she could expect or predict was apparently quite large—began to fail to garner even a momentary rise in galvanic skin response. So for her, if my goal was to increase arousal, we had to build to something, foreshadow a problematic situation (such as purposely making the tie a little bit too loose or in a way that could be perceived as not safe if we were not careful), or otherwise create dramatic tension.

To complement these rises, when her skin responses fell, they would fall deeper and deeper. In short, once she figured me out (she told me when that happened, and I believe her—kinda hot, kinda scary), she used our "down time" to dive into trancy states, falling lower and lower. This allowed us to play with letting her descend, and watching her physiology until it hit a new low point, and then yank her around to create an immediate and dramatic exit from meditative bliss, only to descend once again. It was kind of like shaking a gumball machine to allow the prize to fall lower and lower.

Physiology Meets Humanity

Together we surfed her arousal curve, riding it to higher highs and lower lows. So fun. Until, that is, I ran out of easy tricks. Gentle-ish pushes, balancing tricks, stretches, mild breath restrictions, and such (all planned to not be super intense, as this was our first time tying together) were not cutting it for her now-conditioned arousal system.

So we headed over to a huge wrought iron grating between the living and dining rooms in the hotel room I'd been lucky enough to score. I tied Evie to the grating with feet off the floor, and her arousal response when up immediately—changing the scenery and situation to something new had brought her immediately back to a reasonable level of arousal. And again, the lovely leaning in, letting go. Her arousal then plummeted to its lowest level, as you can see on the chart, and she said she felt spacey in a nice way.

At some point we took off the electrodes and gave ourselves over to the play, and after that she came down, happily fuzzy but intact.

Takeaway Lessons

We learned a couple of things here, and if they apply to one rope bottom, they likely apply to others too:

1. **Staying fresh was important.** Trying new things, whole body movement, unexpected tricks, and so on were important to keeping Evie's arousal response up. And higher arousal rates were complemented by deeper meditative states.

2. **Not doing was as important as doing.** Giving Evie time to let the response level fall, to reflect, was essential. Establishing a rhythm of ups and downs created not a beeline for arousal or a simple meditative state but a more memorable, deeper journey—a hike up and down a mountain that included plenty of time to stop and enjoy the views.

• • •

An ideal outcome of this chapter would be that rope bottoms and tops begin to use insights from neuroscience to make even more of their rope play. Of course, not every insight here will apply to every rope bottom and scene, as each of us and each of our interactions are unique. So, I encourage you to use this chapter to add neuroscience to the understanding of your rope experiences you are already gaining through introspection, good communication, and more rope.

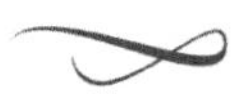

Notes

1. Hooley, JM; Ho, DT; Slater, J; and Lockshin, A. "Pain perception and nonsuicidal self-injury: a laboratory investigation." *The Journal of Personality Disorders.* 2010; 1(3):170-179.
2. Muscatell, KA; Eisenberger, NI; Dutcher, JM; Cole, SW; and Bower, JE. "Links between inflammation, amygdala reactivity, and social support in breast cancer survivors." *Brain Behavior and Immunity.* 2016; 53:34-38.
3. Hughes, S; Jaremka, LM; Alfano, CM; et al. "Social support predicts inflammation, pain, and depressive symptoms: longitudinal relationships among breast cancer survivors." *Psychoneuroendocrinology.* 2014; 42:38-44.
4. DeLeo, JA; Tanga, FY; and Tawfik, VL. "Neuroimmune activation and neuroinflammation in chronic pain and opioid tolerance/hyperalgesia." *Neuroscientist.* 2004; 10(1):40-52.
5. Antonova, E; Chadwick, P; and Kumari, V. "More meditation, less habituation? The effect of mindfulness practice on the acoustic startle reflex." *PLOS ONE.* 2015; 10(5):e0123512.
6. Pichon, S; de Gelder, B; and Grezes, J. "Threat prompts defensive brain responses independently of attentional control." *Cerebral Cortex.* 2012; 22(2):274-285.
7. Carter, CS; Macdonald, A; Botvinick, M; et al. "Parsing executive processes: strategic vs. evaluative functions of the anterior cingulate cortex." *Proceedings of the National Academy of Sciences of the United States of America.* 2000; 97:1944-1948.
8. Leung, YY; Bensmaia, SJ; Hsiao, SS; and Johnson, KO. "Time-course of vibratory adaptation and recovery in cutaneous mechanoreceptive afferents." *Journal of Neurophysiology.* 2005; 94(5):3037-3045.
9. Schwartz, C. "The slip hypothesis: Tactile perception and its neuronal basis." *Trends in Neurosciences.* 2016; 39(7):449-462.
10. Jepma, M; Jones, M; and Wager, TD. "The dynamics of pain: evidence for simultaneous site-specific habituation and site-nonspecific sensitization in thermal pain." *The Journal of Pain.* 2014; 15(7):734-746.
11. Morrison, I; Loken, LS; Minde, J; et al. "Reduced C-afferent fibre density affects perceived pleasantness and empathy for touch." *Brain: A Journal of Neurology.* 2011; 134 (Pt. 4):1116-1126.
12. Ackerley, R; Backlund, Wasling; H, Liljencrantz; J, Olausson H; Johnson, RD; and Wessberg, J. "Human C-tactile afferents are tuned to the temperature of a skin-stroking caress." *The Journal of Neuroscience.* 2014; 34(8):2879-2883.
13. Wittmann, M; van Wassenhove, V; Craig, AD; and Paulus, MP. "The neural substrates of subjective time dilation." *Frontiers in Human Neuroscience.* 2010; 4:2.
14. Sarno, S; Erasmus, LP; Lipp, B; and Schlaegel, W. "Multisensory integration after traumatic brain injury: a reaction time study between pairings of vision, touch and audition." *Brain Injury.* 2003; 17(5):413-426.

15. Williams, LJ. "Tunnel vision or general interference? Cognitive load and attentional bias are both important." *The American Journal of Psychology.* 1988; 101(2):171-191.

16. Dirkin, GR. "Cognitive tunneling: use of visual information under stress." *Perceptual and Motor Skills.* 1983; 56(1):191-198.

17. Van Boven, RW; Ingeholm, JE; Beauchamp, MS; Bikle, PC; and Ungerleider, LG. "Tactile form and location processing in the human brain." *Proceedings of the National Academy of Sciences of the United States of America.* 2005; 102(35):12601-12605.

18. Davidson, RJ. "Affective style psychopathology and resilience: Brain mechanisms and plasticity." *American Psychologist.* 2000; 55:1196-1214.

19. Damasio, AR. The Feeling of What Happens: *Body and Emotion in the Making of Consciousness, 1st ed.* New York: Harcourt Brace, 1999.

20. Wikipedia. *Electroencephalography.* 2016; https://en.wikipedia.org/wiki/Electroencephalography.

21. Cacioppo, JT; Tassinary, LG; and Berntson, GG. *Handbook of Psychophysiology, 3rd ed.* Cambridge and New York: Cambridge University Press, 2007.

22. Suvilehto, JT; Glerean, E; Dunbar, RI; Hari, R; and Nummenmaa, L. "Topography of social touching depends on emotional bonds between humans." *Proceedings of the National Academy of Sciences of the United States of America.* 2015; 112(45):13811-13816.

23. DeGiotto Rope. "07 Japanese Rope Bondage Shibari - Takate Kote." *YouTube video.* 2014; https://www.youtube.com/watch?v=bTyYSXAj9jo.

24. Coan, JA; Schaefer, HS; and Davidson; RJ. "Lending a hand: social regulation of the neural response to threat." *Psychological Science.* 2006; 17(12):1032-1039.

25. Bredfeldt, RC; Ripani Jr., A; and Cuddeback, GL. "The effect of touch on patients' estimates of time in the waiting and examination rooms." *Family Medicine.* 1987; 19(4):299-302.

26. Wilhelm, FH; Kochar, AS; Roth, WT; and Gross, JJ. "Social anxiety and response to touch: incongruence between self-evaluative and physiological reactions." *Biological Psychology.* 2001; 58(3):181-202.

27. Park, G; and Thayer, JF. "From the heart to the mind: cardiac vagal tone modulates top-down and bottom-up visual perception and attention to emotional stimuli." *Frontiers in Psychology.* 2014; 5:278.

28. Thayer, JF; and Lane, RD. "Perseverative thinking and health: Neurovisceral concomitants." *Psychology & Health.* 2002; 17(5):685-695.

29. Aldao, A; Mennin, DS; and McLaughlin, KA. "Differentiating Worry and Rumination: Evidence From Heart Rate Variability During Spontaneous Regulation." *Cognitive Therapy and Research.* 2013; 37(3):613-619.

30. Seo, NJ; Lakshminarayanan, K; Bonilha, L; Lauer, AW; and Schmit, BD. "Effect of imperceptible vibratory noise applied to wrist skin on fingertip touch evoked potentials - an EEG study." *Physiological Reports.* 2015; 3(11).

31. Schirmer, A; Teh, KS; Wang, S; et al. "Squeeze me, but don't tease me: human and mechanical touch enhance visual attention and emotion discrimination." *Journal of Neuroscience.* 2011; 6(3):219-230.

32. Edelson, SM; Edelson, MG; Kerr, DC; and Grandin, T. "Behavioral and physiological effects of deep pressure on children with autism: a pilot study evaluating the efficacy of Grandin's Hug Machine." *The American Journal of Occupational Therapy.* 1999; 53(2):145-152.

33. Wikipedia. *Cognitive Dissonance.* 2016; https://en.wikipedia.org/wiki/Cognitive_dissonance.

34. Festinger L. *A Theory of Cognitive Dissonance.* Evanston, Ill.: Row, 1957.

35. Rothfeld, JM; Gross, DS; and Watkins, LR. "Sexual responsiveness and its relationship to vaginal stimulation-produced analgesia in the rat." *Brain Research.* 1985; 358(1-2):309-315.

36. Schachter, S; and Singer, JE. "Cognitive, social, and physiological determinants of emotional state." *Psychological Review.* 1962; 69:379-399.

37. Wikipedia. *Misattribution of Arousal.* 2016; https://en.wikipedia.org/wiki/Misattribution_of_arousal.

38. Dutton, DG; and Aron, AP. "Some evidence for heightened sexual attraction under conditions of high anxiety." *Journal of Personality and Social Psychology.* 1974; 30(4):510-517.

39. Schick, A; Adam, R; Vollmayr, B; Kuehner, C; Kanske, P; and Wessa, M. "Neural correlates of valence generalization in an affective conditioning paradigm." *Behavioural Brain Research.* 2015; 292:147-156.

40. Whalen, PJ; Kagan, J; Cook, RG; et al. "Human amygdala responsivity to masked fearful eye whites." *Science.* 2004; 306(5704):2061.

41. Dalton, KM; Nacewicz, BM; Johnstone, T; et al. "Gaze fixation and the neural circuitry of face processing in autism." *Nature Neuroscience.* 2005; 8(4):519-526.

42. Diego, MA; and Field, T. "Moderate pressure massage elicits a parasympathetic nervous system response." *International Journal of Neuroscience.* 2009; 119(5):630-638.

43. He, B; Lu, Z; He, W; Huang, B; and Jiang, H. "Autonomic Modulation by Electrical Stimulation of the Parasympathetic Nervous System: An Emerging Intervention for Cardiovascular Diseases." *Cardiovascular Therapeutics.* 2016; 34(3):167-171.

44. Clancy, JA; Mary, DA; Witte, KK; Greenwood, JP; Deuchars, SA; and Deuchars, J. "Non-invasive vagus nerve stimulation in healthy humans reduces sympathetic nerve activity." *Brain Stimulation.* 2014; 7(6):871-877.

45. He, W; Rong, PJ; Li, L; Ben, H; Zhu, B; and Litscher, G. "Auricular Acupuncture May Suppress Epileptic Seizures via Activating the Parasympathetic Nervous System: A Hypothesis Based on Innovative Methods." *Evidence-Based Complementary and Alternative Medicine.* 2012; 2012:615476.

46. Gao, XY; Zhang, SP; Zhu, B; and Zhang, HQ. "Investigation of specificity of auricular acupuncture points in regulation of autonomic function in anesthetized rats." *Autonomic Neuroscience.* 2008; 138(1-2):50-56.

47. Hotta, H; Schmidt, RF; Uchida, S; and Watanabe, N. "Gentle mechanical skin stimulation inhibits the somatocardiac sympathetic C-reflex elicited by excitation of unmyelinated C-afferent fibers." *European Journal of Pain.* 2010; 14(8):806-813.

48. Teng, EJ; Woods, DW; Twohig, MP; and Marcks, BA. "Body-focused repetitive behavior problems. Prevalence in a nonreferred population and differences in perceived somatic activity." *Behavior Modification.* 2002; 26(3):340-360.

49. Uchikune, M. "Study of the effects of whole-body vibration in the low frequency range." *Journal of Low-Frequency Noise, Vibration and Active Control.* 2004; 23(2):133-138.

50. Uchikune, M. "The evaluation of horizontal whole-body vibration in the low frequency range." *Journal of Low-Frequency Noise, Vibration and Active Control.* 2002; 21(1):29-36.

51. Buynitsky, T; and Mostofsky, DI. "Restraint stress in biobehavioral research: Recent developments." *Neuroscience and Biobehavioral Reviews.* 2009; 33(7):1089-1098.

52. Carlson, JN; Fitzgerald, LW; Keller Jr., RW; and Glick, SD. "Side and region dependent changes in dopamine activation with various durations of restraint stress." *Brain Research.* 1991; 550(2):313-318.

53. Meller, E; Shen, C; Nikolao, TA; et al. "Region-specific effects of acute and repeated restraint stress on the phosphorylation of mitogen-activated protein kinases." *Brain Research.* 2003; 979(1-2):57-64.

54. Patel, S; Roelke, CT; Rademacher, DJ; and Hillard, CJ. "Inhibition of restraint stress-induced neural and behavioural activation by endogenous cannabinoid signalling." *The European Journal of Neuroscience.* 2005; 21(4):1057-1069.

55. Wood, GE; Young, LT; Reagan, LP; and McEwen, BS. "Acute and chronic restraint stress alter the incidence of social conflict in male rats." *Hormones and Behavior.* 2003; 43(1):205-213.

56. Bondarenko, E; Hodgson, DM; and Nalivaiko, E. "Amygdala mediates respiratory responses to sudden arousing stimuli and to restraint stress in rats." *American Journal of Physiology - Regulatory, Integrative and Comparative Physiology.* 2014; 306(12):R951-959.

57. Mo, B; Feng, N; Renner, K; and Forster, G. "Restraint stress increases serotonin release in the central nucleus of the amygdala via activation of corticotropin-releasing factor receptors." *Brain Research Bulletin.* 2008; 76(5):493-498.

58. Rademacher, DJ; Meier, SE; Shi, L; Ho, WS; Jarrahian, A; and Hillard, CJ. "Effects of acute and repeated restraint stress on endocannabinoid content in the amygdala, ventral striatum, and medial prefrontal cortex in mice." *Neuropharmacology.* 2008; 54(1):108-116.

59. Padovan, CM; and Guimaraes, FS. "Restraint-induced hypoactivity in an elevated plus-maze." *Brazilian Journal of Medical and Biological Research.* 2000; 33(1):79-83.

60. Becerra, L; Breiter, HC; Wise, R; Gonzalez, RG; and Borsook, D. "Reward circuitry activation by noxious thermal stimuli." *Neuron.* 2001; 32(5):927-946.

61. Dunbar, RI; Baron, R; Frangou, A; et al. "Social laughter is correlated with an elevated pain threshold." *Proceedings of the Royal Society: Biological Sciences.* 2012; 279(1731):1161-1167.

62. Paloyelis, Y; Krahe, C; Maltezos, S; Williams, SC; Howard, MA; and Fotopoulou, A. "The Analgesic Effect of Oxytocin in Humans: A Double-Blind, Placebo-Controlled Cross-Over Study Using Laser-Evoked Potentials." *The Journal of Neuroendocrinology.* 2016; 28(4).

63. Corley, AM; Cano, A; Goubert, L; Vlaeyen, JW; and Wurm, LH. "Global and Situational Relationship Satisfaction Moderate the Effect of Threat on Pain in Couples." *Pain Medicine.* 2016; 17(9):1664-1675.

64. Pieretti, S; Di Giannuario, A; Di Giovannandrea, R; et al. "Gender differences in pain and its relief." *Annali dell'Istituto Super Sanità.* 2016; 52(2):184-189.

65. Johnson, KV; and Dunbar, RI. "Pain tolerance predicts human social network size." *Scientific Reports.* 2016; 6:25267.

66. Defrin, R; Lahav, Y; Solomon, Z. "Dysfunctional pain modulation in torture survivors: The mediating effect of PTSD." *Journal of Pain.* 2016.

67. Kamping, S; Andoh, J; Bomba, IC; Diers, M; Diesch, E; and Flor, H. "Contextual modulation of pain in masochists: involvement of the parietal operculum and insula." *Pain.* 2016; 157(2):445-455.

68. Daly, I; Hallowell, J; Hwang, F; et al. "Changes in music tempo entrain movement related brain activity." *Engineering in Medicine and Biology Society, Conference Proceedings of the IEEE.* 2014:4595-4598.

69. McIntyre, CK; Hatfield, T; and McGaugh, JL. "Amygdala norepinephrine levels after training predict inhibitory avoidance retention performance in rats." *European Journal of Neuroscience.* 2002; 16(7):1223-1226.

70. Streltsova, A; and McCleery, JP. "Neural time-course of the observation of human and non-human object touch." *Social Cognitive and Affective Neuroscience.* 2014; 9(3):333-341.

71. Kihlstrom, JF. "Social neuroscience: The footprints of Phineas Gage." *Social Cognition.* 2010; 28:757-782.

72. Lee, KH; and Siegle, GJ. "Common and distinct brain networks underlying explicit emotional evaluation: a meta-analytic study." *Social Cognitive and Affective Neuroscience.* 2012; 7(5):521-534.

73. Georgiadis; JR. "Doing it...wild? On the role of the cerebral cortex in human sexual activity." *Socioaffective Neuroscience and Psychology.* 2012; 2:17337.

74. Georgiadis, JR; and Kringelbach, ML. "The human sexual response cycle: brain imaging evidence linking sex to other pleasures." *Progress in Neurobiology.* 2012; 98(1):49-81.

75. de Jong, PJ; van Overveld, M; and Borg, C. "Giving in to arousal or staying stuck in disgust? Disgust-based mechanisms in sex and sexual dysfunction." *The Journal of Sex Research.* 2013; 50(3-4):247-262.

76. Borg, C; de Jong, PJ; and Georgiadis, JR. "Subcortical BOLD responses during visual sexual stimulation vary as a function of implicit porn associations in women." *Social Cognitive and Affective Neuroscience.* 2014; 9(2):158-166.

77. Borg, C; and de Jong, PJ. "Feelings of disgust and disgust-induced avoidance weaken following induced sexual arousal in women." *PLOS ONE.* 2012; 7(9):e44111.

78. Wyman, J. *On Symmetry and Homology in Limbs.* Boston: AA Kingman, 1867.

79. Carello, C; and Turvey MT. "Rotational invariants and dynamic touch." *In Touch Representation and Blindness,* edited by MA Heller. Oxford: Oxford University Press, 2000.

80. Tarnecki, R; and Konorski, J. "Patterns responses of Purkinje cells in cats to passive displacements of limbs, squeezing, and touching." *Acta Neurobiologiae Experimentalis (Wars).* 1979; 30:95-119.

81. Fetz, EE; Finocchio, DV; Baker, MA; and Soso, MJ. "Sensory and motor responses of precentral cortex cells during comparable passive and active joint movements." *The Journal of Neurophysiology.* 1980; 43(4):1070-1089.

82. Wang, Y; Wang, JY; and Luo, F. "Why self-induced pain feels less painful than externally generated pain: distinct brain activation patterns in self- and externally generated pain." *PLOS ONE.* 2011; 6(8):e23536.

83. Kubota, S; Endo, Y; and Kubota, M. "Effect of upper torso inclination in Fowler's position on autonomic cardiovascular regulation." *The Journal of Physiological Sciences.* 2013; 63(5):369-376.

84. Harmon-Jones, E; and Peterson, CK. "Supine body position reduces neural response to anger evocation." *Psychological Science.* 2009; 20(10):1209-1210.

85. Strother, L; Mathuranath, PS; Aldcroft, A; Lavell, C; Goodale, MA; and Vilis, T. "Face inversion reduces the persistence of global form and its neural correlates." *PLOS ONE.* 2011; 6(4):e18705.

86. Haxby, JV; Ungerleider, LG; Clark, VP; Schouten, JL; Hoffman, EA; and Martin, A. "The effect of face inversion on activity in human neural systems for face and object perception." *Neuron.* 1999; 22(1):189-199.

87. Stekelenburg, JJ; and de Gelder, B. "The neural correlates of perceiving human bodies: an ERP study on the body-inversion effect." *Neuroreport.* 2004; 15(5):777-780.

88. LaBar, KS; Crupain, MJ; Voyvodic, JT; and McCarthy, G. "Dynamic perception of facial affect and identity in the human brain." Cerebral Cortex. 2003; 13(10):1023-1033.

89. Goldberg, H; Christensen, A; Flash, T; Giese, MA; and Malach, R. "Brain activity correlates with emotional perception induced by dynamic avatars." *NeuroImage.* 2015; 122:306-317.

90. Herrington, JD; Nymberg, C; and Schultz, RT. "Biological motion task performance predicts superior temporal sulcus activity." *Brain and Cognition.* 2011; 77(3):372-381.

91. Trautmann, SA; Fehr, T; and Herrmann, M. "Emotions in motion: dynamic compared to static facial expressions of disgust and happiness reveal more widespread emotion-specific activations." *Brain Research.* 2009; 1284:100-115.

92. Wikipedia. *Emotion Contagion.* 2016; https://en.wikipedia.org/wiki/Emotional_contagion.

93. Massen, JJ; Dusch, K; Eldakar, OT; and Gallup, AC. "A thermal window for yawning in humans: yawning as a brain cooling mechanism." *Physiology and Behavior.* 2014; 130:145-148.

94. Gallup, AC; and Eldakar, OT. "The thermoregulatory theory of yawning: what we know from over 5 years of research." *Frontiers in Human Neuroscience.* 2012; 6:188.

Chapter 4

Warming Up for Bondage

by fuoco

Fuoco is a rope performer, a circus aerialist, and an instructor who has performed and taught all over the world. Visit RopesOnFuoco.com to learn more.

Photo credits

Models: fuoco and SatineAngelic

Photos with shadowy wall by The Silence. Shot at Topologist's studio; learn more at crash-restraint.com.

Photos with plaid rug by iambic9

This chapter isn't by any means a comprehensive guide to warming up for bondage. There are all sorts of stretches and exercises you can do to get your body ready for rope—so if you have a warm-up that works for you already, that's great! But if you feel a bit lost as you look around your local dungeon and see bottoms stretching and moving around in preparation for their rope scenes, then this chapter is for you.

Try to test out these stretches at home before you use them before a scene. Some of them can be very challenging and take a bit of practice. Pay close attention to the images and alignment cues, and always stretch only until you feel a nice stretching sensation.

Warning: Don't stretch too deeply into anything that feels painful, and always back out of any stretch or position that feels like it's causing injury.

If you have questions about any of the stretches here or feel any pain while trying them out, ask a yoga teacher, a personal trainer, or some other movement coach to check your form and see how you might adapt them for your body.

Why Warm Up at All?

The main purposes of warming up for a rope scene are to improve your experience (scene duration, comfort, etc.) and to prevent injury. We want to increase blood flow to our tissues (both muscles and joints) and "wake up" some of the muscles that we might not have used throughout the day. If you spend a lot of time seated at a desk, it's highly likely that blood flow to certain areas of your body decreases throughout the day. And this is normal. Your body doesn't need every single muscle to be functioning optimally to sit in a chair for an extended period of time. But it can greatly benefit from restoring that blood flow if you want to roll around on the floor in bondage or hang from the ceiling from a few pieces of rope!

Bondage, especially suspensions, can be a strenuous activity requiring a lot of effort. (Obviously we're not talking about something like a nice decorative chest harness or your wrists tied gently to the bed here.) To make strenuous bondage—where you'll be put in taxing positions or those requiring stamina—more fun and to reduce your risk of injury, you're going to want to make sure that all of the muscles and joints involved are healthy, happy, and experiencing lots of good blood flow.

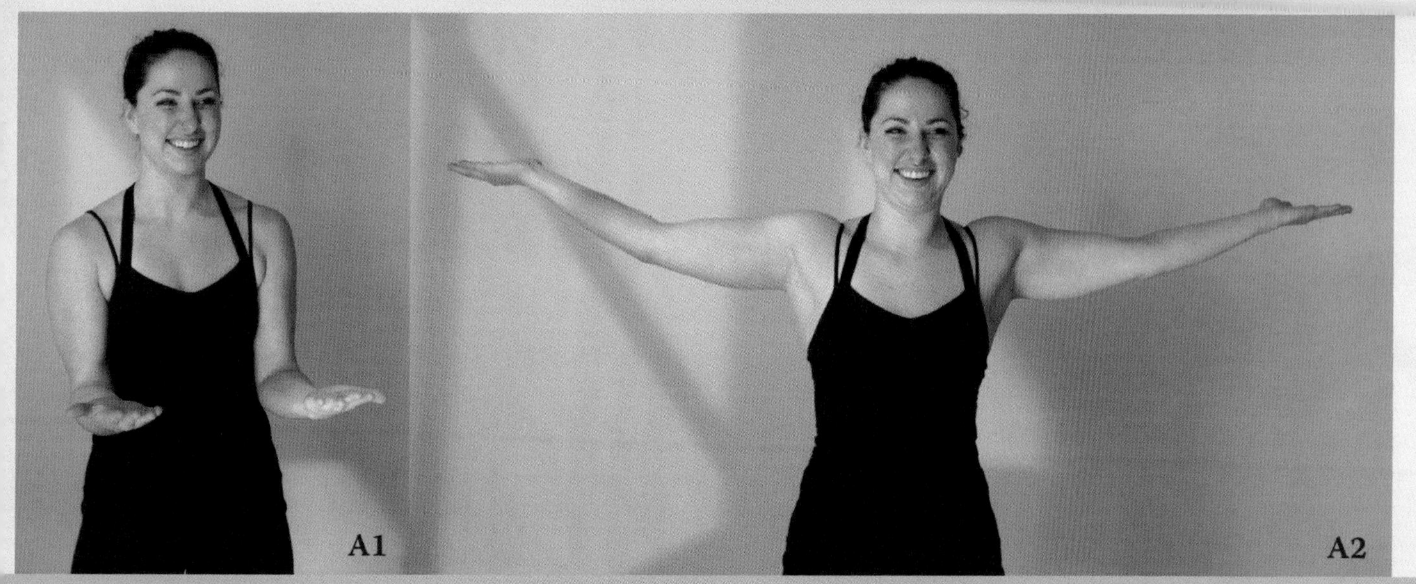

What *Not* to Do

The point of your warm-up is not to become more flexible five minutes before a rope scene. I see bottoms doing this all the time: They prepare to be tied up by sitting in the splits or pushing into their backbend as much as they can. But stretching like that—for the purpose of developing flexibility—is a totally different practice, and could actually decrease your ability to use your muscles effectively during your rope scene. Remember that all we're trying to do here is wake up the muscles and get the blood flowing. In fact, a well-rounded pre-scene sequence may even take less time and be gentler than you think!

If you do want to enhance your flexibility outside of pre-scene warming up, by the way, talk to a yoga teacher, a dance teacher, a circus teacher, or some other type of movement specialist. Some cities even have dedicated flexibility coaches. Just remember that flexibility training is different than warming up for a scene.

So how should you be warming up? Briefly and gently moving your major joints through a range of motion, and then stretching the important muscle groups, is a great idea. This combination of easy muscle activation and passive stretching should be enough to get the blood flowing and the muscles working.

The Exercises

The major areas I'd encourage rope bottoms to focus on are the shoulders, spine, and hips. Let's talk about each of those spots.

The Shoulders

Warming up the shoulders is super important, especially if you're going to do a bondage scene that uses any harness that includes the arms. Takate-kotes (box ties), strappados and armbinders, teppous—all of these ties put a lot of load on the shoulders, and it's important that the shoulder joint and all of the muscles that support it are warm and in good working condition. The two warm-ups below are followed by some shoulder stretches.

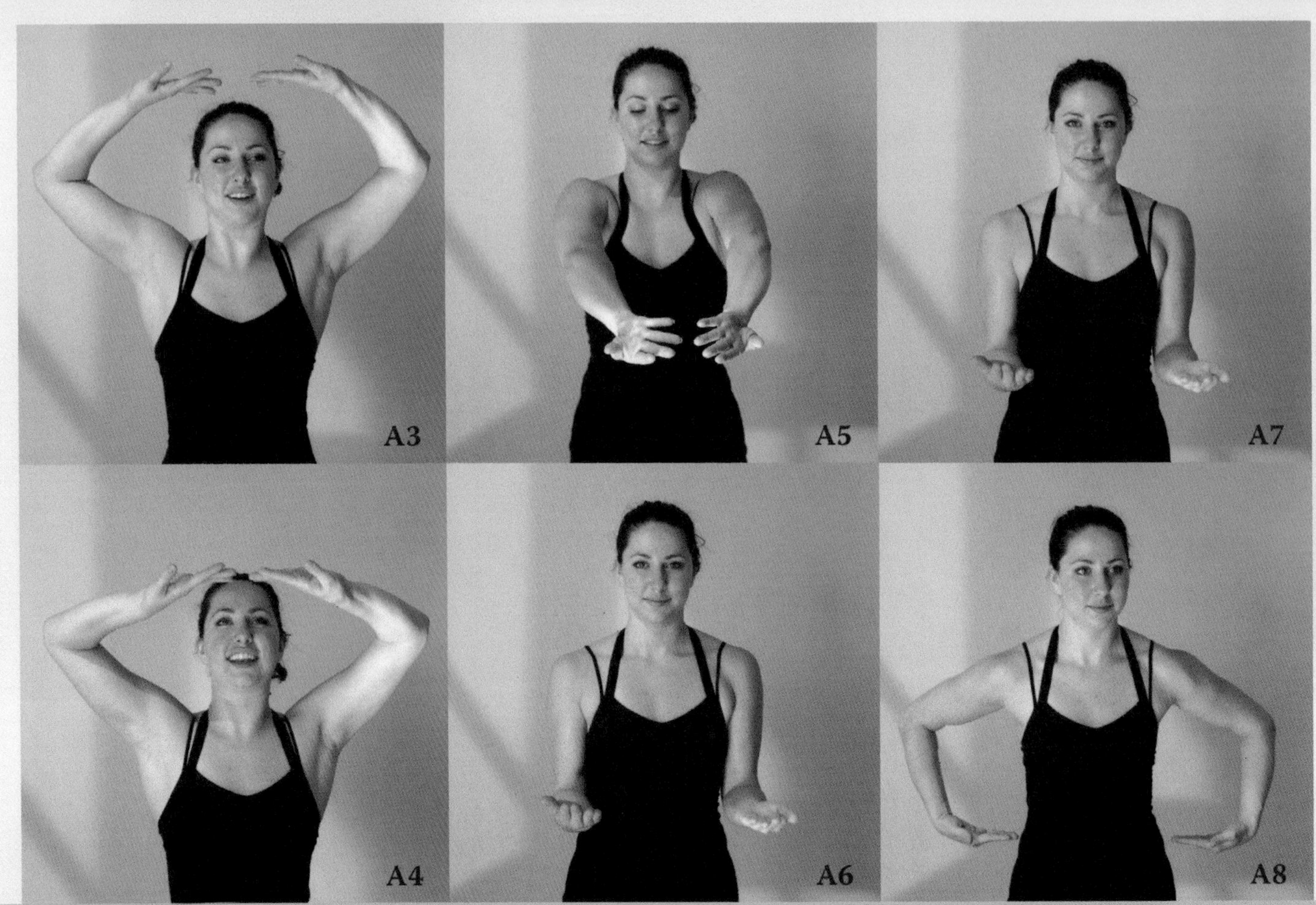

1. Teacups

My favorite way to get the shoulders warm is through an exercise called Teacups. Bring your elbows in toward your waistline with your palms up (A1). Your forearms should be parallel with each other and with the floor. Now you're going to imagine that in your upturned palms, you're holding teacups filled with very hot tea. Try not to spill your tea as you do this exercise!

First bring your arms out in front of you, then move them upward and back in a wide circle (A2), so that your hands end up over your head (A3). Now for the tricky part: With the palms continually facing up, move the hands down and in front of you in a swimming motion (A4 and A5) until your fingertips are pointing forward and your arms are parallel to each other and the floor again (A6). You've probably spilled tea all over yourself by this point. Don't worry! It's imaginary, so just give yourself a refill and try again. This time, try to focus on moving only your shoulders. Try not to bend backward or forward—even if that means spilling more tea.

When you've done this two or three times in one direction, try moving in the other direction. You'll start in the same spot (A7), but this time wing your elbows out and rotate your hands in (A8) so that your fingertips point to your waistline. Keep rotating as the palms spin under (A9) and move to the front of your body (A10). Your arms will come overhead from front to back (A11) and spiral out (A12), making their way back to where they started (A13).

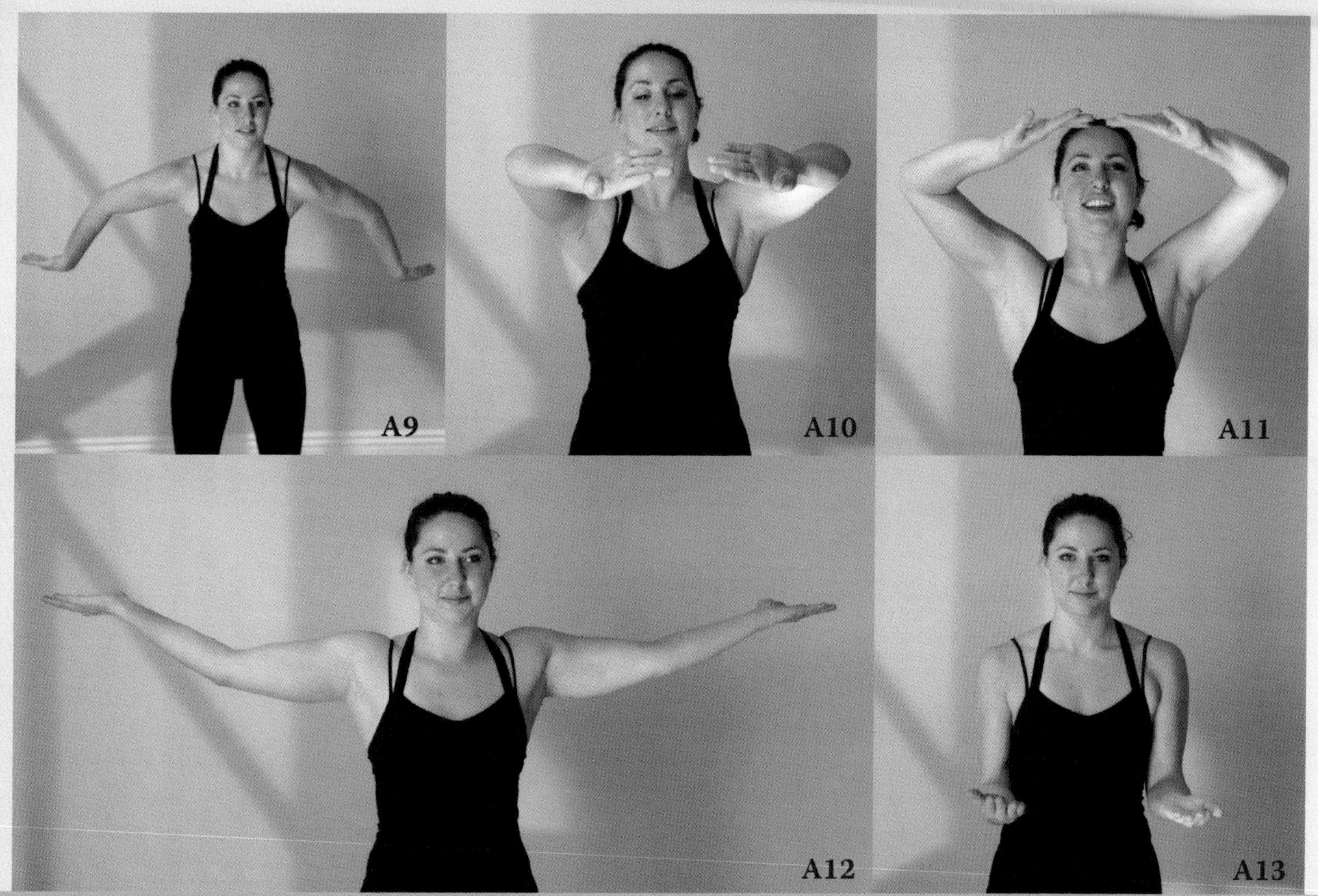

2. Scapular Push-Ups

Make your way into a push-up position on your toes or on your knees. You're going to try to achieve the motion of a small push-up, without bending your arms at all. Keep your torso tight (no sagging hips or butt stuck up in the air), and then move your shoulder blades toward each other (B1), like you're trying to pinch a pencil between your shoulder blades on your back. Then push into the floor and push the shoulder blades away from each other hard (B2). Try doing two sets of eight of these.

Stretches

Now that your shoulders are warm, let's stretch them out a little bit. Most rope bondage harnesses that load the shoulders do so with the shoulders internally rotated. Most shoulder stretches stretch the shoulders in external rotation. So we want to make sure that we're doing both. If you don't know the difference, then do these two exercises:

1. Bring your arms down by your sides and then rotate the hands so that the palms are facing forward and your thumbs are pointing out, away from your body. This is external rotation. If you turn your hands so that your palms are facing to the back and your thumbs are pointing in toward your waistline, this is internal rotation.

2. Now do the same thing but bring your arms straight up over your head. Turn the palms away, so that the pinkies rotate in toward each other. This is actually external rotation! Don't believe me? Keep your hands in exactly the same position and bring the arms back down to your sides. You'll be right where you started—with your palms facing forward.

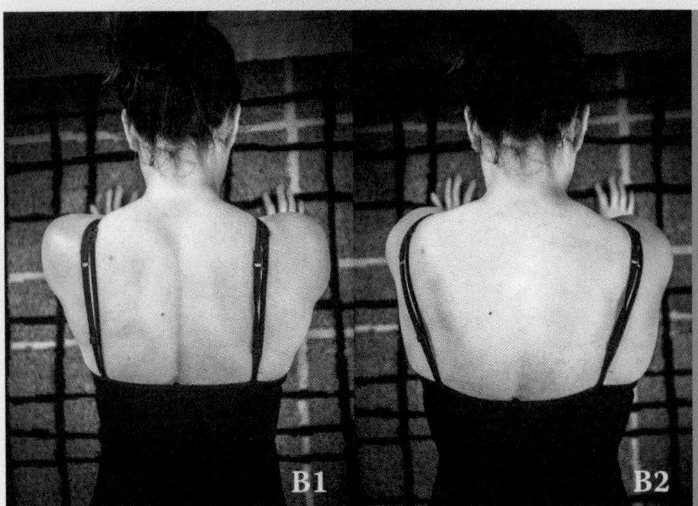

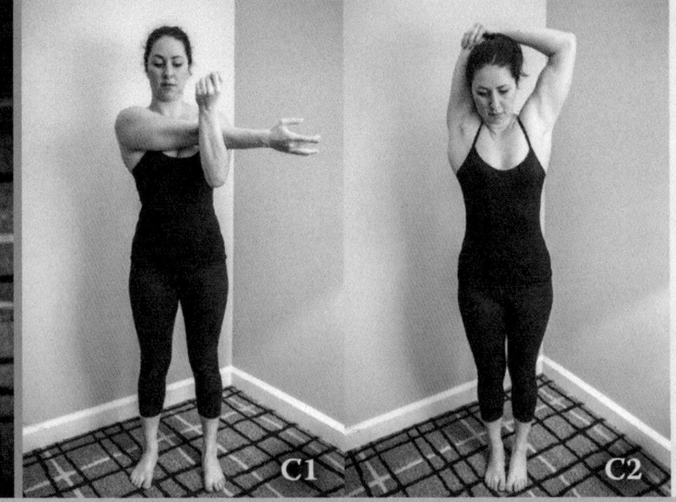

1. External-Rotation Shoulder Stretches

Start with gently stretching each shoulder in external rotation (C1 and C2). You should remember these from gym class. Don't throw your arms into position or tug on yourself too hard. Slowly and gently pull your arm into each stretch and hold it there for about five breaths. Then switch arms and repeat. The second exercise stretches the triceps as well as the shoulder.

2. Internal-Rotation Shoulder Stretches

Now for a few internally rotated stretches. Face a wall and place one straight arm on the wall, up at about the two o'clock position (D1). Think about pushing the very top of the shoulder (where your collarbone and shoulder meet) in toward the wall as you turn your body away from the wall, over your extended arm (D2). You should feel a stretch through the front of the shoulder and maybe into the chest.

Now do the same thing again, but with a bent elbow that sits at three o'clock (D3 and D4). If this feels OK and you want more of a stretch, then move the butt down toward a seated position (D5).

Switch to the other arm and repeat both exercises for the other shoulder.

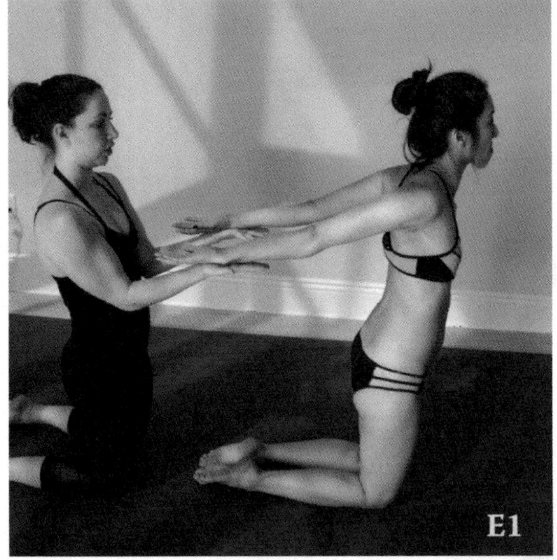

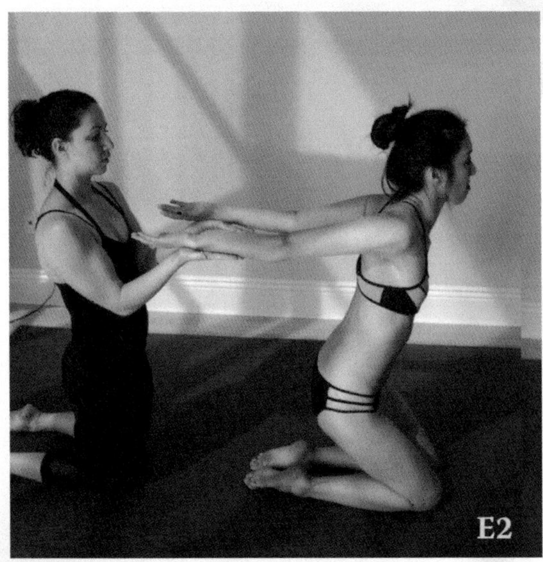

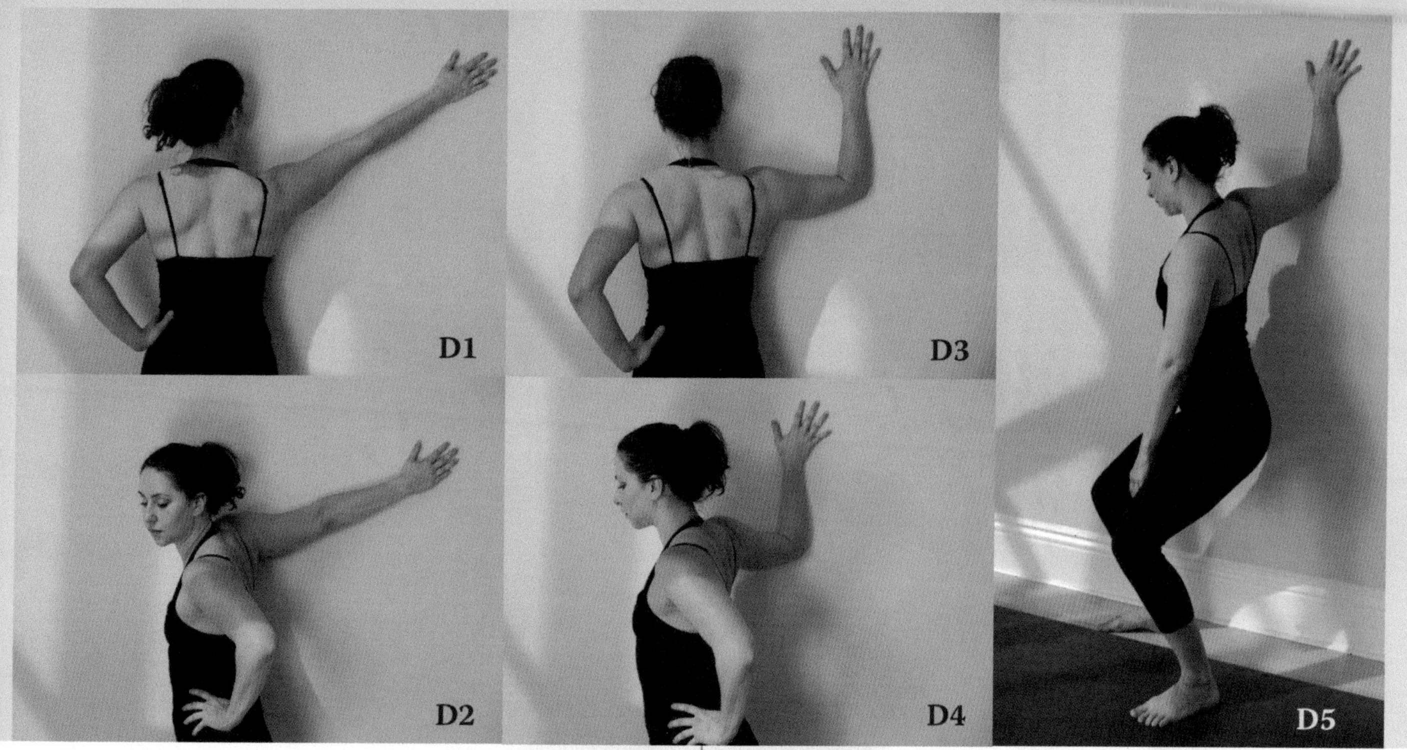

3. Partner Shoulder Stretch

Stretching with a partner can be very effective and a fun way to start connecting. Kneel straight up in front of your partner with your arms out behind you and your palms up. Have your partner place their palms under your palms and onto your forearms and brace you (E1) while you sit your butt down to deepen the stretch as far as is comfortable (E2).

SatineAngelic has quite flexible shoulders! Don't worry if your stretch doesn't look like hers in E1 and E2—just go until you feel a gentle stretch, and remember to communicate with your partner.

The Spine

We're going to gently warm up and stretch the muscles that support the spine all in one go. Warming up and stretching the spine require several sorts of movements: forward bending, backbending, side bending, and twisting.

1. Neck Stretch: Side to Side

It's a good idea to warm up the spine from the top down, so start with your neck. Let your body be still and comfortable (try not to bend into these stretches too much—keep everything below your neck neutral), and drop one ear toward your shoulder (F) and then the other. If you'd like to make this stretch a bit deeper, flex the opposite hand and push it toward the floor.

2. Neck Stretch: Front and Back

Slowly look up (G1) and then look down, moving your chin toward your chest. Make sure that as you look up, you feel like you're reaching your jaw toward the ceiling and not crunching your spine at the base of your neck (G2).

3. Cat-Cow

Some Cat-Cows to follow this up should feel nice and will increase blood flow to the spine and supporting tissue. Come to a tabletop position (Bharmanasana, or Table Pose, in yoga), with your palms directly

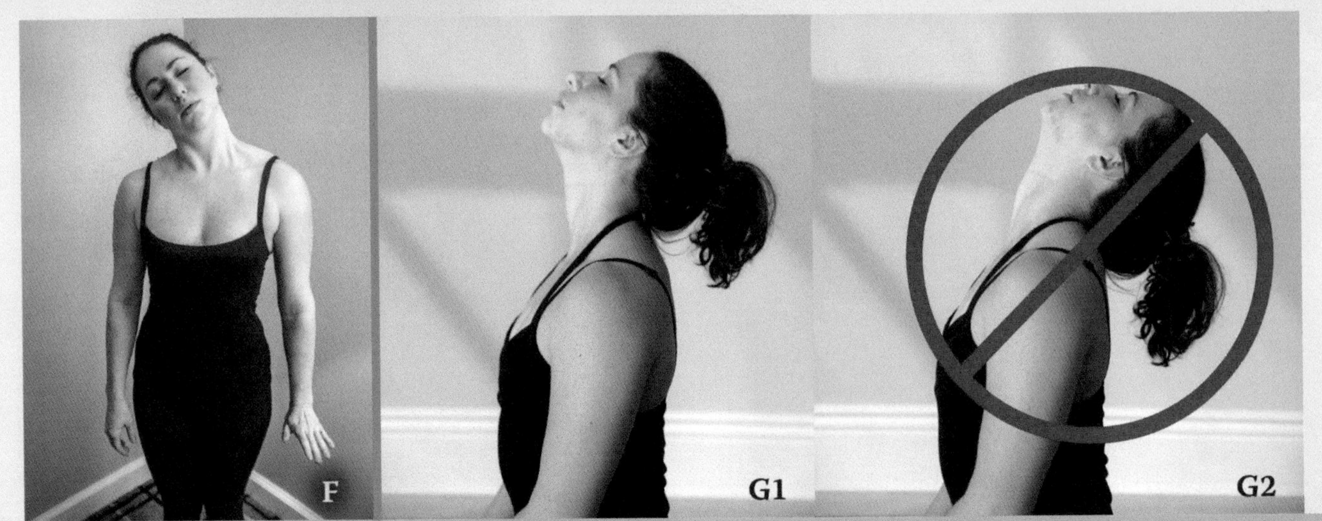

under your shoulders. Keep your arms straight and strong as you inhale and let your belly come down to the floor—imagine a cow udder (H1). Then as you exhale, push the floor away, feel your shoulder blades move away from each other, and round your back like a scared cat (H2). Do this a few times, trying to move on the inhalation and exhalation.

You can do this at the wall as well. H3 shows the cow position, and H4 shows the cat position.

4. Side Stretch

Standing poses are a great way to gently stretch your muscles while activating others, since you need to balance and support your weight in these positions. Stand with your feet about hip width apart, and then reach up overhead and grab one of your wrists (I1). Pull on that wrist as you push your hips in the opposite direction (I2). Try to imagine that you're side bending in between two panes of glass, so you don't tilt forward too much or bend backward too much.

Do this for five slow, steady breaths, then repeat on the other side.

Repeat any of these exercises if your spine still feels tight and stiff, or add any spinal exercises of your own that you know and like. Sun Salutations are an excellent way to warm up the spine. You can find many great video tutorials on the Internet, or head over to your local yoga studio—it's way easier to learn the whole flow in motion in person with an instructor.

The Hips/Lower Body

We use our hips and the muscles in our lower body a lot in rope. Hanging in a hip harness will feel much better if you've moved your hips through a range of motion already. And your ability to support your weight in a futomomo suspension will be greater if you've made time for a good warm-up. So last but certainly not least, let's warm up the hip flexors and lower body.

Warm-Up

We'll just do one warm-up before getting into the stretching, but it has three parts.

Leg Pulses

Use a pole, wall, or chair for stability if you like. Bring your leg in front of you and lift it as high as you can while still keeping your hips level (J1 and J2). Keep the standing leg firm and strong, but don't lock your knee. Using very small movements, pulse the leg up 10 times, and then hold it up a tiny bit higher than where you started for 10 seconds. Switch legs and repeat.

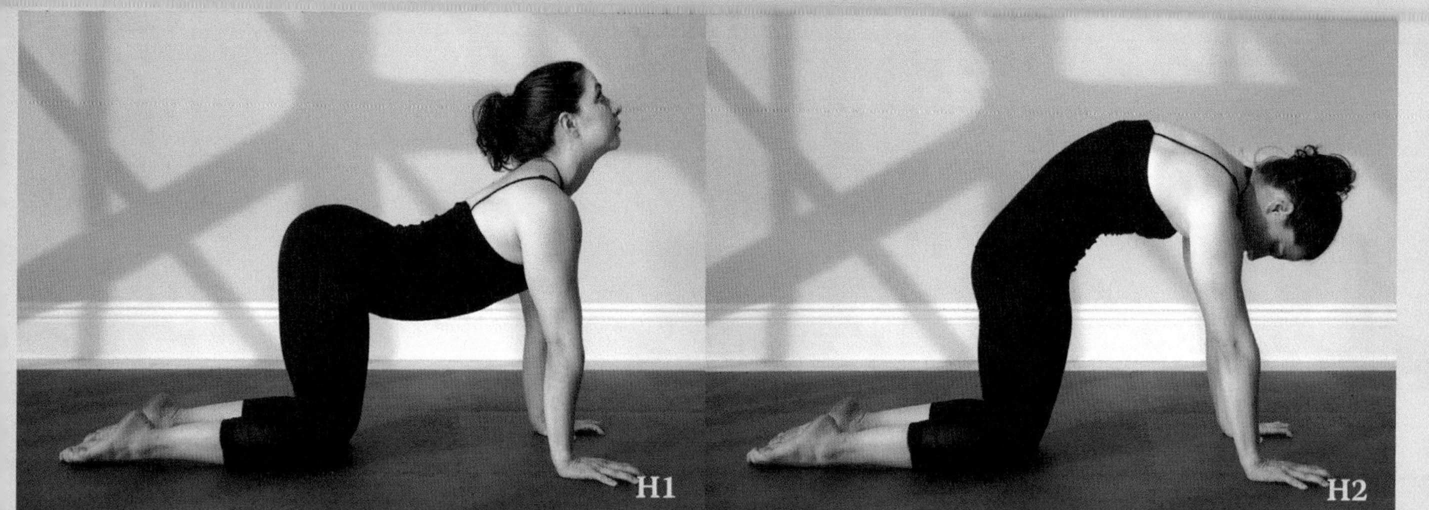

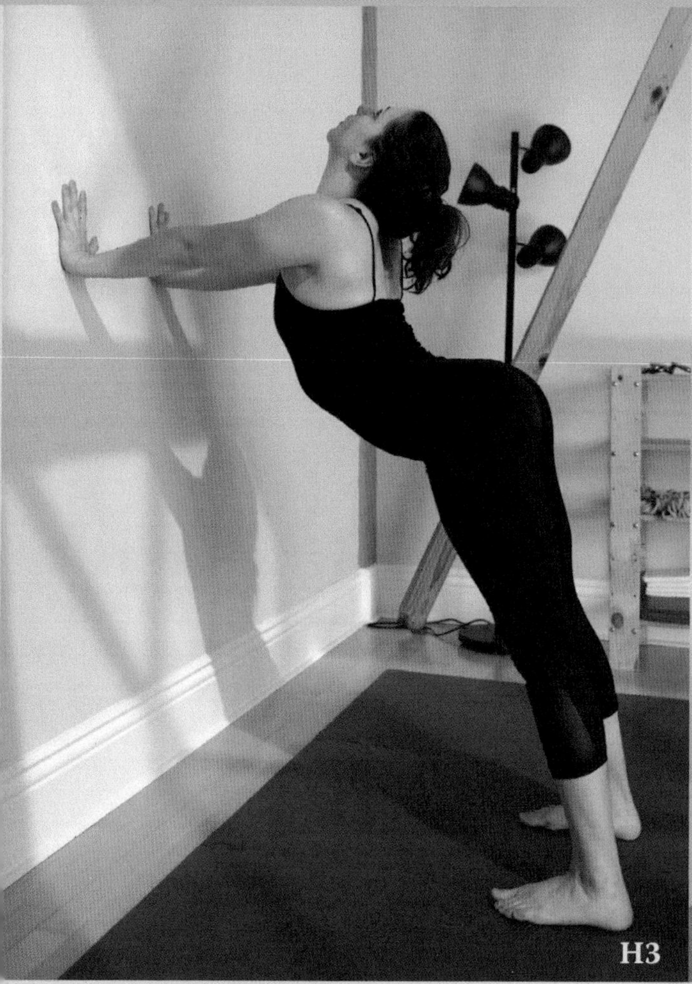

H3

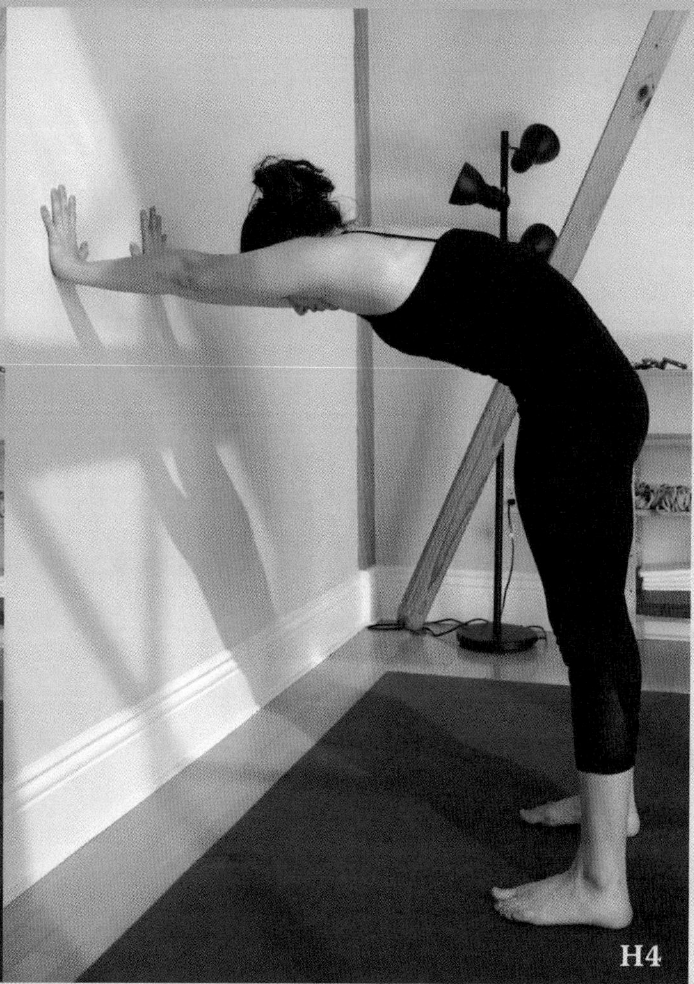

H4

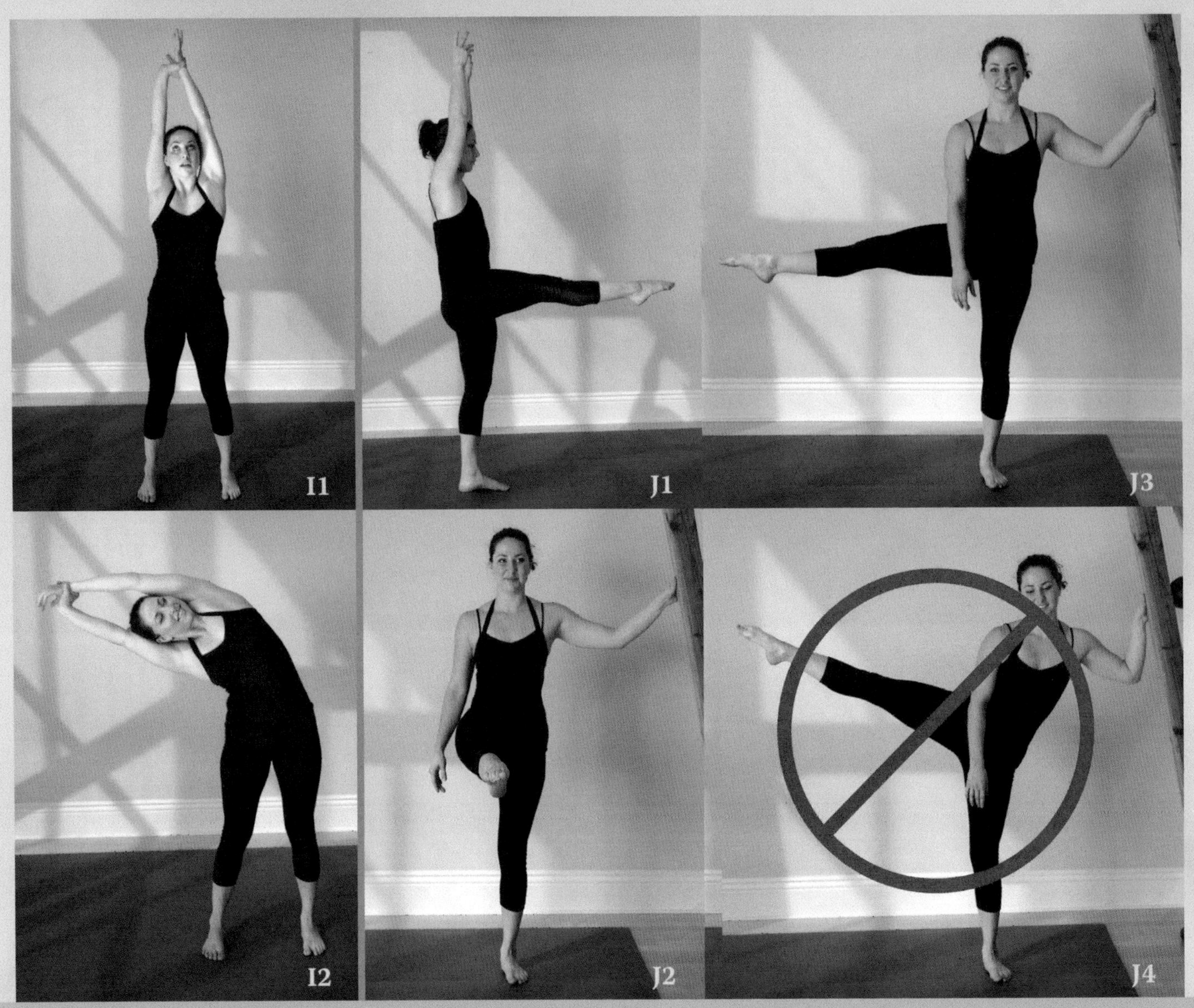

Doing this without support (J1) will help you work on your balance, but hold on to something (J2) if you need the extra stability.

Next, do the same thing (10 pulses and a 10-second hold) with your leg out to the side (J3). Make sure not to raise your leg above hip level (J4).

Lastly, do the same thing (10 pulses and a 10-second hold) with your leg extended out behind you (J5). Keep your hips square and try not to arch your back too much when the leg is behind you. J6 shows uneven hips.

Stretches

Lower body feeling warm? Let's start stretching the hips, hamstrings, and quadriceps.

1. Easy Lunge (Hips)

Make sure that your forward knee is stacked over your ankle, to avoid knee problems, and that the tops of both hip bones are pointing forward (K1). In other words, if you were to look at your profile in a mirror, you would want to see your shinbone in a straight line, not at an angle (K2), and see only your silhouette, and not the front of your pelvis or butt cheeks. Moving the

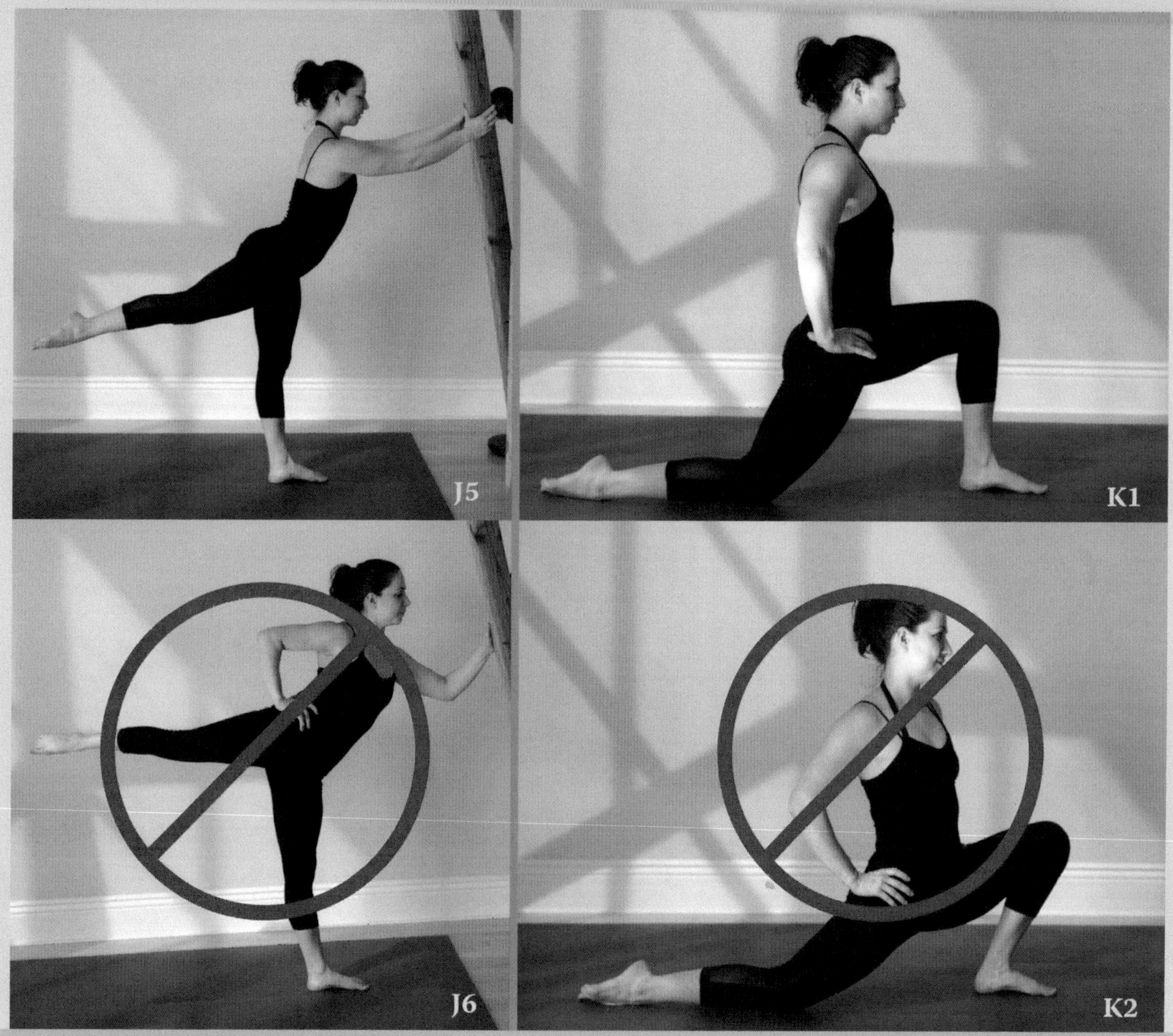

knee past the ankle, as in K2, is no good for that knee joint. My hips are also open toward the camera in K2, and you can see my pelvis—also not good.

You can place your hands on the floor, rest them on your forward knee, or place them on your hips. Whichever you choose, lower your pelvis toward the floor until you feel a gentle stretch through the back hip and the quadriceps of the back leg.

2. Half Split (Hamstrings)

From the lunge position, push the forward leg straight until the hips are stacked over the back knee (L1). You should feel it stretching out the hamstrings, the muscle that runs down the back side of the front leg.

Try to maintain a flat back and bend forward, thinking about lining up your sternum with your shinbone. As with the lunge, keep both hip points pointing forward. If it helps, you can think about pushing your back hip toward your forward knee.

Notice in L1 that both hip points are forward, and that there's a straight vertical line from my knee to my hip. In L2 my back hip is opening up and I'm sitting my butt down instead of keeping it stacked.

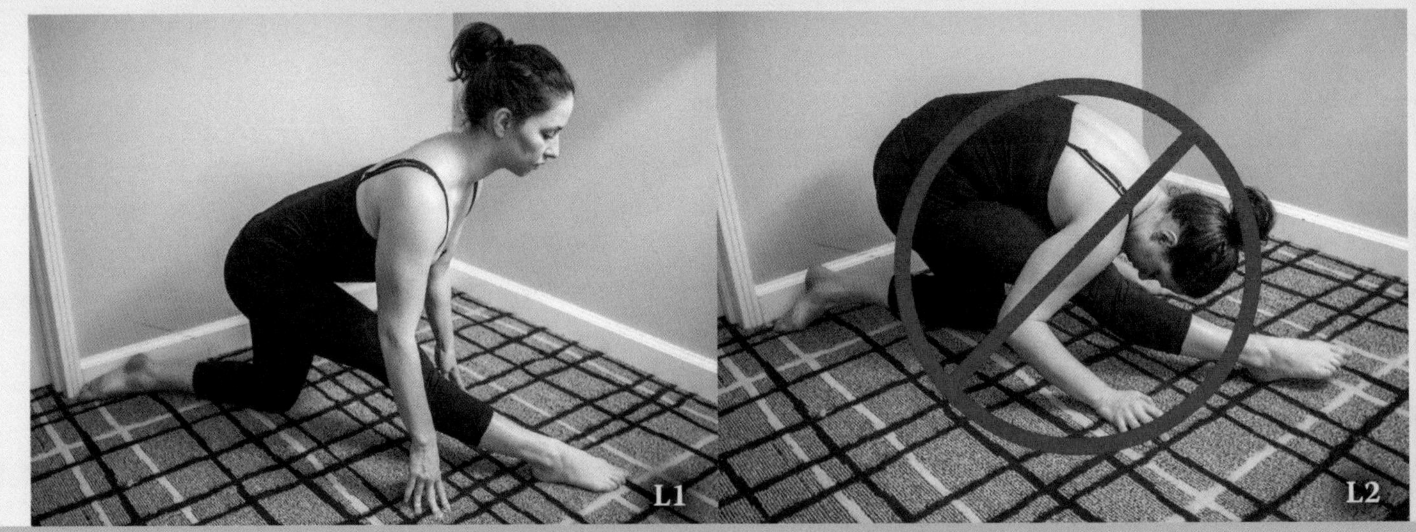

3. Quadriceps Stretch

The quadriceps make up the big muscle group on the top part of the leg (above the knee). You can do this stretch on the floor or standing. If you're doing it on the floor, be very careful to go only as far as is comfortable, even if that means leaning only an inch back.

Kneel down with your knees close and your feet a bit wide. If this position hurts your knees at all, you can bring your feet together so that they rest under your butt—or try the standing version. Start to sit down in between your feet and lower your upper body down (M1). Maybe you just lean back a bit, maybe you lower down to your elbows, or maybe you go further toward the floor or lie fully on your back (M2). You can have your hands at your sides or on your chest, or bring them overhead.

If you're all the way lying down and still don't feel a stretch, focus on the arch in your lower back (M3) and try to flatten it out, minimizing the distance between your lower back and the floor (M4).

Standing variation: Use a pole, wall, or chair to stabilize yourself. Reach back for your foot behind you, grab the ankle or the top of the foot on the same side as your hand, and pull it gently toward your butt (N). Try to keep the spine neutral—it may want to arch into a backbend here.

Don't worry about getting your foot as close to your butt as mine is in N. Focus more on keeping your spine neutral (maybe even tucking your pelvis a little bit) while you gently pull the foot closer toward your body.

To Complete Your Warm-Up

Hopefully now your muscles are "awake," you feel a bit looser, and your blood is flowing nicely. A complete warm-up, however, starts well before you're eyeing your partner's ropes in anticipation. Drink lots of water and eat the right amount of good food for you throughout the day beforehand. (Eating too much or too heavy a meal right before getting tied up can make you feel sluggish or nauseous, while eating or drinking too little can make you feel lightheaded, dizzy, or just distracted.) Avoid drugs and alcohol, which can impair your judgment in all areas—and alcohol can dehydrate you as well. And especially if you've been drinking lots of water, hit the bathroom before you hit the ropes.

Consider bringing a yoga mat or blanket with you to the playspace so that you'll have a clean surface to warm up on too. And having a rope bottoming bag with snacks, water, medications, and anything else

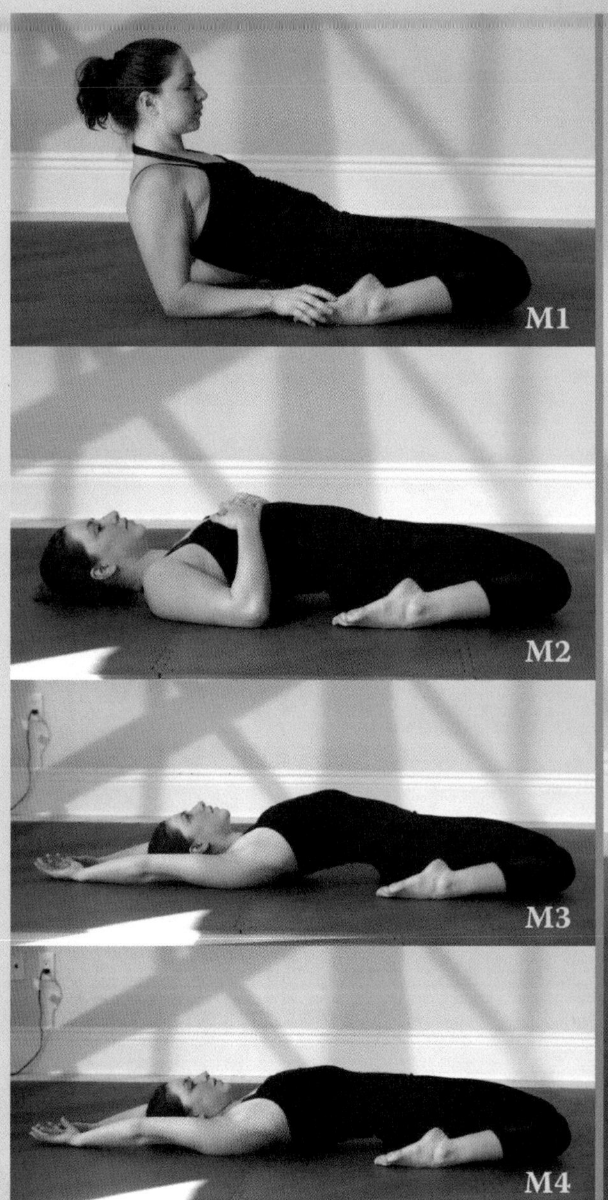

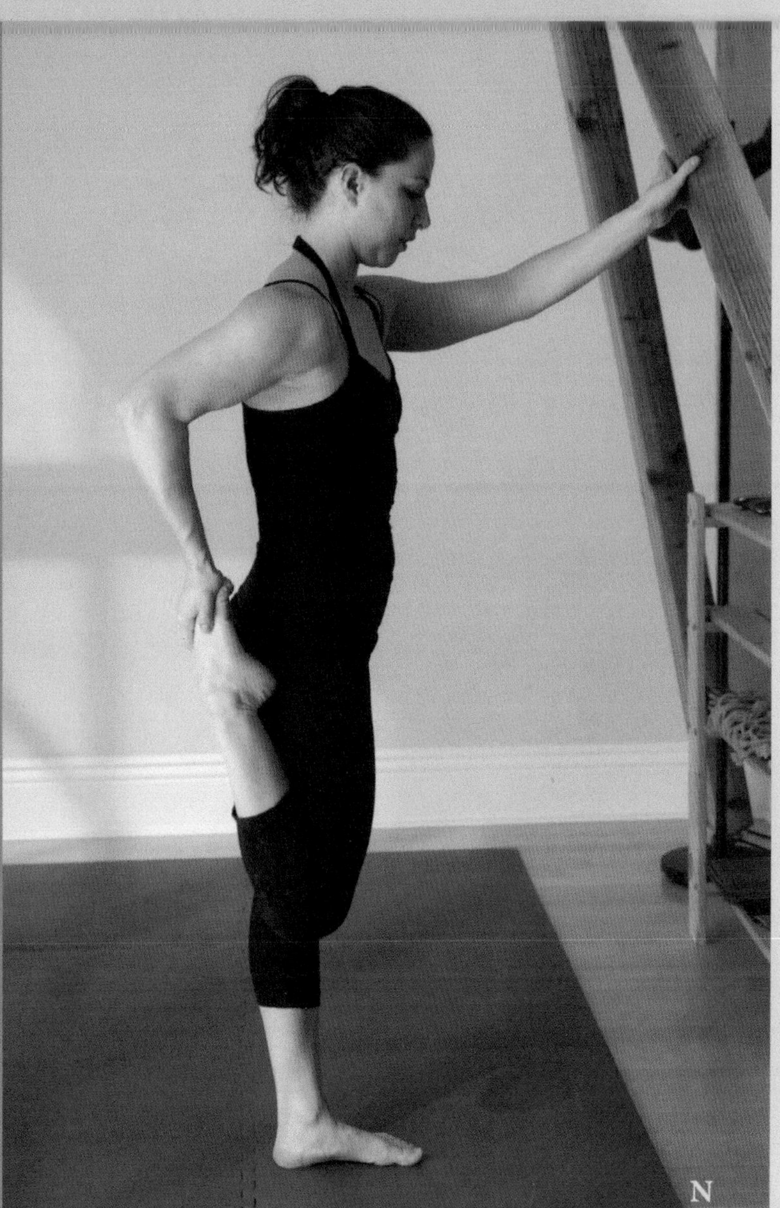

that will make the experience better or help keep you safe is a good idea.

And to reiterate, please do find someone in your community to talk to—a yoga teacher, a personal trainer, a movement coach—face to face if you have any questions about anything in this chapter. Everyone's body is different, and some of these stretches and exercises may work better for you than others, or you may benefit from modifications not shown here. A professional you see in person will be able to assess where you're at and suggest modifications or alternate exercises to better suit your needs.

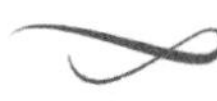

Happy roping!

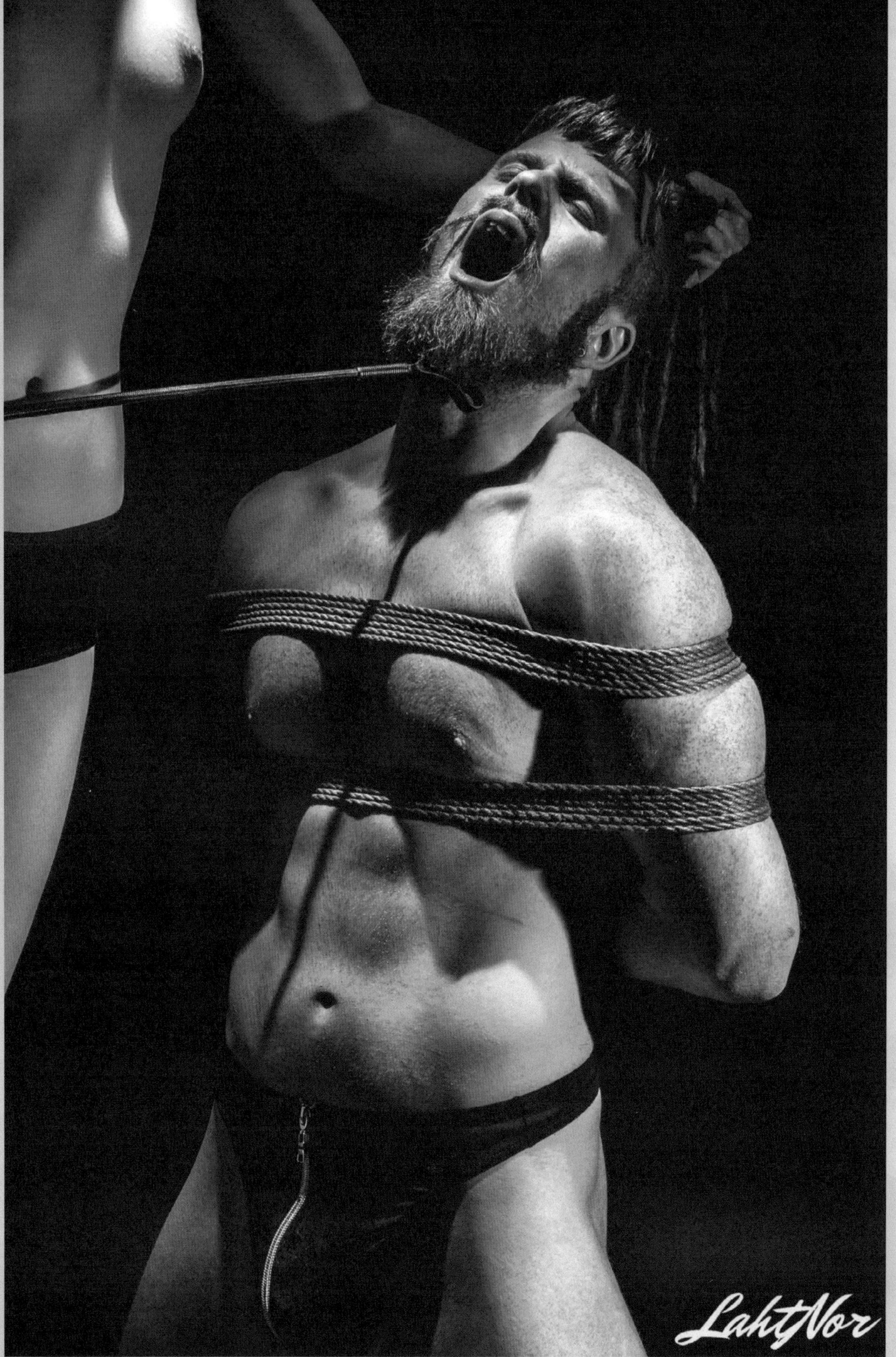
LahtNor

Chapter 5

Pain Processing and Breathwork

Bondage without pain, for me, is like a birthday party without cake—it just doesn't feel complete. If you're only into decorative bondage that feels like a hug, or having your wrists gently tied together with silk rope, you may want to skip this chapter. If the thought of gasping, moaning, crying, or begging for mercy turns you on, you're in the right place.

What exactly is pain, for starters? The International Association for the Study of Pain defines it as "an unpleasant sensory and emotional experience associated with actual or potential tissue damage, or described in terms of such damage."[1] But that doesn't quite work for our purposes, does it? For one thing, are all you masochists snickering at "unpleasant"? And anyone who's been in bondage knows that you don't actually need to experience actual tissue damage or the thought of it to be in pain.

Rope bottoming isn't simple, and neither is pain, so I think this multifaceted description from Margaret A. Caudill, MD, PhD, is better for our purposes:

- *Biologically,* pain is a signal that the body has been harmed.
- *Psychologically,* pain is experienced as emotional suffering.
- *Behaviorally,* pain alters the way a person moves and acts.
- *Cognitively,* pain calls for thinking about its meaning, its cause, and possible remedies.
- *Spiritually,* pain may be a reminder of mortality.
- *Culturally,* pain may be used to test people's fortitude or to force their submission.[2]

All of those aspects may come into play in a single rope session! So when we talk about pain processing for rope, we're actually talking about a deeply complex process that goes well beyond the body. And the experience of pain is *highly subjective.* That subjectivity and those nonbody aspects are good news for rope bottoms, because while most of us can't control our physical sensory reaction to a painful stimulus, we can change how we *perceive* that stimulus. How? The brain gives meaning to the pain messages it receives, and we can cause other messages to be sent simultaneously to the brain that affect the meaning. We can also affect the context in which we experience the pain—setting up our environment, drawing on a supportive partner connection, and so on—to change how we perceive it.

Unlike those people who use meditation, breathwork, a hypnotic trance, or whatever else to put their entire body in a state where it doesn't register pain at all (like for having their chest cut open on an operating table without being "put under" by anesthesia), we actually *need to stay aware of pain* on some level. Why? Because monitoring pain and other sensations can help us avoid nerve damage and other kinds of injuries and issues. Plus, being completely outside the body would pretty much defeat the whole purpose of why we do rope, right?

As for why we might actually want pain at all in a rope scene, that's also highly subjective. I like it in

Lahtnor in self-bondage. Photo by Lahtnor: facebook.com/lahtnor

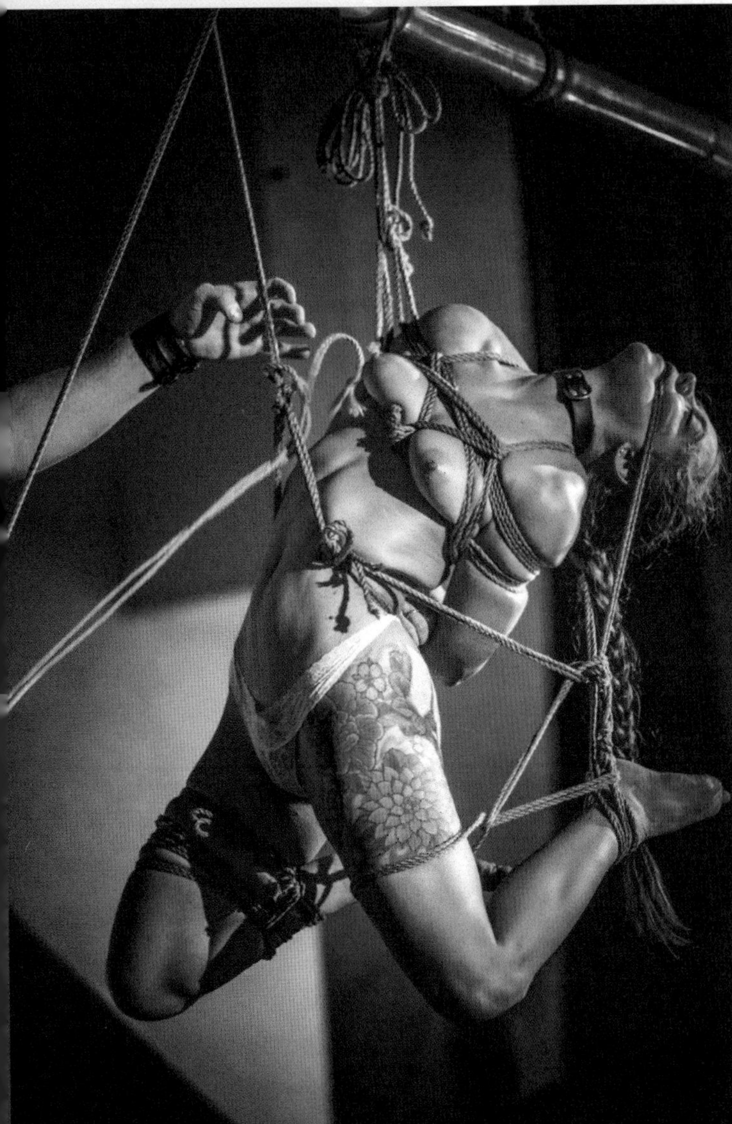

Cat. Bondage by -EM-. Photo by iambic9

part because it helps put me into a trancy ropespace and because it makes me feel more connected to my partner, like we're going through something deep and intimate together. Pain can also help us feel a sense of accomplishment—overcoming a challenge—or it can be cathartic, helping us release emotions we've been storing up. And for some people, pain is directly associated with pleasure, so it's reason enough all by itself.

"How Do I Know Whether the Pain Is Good or Injury-Causing?"

That's the million-dollar question, isn't it? And it's definitely important to learn to distinguish between pain that indicates current or impending injury and pain that's to be expected for the tie and your body. Although some warning signs of nerve damage include numbness, tingling, a zapping feeling, burning, and coldness, sometimes those indicate less worrisome circulatory issues instead. And it's possible to get nerve damage without any warning signs. I've gotten sensory nerve damage (no feeling on a surface area of skin) several times on my thighs and not realized it until I was putting my pants back on.

So how do you tell the difference? There's no hard and fast answer. Every body is different, and even the same body doesn't necessarily experience pain the same way from day to day. You'll just have to learn over time—gaining knowledge of how your body reacts as well as knowledge of how ties work. If you're suspended by a single leg in a super-tight futomomo, for example, and your entire foot gets tingly, cold, or numb, it's more likely a circulatory issue (because the blood supply is being actively impeded and because you're upside down) than impending nerve damage.

Jay Wiseman does offer this nugget of wisdom, however, and it's easy to remember even during those times when your brain feels short-circuited:

"Good pain good; bad pain bad."

If it feels wrong, it's wrong, and you should tell your rope partner.

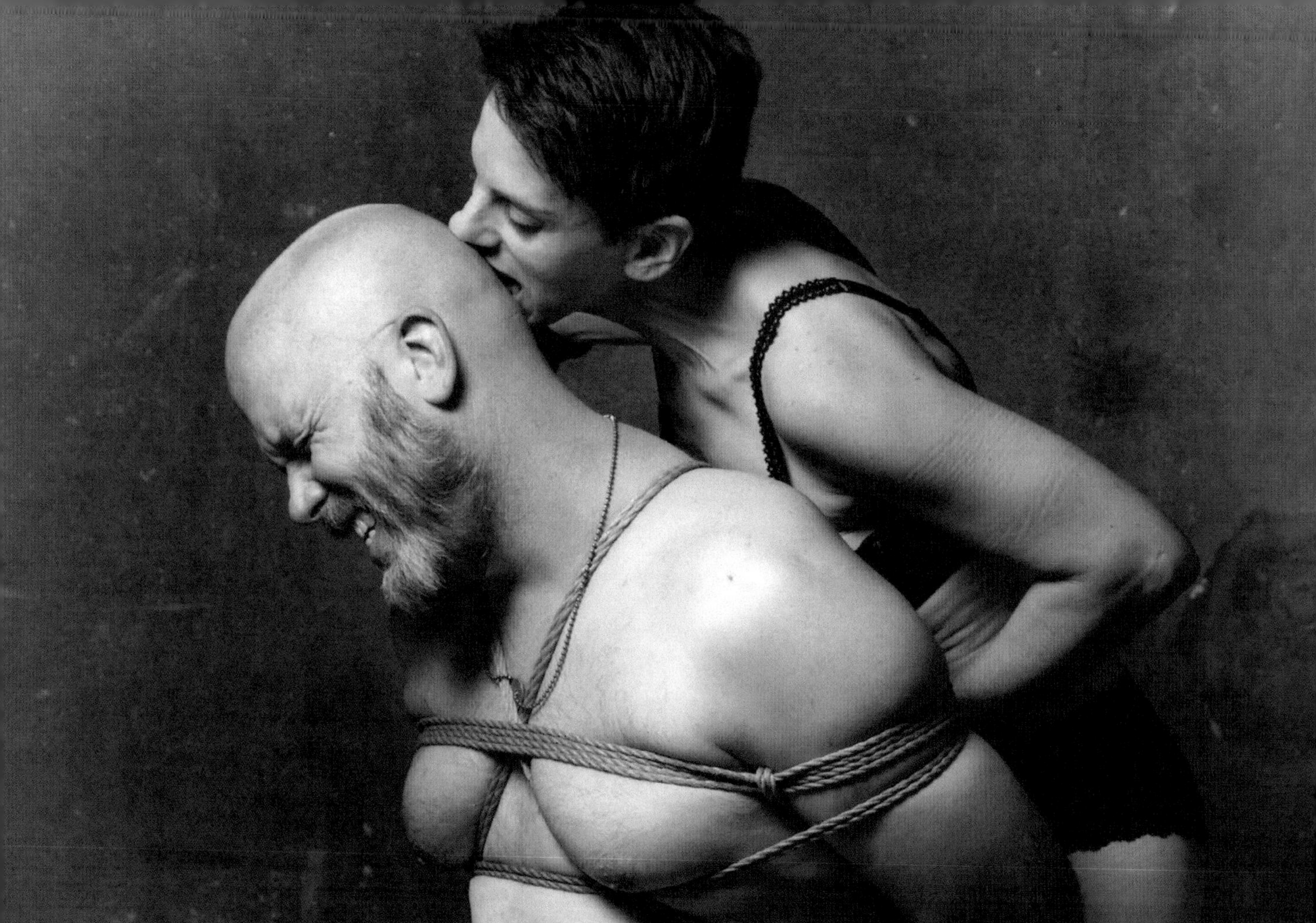

Ojipan and goodmosttimes. Bondage by goodmosttimes. Photo by LiquidErotica; liquiderotica.net

A Little Background

First, I have no professional medical training or training in pain management. Everything here is based on my research and experience as related to rope bottoming. The ideas may or may not work for you, but they'll at least serve as a basis for your own exploration. Please do not do anything that isn't right for you! Especially regarding pain, I urge you to be cautious in your explorations, as pain can obviously be a sign of impending or occuring damage.

Second, "pain processing" seems to imply an internal process: visualization, breathwork, and so on. But here we'll also cover more external methods of affecting the experience of pain, such as being caressed by a partner and listening to music. So really this chapter is about pain management in rope, but a) that sounds too medical and negative, like dealing with a chronic bad back, and b) "pain processing" is the standard term used for BDSM scenes.

Third, SubmissiveGuide.com has a whole series of helpful articles on pain processing.[3] Some of the ideas here and there overlap, but I've found pain processing in rope play to be quite different from pain processing in kinky impact play (like flogging, caning, whipping). In many impact scenes, the pain is localized and comes in bursts, and there can be time to process between the bursts—like, you shriek and your leg curls up, and your top stops to caress you. There's also often a warm-up in impact play that increases the body's ability to take pain, and you can often move at least somewhat, like wiggling or stamping your foot.

In rope, the pain can be localized, in multiple areas, or even all over, and it can happen slowly or in one fell swoop. There's often a higher degree of sustainability required in rope—especially in suspensions, even if there are transitions. And your movement may be completely restricted. Plus, a partner with an impact toy can stop giving pain on a moment's notice, whereas a rope bottom may have to keep enduring pain during untying. Lastly, some rope bottoms don't actually identify as submissive.

So the methods here are ones that I and other bottoms have found useful specifically for being in rope, with and without being submissive. But I do recommend reading that series on SubmissiveGuide.com to see if anything resonates with you, and because it contains interesting information about pain and masochism not included here. And check out Chapter 3, written by Neuromancer28, especially the section "Not Just the Rope," which talks about factors affecting our perception of pain.

OK, now let's dig in! Assuming you're dealing with the good kind of pain, how do you process it to go deeper into your rope experience instead of begging to get out?

Breathwork

Breath is life. In the simplest terms, we breathe to get oxygen to our cells on the inhalation, which then create the energy that keeps us alive, and to rid our body of waste products like carbon dioxide on the exhalation. Oxygen deprivation can cause brain damage after about three minutes in most cases and, not too long after that, death. So until scientists perfect the technology for injectable oxygen-filled microparticles,[4] we'll have to keep breathing the old-fashioned way to live.

But there's way more we can do with the breath than just using it to, you know, stay alive. Deep, slow breathing is well known to activate the parasympathetic (calming) nervous system, lowering our blood pressure and heart rate.[5] *Yoga Journal* goes so far as to say that "deep, slow, rhythmic breathing can reduce anxiety, fear, pain, and depression; activate your immune system; increase your ability to concentrate; and release healing and 'feel-good' hormones, such as serotonin and oxytocin."[6] And sex and intimacy coach Xanet Pailet even says females can learn to breathe themselves to orgasm—no genital touching required.[7]

So let's make use of some of those amazing powers of the breath! We'll start with some simple breathwork techniques.

Before Rope Play: Alternate Nostril Breathing

Yogis have been using this breathing technique for thousands of years to calm the mind and create balance in the body. If you practice it before rope play, it can help you be more present and in a clearer state of mind to be receptive to the pain processing techniques we'll discuss later. The Sanskrit name for Alternate Nostril Breathing is Nadi Shodhana Pranayama (*nadi* = energy channel; *shodana* = cleansing or purification; *pranayama* = breathing technique). Here's why it works, on a basic level:

At any given moment, we breathe mostly through one dominant nostril, left or right. (See for yourself:

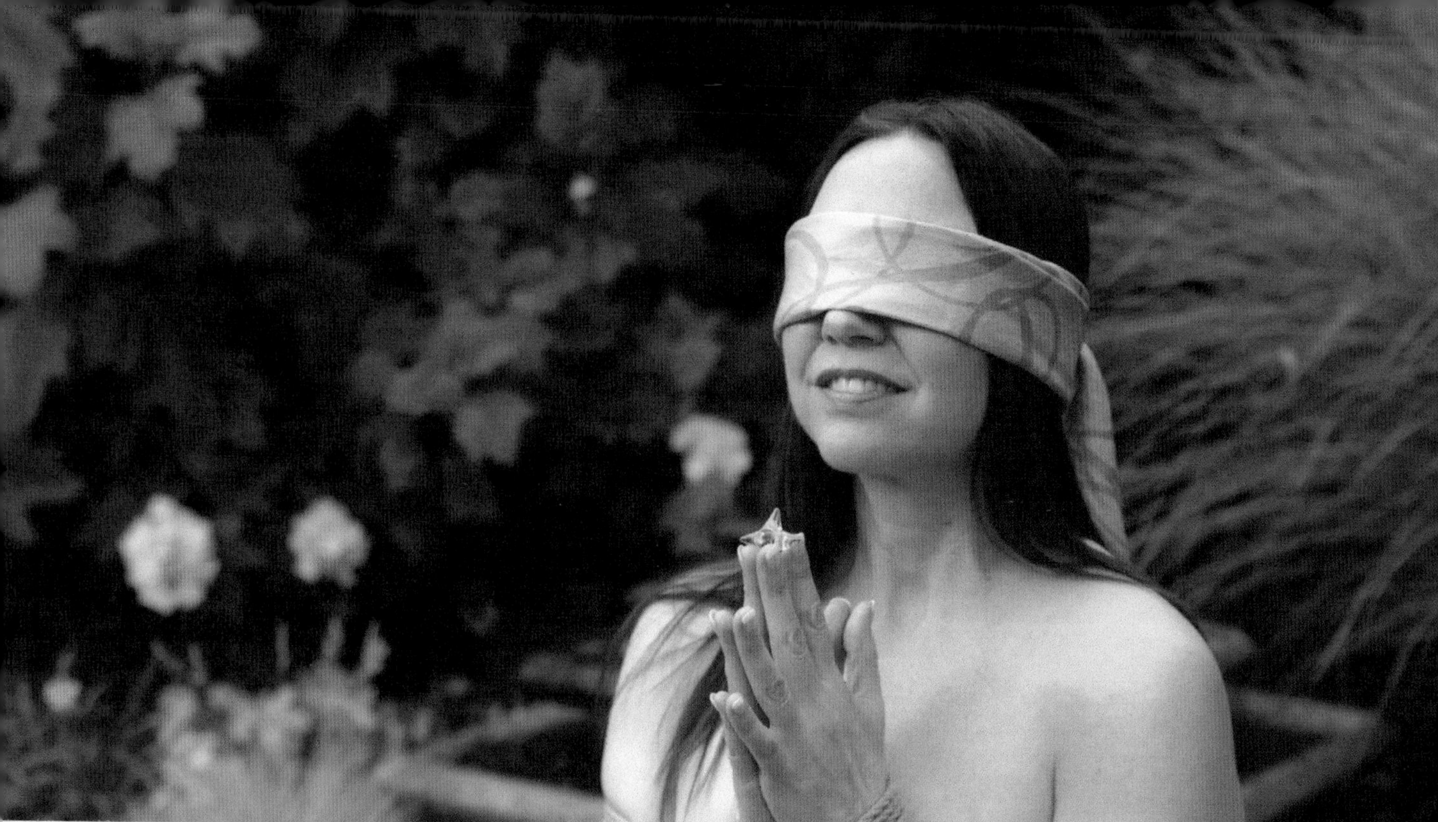

*Evie Vane. Bondage and photo by The Silence. Glass jack by RPG (Rottn Priks Glass), available at www.mocojute.com. Location courtesy of _impysh_*

Close each nostril alternately with a finger and see which one you can breathe through more easily.) The dominant nostril switches every few hours in most people. And which nostril is dominant affects whether our sympathetic (fight-or-flight) or parasympathetic (rest-and-digest) system is dominant. For instance, there is "evidence that right nostril breathing increases the generalized sympathetic tone of the body."[8] When you practice Alternate Nostril Breathing, you're counteracting the dominance of one side, thus equalizing the systems and creating balance.

You can also experiment with single nostril breathing to change your energetic and mental state (search online for techniques and cautions). But here we'll just focus on Alternate Nostril Breathing.

Warning: Approach *all breathing practices* with caution, especially if you have a respiratory condition, high blood pressure, or any other medical condition that could be negatively affected. It's best to work in person with someone trained in breathwork until you gain experience, but at the very least, work within your abilities and stop if you feel dizzy or faint.

There are plenty of videos online that can show you how to do Alternate Nostril Breathing, and you'll find some variations. It's super easy once you do it a few times. Here's my preferred technique:

1. Sit in a comfortable position with your shoulders relaxed and your spine straight. You can sit cross-legged on the floor (on a pillow if you like) or in a chair. Relax your face or smile softly.

2. Rest your left hand, palm up, on your left knee, with the tips of your index finger and thumb touching (Chin Mudra in yoga).

3. With your right hand, rest the tips of your index finger and middle finger between your eyebrows.

Put your ring finger and little finger lightly on the left nostril and the thumb lightly on the right nostril.

4. Close your eyes and breathe in deeply through both nostrils. Press your thumb on the right nostril and gently breathe out through the left nostril.

5. Without moving your fingers, breathe in through that same (left) nostril. Then press the left nostril closed with your ring finger and little finger, lift up your thumb, and breathe out through the right nostril.

6. Breathe in through that same (right) nostril, press the right nostril closed, lift up your ring finger and little finger, and breathe out through the left nostril. That's one complete round, because you're back where you started.

Most sources recommend doing five to 10 cycles, or about three to five minutes.

Box Breathing

Since you don't need your hands for this one, you can use it to help you process pain while in bondage, in addition to calming and centering yourself beforehand. The very act of focusing on your breath will help take your attention away from the pain (which your body may adjust to while you're doing it), plus you'll be getting the relaxation benefits of controlled breathing. I first heard about box breathing from Graydancer; it's also called square breathing or four-square breathing. Here's how to do it:

1. If you're not tied up, sit cross-legged or on a chair with your spine straight and your shoulders and face relaxed. If you're tied up, skip to Step 2.

2. Close your eyes and your mouth, then breathe in slowly through your nose for a count of four. Hold your breath for four seconds.

3. Open your mouth slightly and exhale for the same count of four. Then hold for another four seconds. Repeat for up to a few minutes if you like.

Tips: On the inhalation, expand your belly if it's available to you. If it's not, expand into whatever body part isn't restricted. If your mouth is blocked (by a gag, say), inhale and exhale through your nose. Even if you don't follow the exact method above, you'll still be drawing on the benefits.

Counting Breaths

This may be the simplest of the three breathing practices to use when you're in that bondaged state where you can barely remember your own name. Like the box breath, it can help take your attention away from pain while calming your mind.

1. Inhale while thinking "1." Exhale while thinking "1."

2. Inhale while thinking "2." Exhale while thinking "2." And so on. Repeat for up to a few minutes if you like.

Tip: Don't worry if you get distracted. Just notice the thought and go back to counting where you left off.

Breathing Into Different Parts of the Body

Abdominal breathing, also called diaphragmatic breathing, comes naturally to infants and even young children. As we get older, this generally gets replaced by chest breathing. There are a number of possible reasons for the switch (the way our bodies develop, stress, societal pressure to have a flat stomach, and so on), but we can still consciously choose which places to breathe into.

kitteninlimbo. Bondage and photo by Sean Grey; MrSeanGrey.com

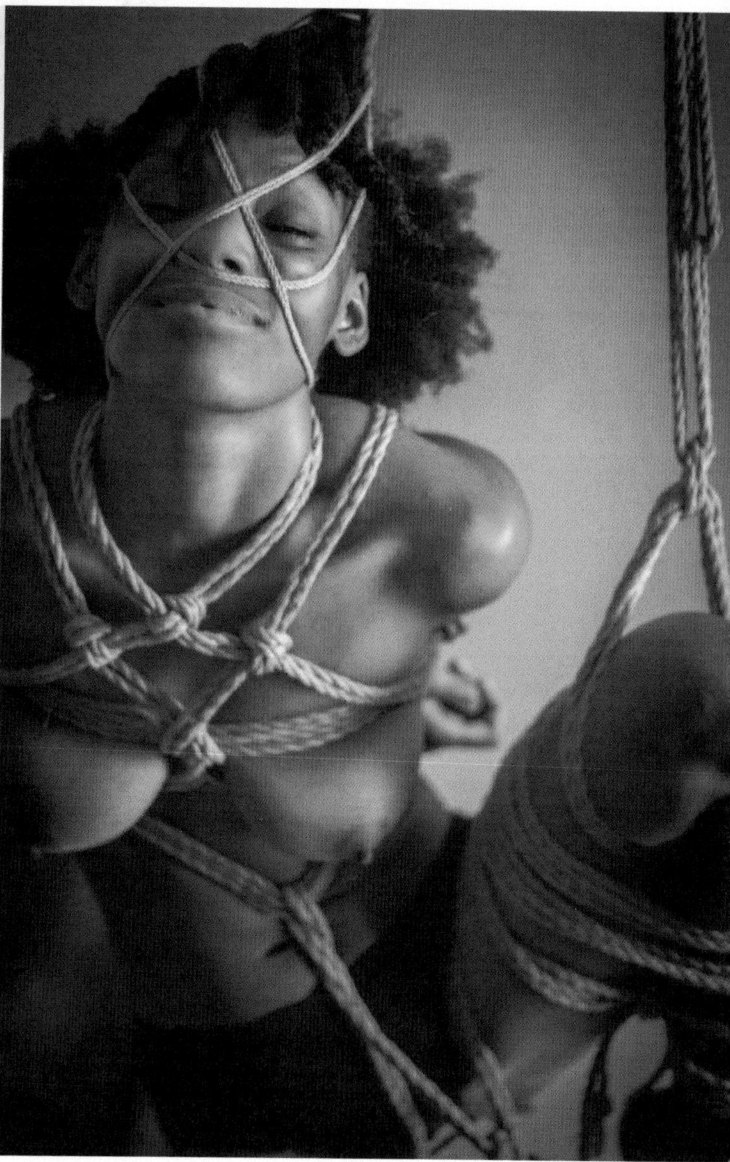

This is good news for rope bottoms, since many ties (notably the takate-kote) constrict the chest. The more practice you have breathing into different body parts, the more options will be at your disposal when you're in a tie that restricts the breath.

Myth: If You Can Talk, You Can Breathe

I've been told more than once in bondage that if you can talk you can breathe, but it just isn't true. In a well-publicized case in 2014, Eric Garner reportedly yelled "I can't breathe" 11 times while in a chokehold by a New York police officer before losing consciousness and dying. (Asthma was reportedly a contributing factor.)[9] And in 2013, Jorge Azucena died in police custody in Los Angeles, reportedly after his repeated pleas for help—"I can't breathe," "I have asthma," and "help me"—went unheeded, and he stopped breathing.[10]

In terms of asthma, the Mayo Clinic advises seeking emergency medical treatment if you have signs or symptoms including "the inability to speak more than short phrases due to shortness of breath."[11] That seems like a reasonable guideline for bondage that restricts your breath, either through direct rope pressure on the chest or through the body's being torqued or contorted. If you feel like you can't breathe and you can't speak more than short phrases, communicate that to your partner so they can alleviate the restriction—another point in support of having nonverbal signals even if the mouth is available.

Upper-chest (thoracic) breathing. You probably don't need to practice this, because it's the way most grown-ups naturally breathe. Place a hand on your chest and watch it rise and fall as you breathe into the upper chest.

Abdominal (diaphragmatic) breathing. You can do this sitting in a chair, but if you've never tried it before, lying down is easier. Lie on your back with your head supported and your knees bent. Put a bolster or

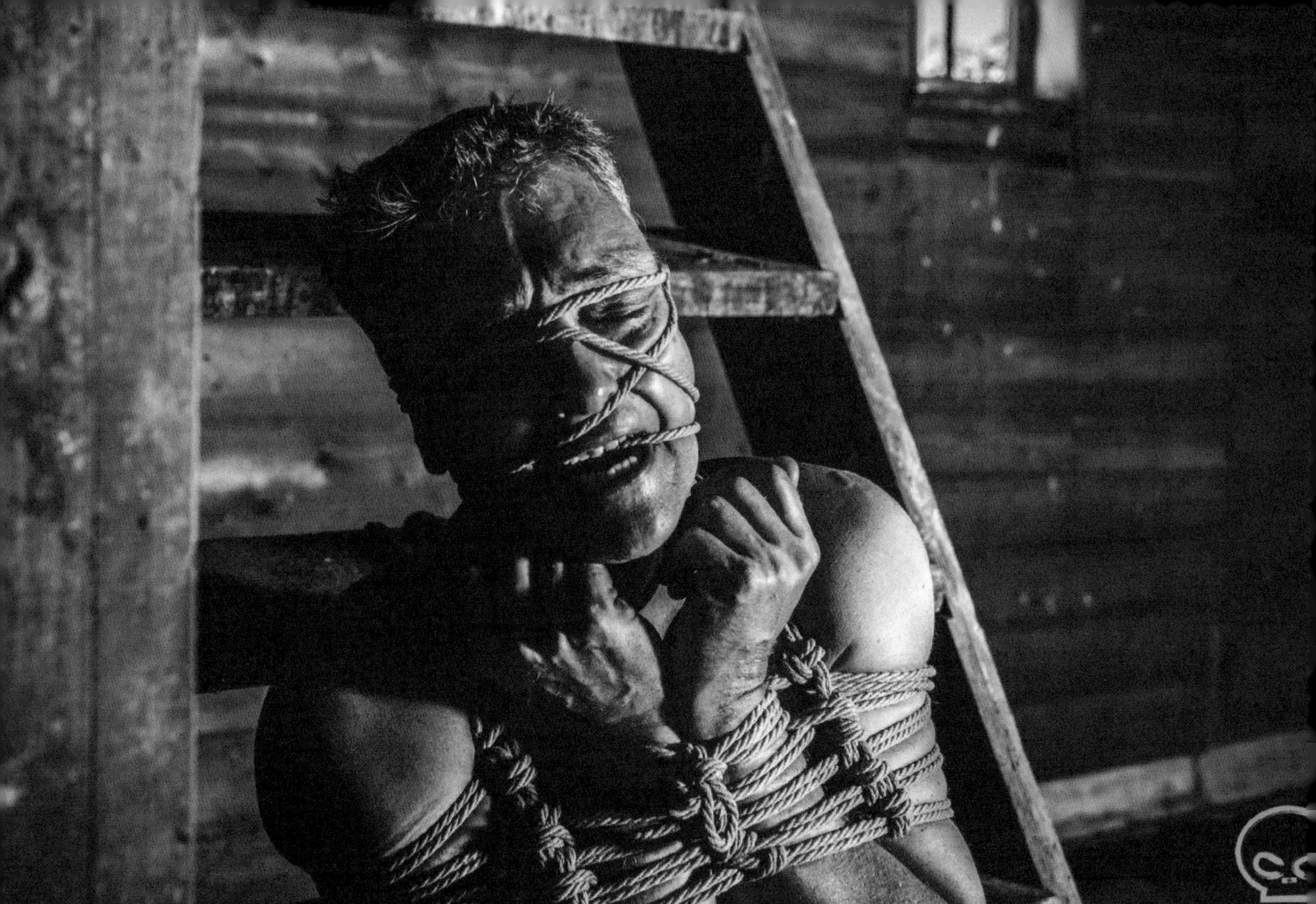

Proteus_AKT1. Bondage by Heidi. Photo by Sir_Kraska/Matthew Kraska, Branded Skull Photography

a pillow or two under your knees if you want more support. Place one hand below your rib cage and the other on your midchest. Breathe in slowly so that the hand under your rib cage rises while the hand on your chest stays still.

Clavicular breathing. If there's rope constricting your diaphragm as well as your chest (and one strand on each is all it takes), your breathing will have to take place in the top one-third of the lungs, meaning it's very shallow. Place your hand on your clavicle (collarbone) and try to breathe into only this area. You may find your shoulders rising too.

While this may be so hard to do without rope on that you feel like it's only an energetic practice (like trying to feel the space behind your eyeballs expand), your lungs are actually working. They do extend above the clavicle, though there are differences of opinion as to how far.[12] Very shallow clavicular breathing can happen during panic attacks, shock, and hyperventilation, among other conditions, and you may have to consciously override the mental association—for instance, you may have to remind yourself that you're not panicking just because you're breathing so shallowly.

Also, if you do find your shoulders rising when you're breathing at the clavicle, be extra cautious about nerve damage, because you could be compressing nerves in the brachial plexus. Those nerves run all the way down the arms to the hands, so compressing them could cause things like wrist drop or other loss of motor function.

Back breathing. This is another one that may feel only energetic at first but is physically possible. I love this description from Sonia Connolly of Sundown Healing Arts:

"Shallow chest breathing takes up as little space as possible. Deeper belly breathing pushes out into the world. Back breathing claims the space that is already yours, the three-dimensional cathedral arch of ribs, spine, and sternum waiting to be filled and emptied and filled again by your own breath."[13]

Here's her description of how to practice it for yourself:

"Put your hands on your waist, thumbs to the back, and then move your hands as far up and back as you comfortably can. Let the bones of your thumbs connect with the bones of your ribs with light pressure. As your breath flows in, allow those back rib bones to push your thumbs apart."[14]

Can you feel your back expand with the breath? If not, don't give up. Just keep practicing, or maybe try it with a partner putting their thumbs on your back, and eventually you may be able to feel it.

Other body parts. Here's where we get into the energetic stuff, requiring visualization. Depending on how in tune you are with your energy body, you may find that visualization works or you may think it's total hogwash. One idea is just to send your breath to whatever body part is in pain, creating a feeling of more space there. Another is to imagine that you're inhaling pure white light into the body part to create lightness and ease, and exhaling all the muck of tension or pain.

These techniques are just for pain processing and not actual breathing, of course. No amount of practice will allow you to literally breathe using your eyeballs or your feet—or any other body part not involved in the respiratory system.

Now that you're nice and relaxed thanks to all of these breathing practices, let's move on to the pain processing portion.

Pain Processing

As mentioned above, there are internal and external ways to help change your experience of pain. There are also factors that affect your experience of pain that you may or not be able to do anything about. Let's start with the latter.

Bodily and Environmental Factors

Certain medications and hormonal factors can make you more or less sensitive to pain—females may feel pain more intensely right before their period, for instance. Being short on sleep or hungry or thirsty can have an effect too. Then there's the space you're tying in: Is it too warm or too cold, too light or too dark, too quiet or too noisy? Does the music set your teeth on edge? All of those factors can affect your pain perception. Consider keeping a log of your experiences in various settings, noting any bodily or environmental factors that came into play and how they affected your experience of pain. Then you can possibly figure out ways to mitigate them in the future.

While we're on the subject of medications...drinking alcohol or taking drugs can certainly reduce the feeling of pain in the short term. But they're a really bad idea with rope, because 1. They affect your judgment and your perception, which can be highly dangerous in rope bondage, and 2. You run the risk of missing signs of impending injury. Make the smart choice.

Be aware of the body's own chemicals too. Endorphins, which are hormones released in response to pain (among other things), act as natural opioids, meaning they reduce the feeling of pain and increase the feeling of pleasure—even to the point of euphoria. It's worth keeping that in mind as you monitor your body for potential nerve damage or other injury.

Taking over-the-counter pain relievers, such as acetaminophin (Tylenol), ibuprofen (Advil), or naproxen sodium (Aleve), before a scene is a personal decision. But it's worth researching them and learning about the side effects (such as stomach upset, increased blood pressure, and mild blood thinning) and contraindicated medicines (such as blood thinners) to make an educated decision about your use of them for rope play.

Now let's look at some factors you may have more control over.

External Pain Modifiers

Music. I can't get the story out of my mind of a guy, Vijay Welch-Young, who had his chest cut open and his ribs pulled apart without anesthesia and without "leaving" his body through any trance-induced state.[15] He said one of the things that helped him was music, and he mentioned a study of patients after open-heart surgery that "showed music to significantly reduce pain intensity."[16] Those patients got to choose their own music, which is one reason it may have worked, while that elevator music being piped in at the dentist's chair might not.

Anecdotally, I can tell you that the music Kanso plays at our BARE (Bay Area Rope Exchange) parties definitely allows me to go through more challenging ties than if I were doing them in a perfectly quiet or even chatter-filled room. The music is sexy and there's something trance-like about it, although it doesn't all fall in the genre of trance. It puts me in another world in rope, one where the experience of pain is less something to endure and more a path to transcendence.

Cherise33 and _Rae_. Bondage by _Rae_. Photo by -CG-

Sexual pleasure. This is such a well-known one that I'm surprised Welch-Young didn't try to have someone give him a BJ during that surgery (maybe it would have distracted the surgeon too much). In Chapter 3, Neuromancer28 cites a study on rats, but anyone who's ever had a vibrator applied to the right place while undergoing something painful knows that it can easily take your mind off whatever's hurting. For this reason, it's a good idea to be extremely careful about mixing sexual stimulation with rope play, to avoid nerve damage and other injury.

Changing your stance. Harvard Business School professor and researcher Amy Cuddy gave a TED talk on how "power posing"—standing in a position of confidence—can change other people's perceptions of us, our own self-perception, and even our body chemistry.[17] She started by talking about nonverbal signs of power: how becoming expansive (spreading arms and wings, for example) is a sign of dominance in the animal kingdom, and how people who win physical competitions tend to raise their arms in an outward V shape and lift their chin. In contrast, when we're feeling powerless, we close in on ouselves and make ourselves small.

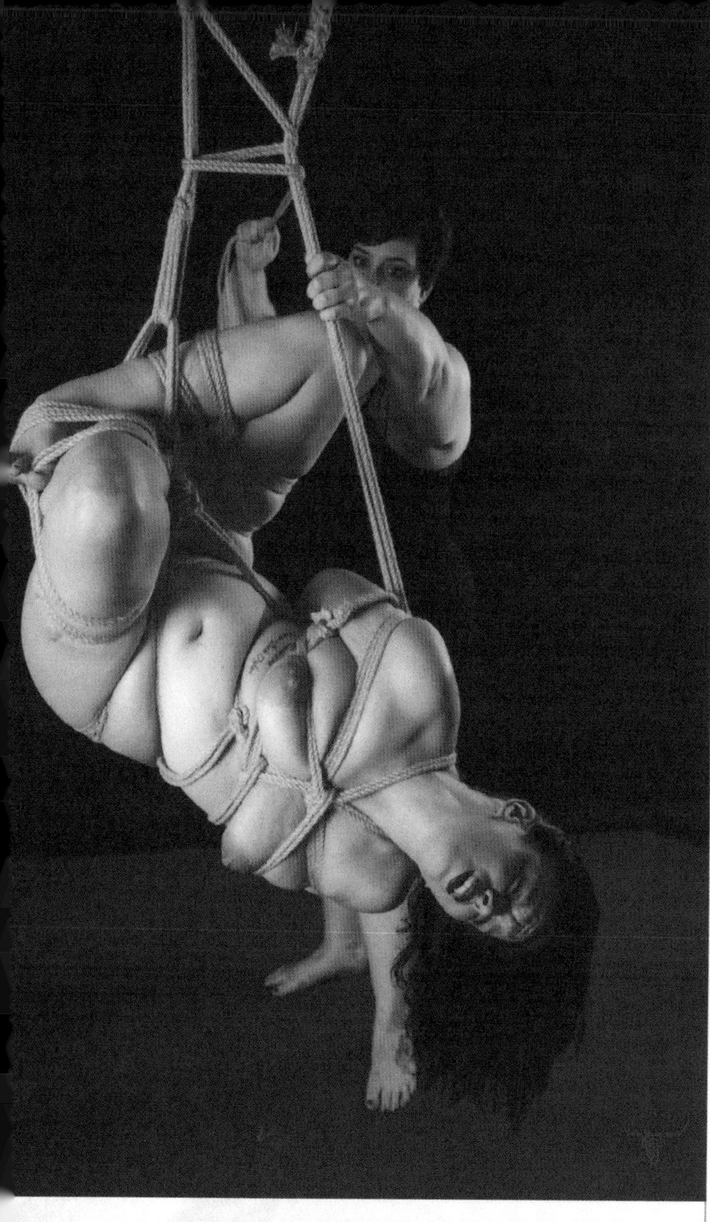

Interestingly, her research showed that adopting a power pose of expansiveness can actually increase our feeling of power—more than "faking it till you make it," it's actually faking it *to* make it—and can both raise testosterone and lower cortisol (stress hormone) levels.

"But hey," submissive types might be thinking, "what does this have to do with me? I don't want to get all up in my partner's face with a power pose and be acting all dominant." Here's the thing: I've been subconsciously using this technique in rope for years, and I can tell you that what you're actually doing is showing the pain—not your partner—who's boss. You're adopting a position of strength to face your rope challenges and any pain head-on, as opposed to cringing and cowering and letting them get the better of you.

The power poses Cuddy shows would probably feel silly in bondage even if your arms are free. Instead, I lift my head, jut my chin out, lift my chest, and maybe even move my shoulders back. I also try to expand into a pose, radiating my energy outward, as opposed to sinking down into it. You might be surprised how subtle bodily and energetic shifts like this can affect your experience of pain in rope.

This is not to be confused with "powering through" a pose when your instinct is telling you it's bad for you, by the way. Powering through when you really think you need a transition or to come out is a good way to get injured.

Pressure or rubbing. Some sensory nerves carry pain messages, and some sensory nerves carry other messages. Rubbing, pressing, or caressing near the painful area can send information to the brain that competes with the pain information, and depending on the level of pain, that other info can "win out." If you've ever had a bikini wax and the waxer rubbed your inner thigh right after ripping out the hair, now you know why.

Usually you don't have the ability to rub yourself in bondage, but it sure can be a nice thing to let your partner know about if they don't already.

Trusting your partner. Fear and mistrust can both magnify our experience of pain. Imagine you need to get two teeth pulled. For one extraction, a friendly, professional-looking dentist with framed degrees on

Clover

Sharing the Journey

Clover is a world-renowned bondage educator, performer, and model, and the author of "A Guide for Rope Bottoms & Bondage Models." Visit kinkyclover.com to learn more.

I love Kinbaku and often find myself in the conflicting position of loving rope but hating pain. I do not identify as a masochist; I have to work to enjoy pain, but every moment is worth it. Enjoying rope and the sensations it offers, the psychology of my situation, and the fact that I regularly tie with someone I trust really help my brain translate those negative sensations into pleasure. We are all unique, and our bodies will perceive and interpret sensations differently.

Everyone will have a different relationship to pain, and that relationship can change and develop over time. Things I found difficult to sustain or even impossible to achieve years ago are often part of my favorite scenes today. Knowing that the pain my rigger puts me through is controlled and deliberate helps me to relax in rope and submit to the pain. While this is important, I have learned that trusting myself helps more with my pain processing: trusting my judgment of my limits in the moment, confidence in understanding I can communicate with my rigger, and feeling safe to explore my limits without fear.

I enjoy challenging my body and feel a sense of achievement when I can sustain a difficult predicament position or painful tie. My approach to pain processing is to focus on the pain itself, make a judgment if I am being harmed or it is just pain due to stress. Depending on the situation I will move against it, engaging the areas that hurt; not only does this check for any sensory damage, but it helps me to connect with the pain and make it more intense. At this point I imagine the pain is "white pain." Then I relax and submit to it—the pain feels less intense, and I imagine it is warm and spreading through my body. I manage my breathing; if it has quickened, I slow it right down or stop it altogether, starting again slowly. If the position I am in allows, I will breathe deeply, close my eyes, and imagine with each exhale the pain is leaving my body. By this point I am typically calm, riding the waves of warm, gentle pain.

If pain in rope is new to you, it can be easy to meet the "panic spiral." Panicking in rope is often caused by fear, having doubts about your abilities, putting pressure on yourself to succeed in a challenging situation. When I have experienced this, I have asked my rigger to try something similar again another day. Sometimes experiencing something once makes the second attempt easier; knowing what sensations to expect can help you mentally prepare. Sometimes it works and other times it won't. Try again—rope bottoms need practice and lab time too, and I am sure your rigger will be happy to tie again.

Expand your objective knowledge by reading factual information on anatomy etc. Read articles on rope bottoming and see if they relate to you. Keep in mind that you may have a different view on subjective matters.

Keep trying, gain experience and body awareness, listen to what your body is telling you. If you can, discuss your experiences with your rigger and try different approaches to things you are struggling with. Different transitions, moods, and even just a different day can make a huge difference.

Have you ever noticed that tie you love but haven't done in a long time feels different than the way you remember it and may even feel more intense? You will naturally build a tolerance to rope. I recall the first time I was suspended in a futomomo tsuri (thigh suspension), I had bruises a few hours later; now I don't bruise at all. Similarly, if you are out of practice, your body will lose that tolerance; however, it's quite easy to develop it again.

Be patient with yourself and embrace pain on your terms. Have fun with rope as a well-educated, confident rope bottom!

Clover. Bondage by WykD Dave. Original image by Suffering4Art. Painting by RavenArt

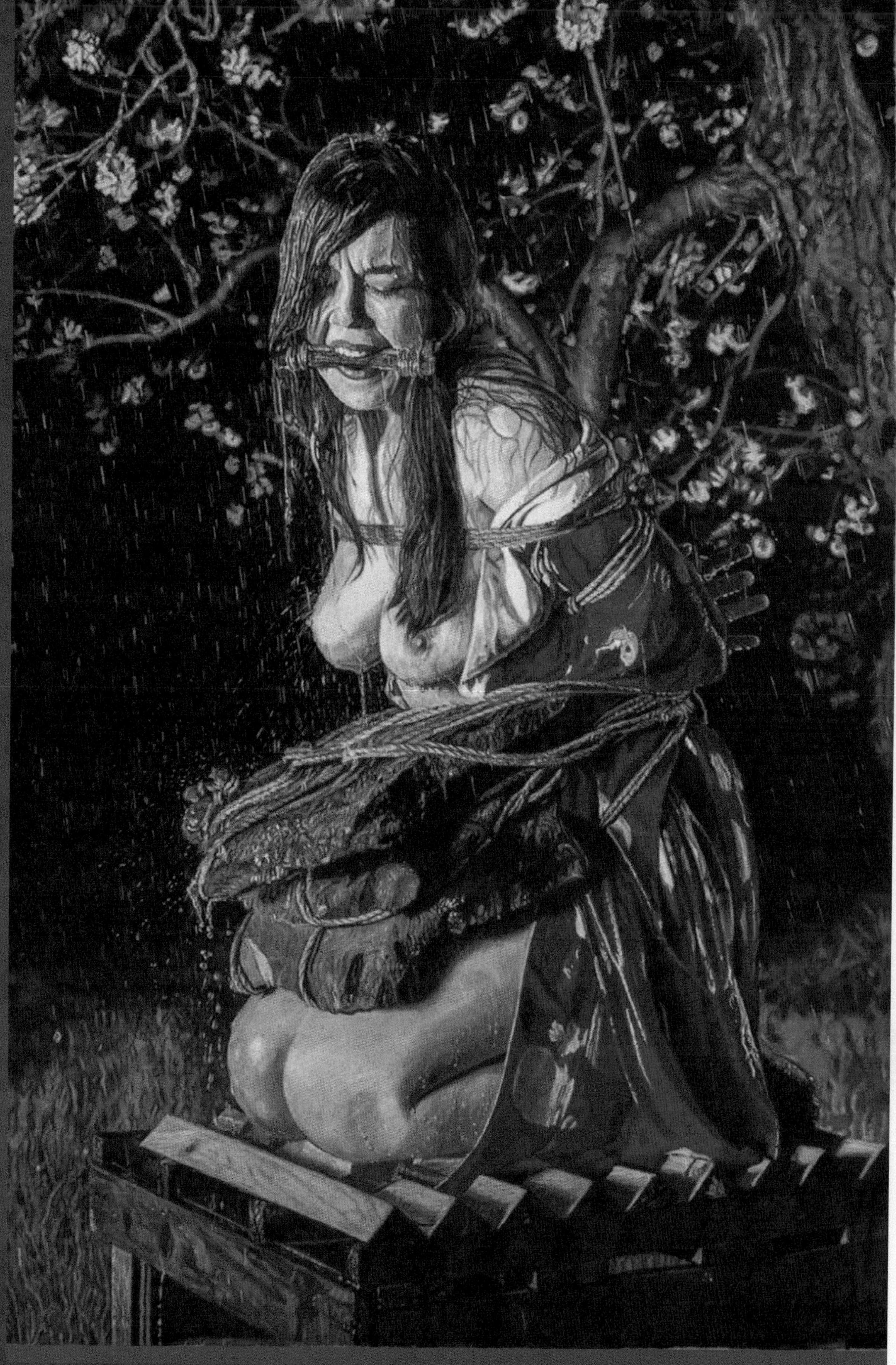

the wall and an assistant in a clean office explains the procedure (and maybe puts on some nice music of your choosing). For the other extraction, you're shown into a sketchy-looking office where the dentist is wearing ripped jeans and has shaky hands, and the assistant looks like they moonlight as a drug dealer. Even if the procedure is exactly the same, you can guess which one you might actually perceive as more painful.

For rope play, talking with your partner thoroughly about their bondage education and experience, and negotiating thoughtfully so you know what to expect (good ideas even without any pain-management motives), can help you feel more trusting and relaxed, which in turn may positively affect your pain experience.

Knowing when it will end. One of the most challenging scenes I ever did involved bamboo and a number of transitions, in a "playformance" situation. I had never been tied with bamboo before, had never played with this partner before, and it was past my usual bedtime and also after doing rope with other people. It got harder and harder, and involved some screams, until "NononoIcantdoitIcantdoit!!" came out. My partner seemed entirely unruffled by this and said (possibly even with a note of humor in his voice) something like, "Hmm, really? Can you count to 30 for me? It will be better by then."

It was actually better by 20, and we went on to do still-challenging things that still involved some screaming, and it was one of the best rope experiences of my life. Being "counted down" made all the difference, because I knew the pain would end within an exact amount of time. If he had said something like, "Can you stay in it just a little while longer?" I would have said no way. But knowing specifically how long I had

Evie Vane. Bondage by MrKiltYou. Photo by The Silence

to endure, and having the counting to focus on instead of the pain, made it endurable.

It's worth noting also that I had researched him and known him to be highly skillful. And when I told him I couldn't do it, he stayed entirely calm. Both of those things increased my trust in him, which likely affected my pain experience as well.

Knowing what's happening or coming. When you go to the doctor's office to get a shot, the person doesn't just sit you down and stick the needle in. They say something like, "You're going to feel a sharp prick, and the area may feel a bit tender or achy afterward." Knowing what's happening to us allows us to process the pain better, and also to draw on similar previous experiences: "Ah, right, I remember getting a shot last year and it wasn't so bad." The known is also less scary than the unknown, and less fear can mean a reduced pain perception.

For rope play that you expect to be especially painful, you could talk to your partner about what tie(s) you'll be doing and how long you might be in each one. Or, if you'd rather be surprised, and there's no music or vibrator around, you could try the following "internal" pain processing methods.

Internal Pain Processing

Sitting with the pain. Obviously you won't always be sitting when you're tied up—you might be standing, lying down, in the air, on your knees... "sitting" with the pain simply means allowing it to happen, not resisting it. BDSM and meditation ex-

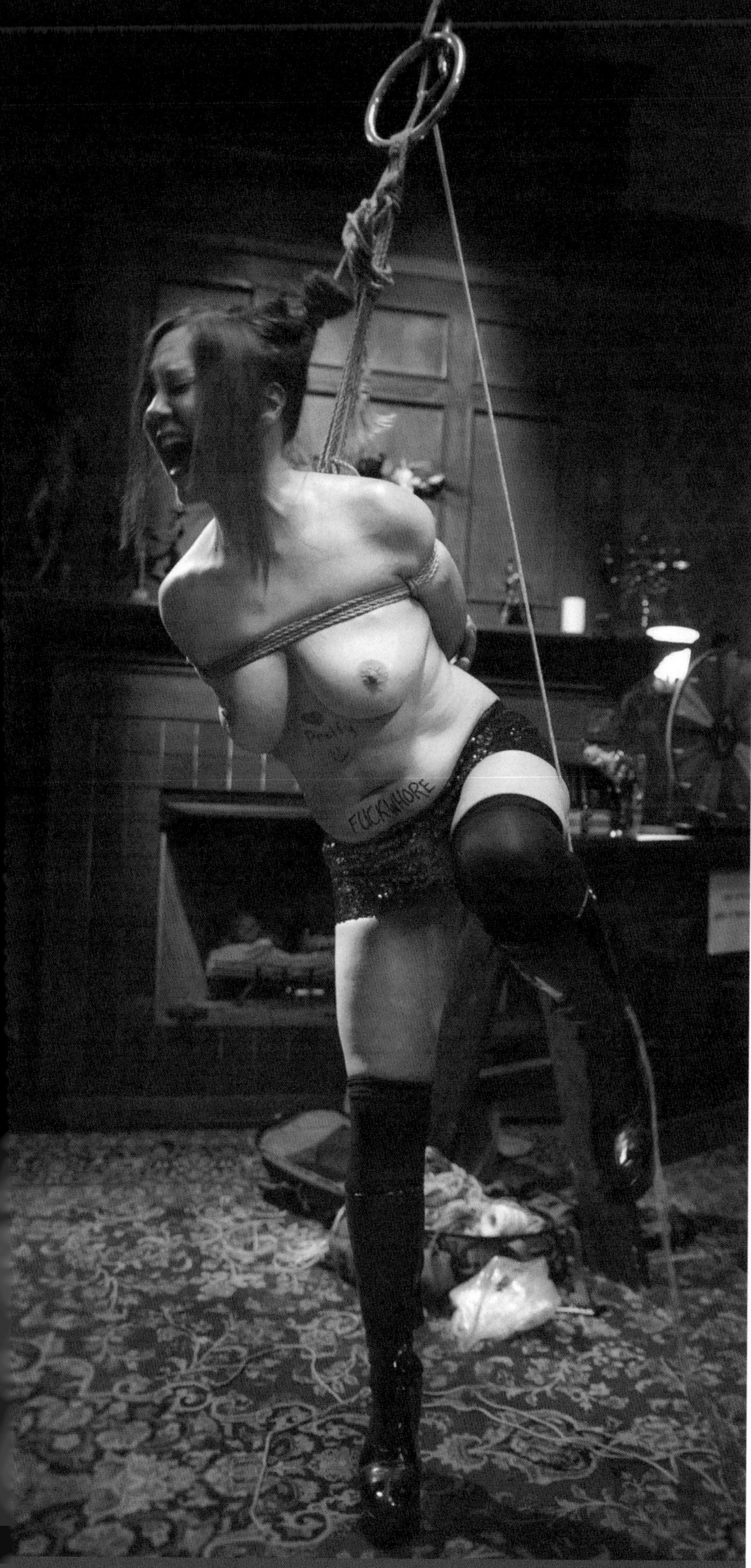

pert Ian Snow leads an illuminating exercise in one of his classes that helps teach this: You take a clothespin and attach it in a reasonably but not unbearably painful location. (I put it on my tongue; others in the class did nipples, arms, thighs.) Then for about five minutes you just sit still and observe the sensation. Is it like heat? Pressure? Burning? Does it change? Does your consciousness of it ebb and flow, so that there are moments when you don't even feel it? You're just observing here, not trying to change anything or judge any part of the experience.

You might want to notice your emotions too. Fear? Anger? Resignation? Maybe even contentment? Again, you're just observing, not judging or changing anything. If you have a thought that's beyond observation, just notice it, let it float by like a cloud, and resume noticing the sensations and emotions.

I found two things most interesting about this exercise:

1. The *pain became the meditation.* Just like focusing on something external, such as a candle flame, focusing on my internal experience of pain shut out a lot of that annoying mental chatter. And when

the five minutes were up, I felt as calm, relaxed, and focused as if I'd been chanting or doing yoga.

2. After the first minute of "Ow, holy fuck, I'm not going to last five minutes!" my thoughts slowly settled into noticing, and the *act of noticing changed the sensation* into something less painful and even interesting. From there the pain came and went sporadically, but even when it was there, observing it instead of being consumed by it changed the nature of it into something more tolerable.

This kind of sitting with the pain is the internal method that works best for me in challenging ties. On a physical level, it keeps me focused and in my body, which in turn makes me feel completely present. But it also becomes a metaphor for life that has emotional effects. When life throws something challenging or painful at me, or I experience painful emotions, am I going to run and hide? Or am I going to accept the pain, face it, and not let it ruin me? Knowing I've sat with pain in a rope tie gives me the confidence and courage to feel and face discomfort and pain in the rest of my life, to accept them and move on.

Ian Snow's exercise is enlightening whether you're a novice or an experienced rope bottom. Try it and see for yourself.

Separating yourself from the pain. Phenomenalist philosophers believe that nothing actually exists outside of our perception of it (perception being the information presented to our senses). It's one of those mind-blowing concepts, like life is all a dream, that dropping LSD makes easier to understand. It also has interesting applications for pain processing. If your laptop ceases to exist when no one is seeing it, then theoretically, pain should also cease to exist when no one is noticing it.

We've already talked about how music, sexual pleasure, and focusing on the breath can take your attention away from pain. Now here are three ways to actually visualize detaching your pain from yourself and putting it in a place where you won't notice it unless you choose to.

1. Visualize gathering the pain into a ball and dropping it over a fence. You can reach over and pick it up again anytime you want, but for now, you're separated from your pain by the fence.

2. Visualize gathering the pain up and placing it in a box. Put a lid on the box. Place the box in a closet and close the door. You can open the door and take the box and the pain out later.

3. Visualize the pain pouring from your body into a jar or bottle. Then put a cap on it and place it in a cabinet. You can open the cabinet and take the jar out later.

Spreading the pain out. This is another visualization technique. You locate the center of the pain and then feel the pain spreading out, like an ice cube melting or a pool of light dispersing. It doesn't necessarily change the overall amount of pain you feel, but it makes it feel less intense because energetically the pain is being spread out over a greater area.

Letting it out. This is a mix of internal and external. There's a reason martial artists shout (called a *kiai*) when they punch, chop, or kick something. It helps with proper breathing, but it also helps maximize the energy being directed at the opponent. Weightlifters, tennis players, and other athletes also tend to grunt while exerting effort, and it isn't just to sound badass. One study showed that yelling increased the force generated by 10 percent[18]—meaning it actually makes you *stronger*.

Also, if you think of the pain as energy, then screaming, yelling, laughing, cursing, crying, and so on can help release that energy from your body. I now ask partners before a particularly challenging scene, "Do you mind if I yell at you that you're a fucking motherfucker?" So far, no one has minded.

Fantasizing. Pain can seem more tolerable if it's an expected part of a fantasy or role-playing scenario. And your partner doesn't even need to be in on it. Sometimes I'll think, "Well I've been kidnapped and I'm totally at their mercy, so there's nothing I can do about it." (Of course something can be done about it in reality.) My partner doesn't even know about that backstory, but it helps me process the pain more easily. Maybe your fantasy is that you're being tortured for information or punished for driving your partner to utter distraction with your hotness.

• • •

Which of these external and internal pain processing methods is right for you? The only way to know is to try them out. Consider requesting lab time with a partner if you don't want to experiment during actual scene time.

Notes

1. Merskey, H; and Bogduk, N. "Classification of chronic pain." IASP Task Force on Taxonomy. Seattle: IASP Press, 1994.

2. Caudill, Margaret A, MD, PhD, MPH. *Managing Pain Before It Manages You*, 4th ed. The Guilford Press, 2016.

3. http://www.submissiveguide.com/2011/04/processing-pain-in-play-what-is-the-natural-process/

4. Kheir, JN et al. "Oxygen Gas-Filled Microparticles Provide Intravenous Oxygen Delivery." *Science Translational Medicine.* 2012; vol. 4, no. 140:140-88

5. http://www.health.harvard.edu/blog/stress-raising-your-blood-pressure-take-a-deep-breath-201602159168

6. Miller, Richard, PhD. "Tune in to your breath to find inner peace." *Yoga Journal*, Oct. 2016:20.

7. http://powerofpleasure.com/freeing-the-female-orgasm-breathe-your-way-to-orgasm/

8. Shannahoff-Khalsa, David. "Lateralized rhythms of the central and autonomic nervous systems." *International Journal of Psychophysiology.* 1991; 11:225-251.

9. http://www.nbcnewyork.com/news/local/Eric-Garner-Death-Chokehold-Investigation-272043511.html

10. http://www.newsweek.com/man-died-asthma-lapd-ignored-his-pleas-report-266611

11. http://www.mayoclinic.org/diseases-conditions/asthma-attack/basics/symptoms/con-20034148

12. Bergman, Ronald A, Ph.D., et al. "Atlas of Human Anatomy in Cross Section: Appendix: Topography of the Thorax and Abdomen." http://www.anatomyatlases.org/HumanAnatomy/Topography/Lungs.shtml

13. http://traumahealed.com/articles/claim-your-space-breathe-into-your-back/

14. Ibid.

15. http://www.cracked.com/personal-experiences-1604-major-surgery-with-no-painkillers-5-things-i-learned.html

16. Jafari, Hedayat, et al. "The effects of listening to preferred music on pain intensity after open heart surgery." https://www.ncbi.nlm.nih.gov/pmc/articles/PMC3590687/

17. https://www.ted.com/talks/amy_cuddy_your_body_language_shapes_who_you_are?language=en

18. http://www.newsworks.org/index.php/local/the-pulse/64326-the-science-of-grunting-while-weightlifting

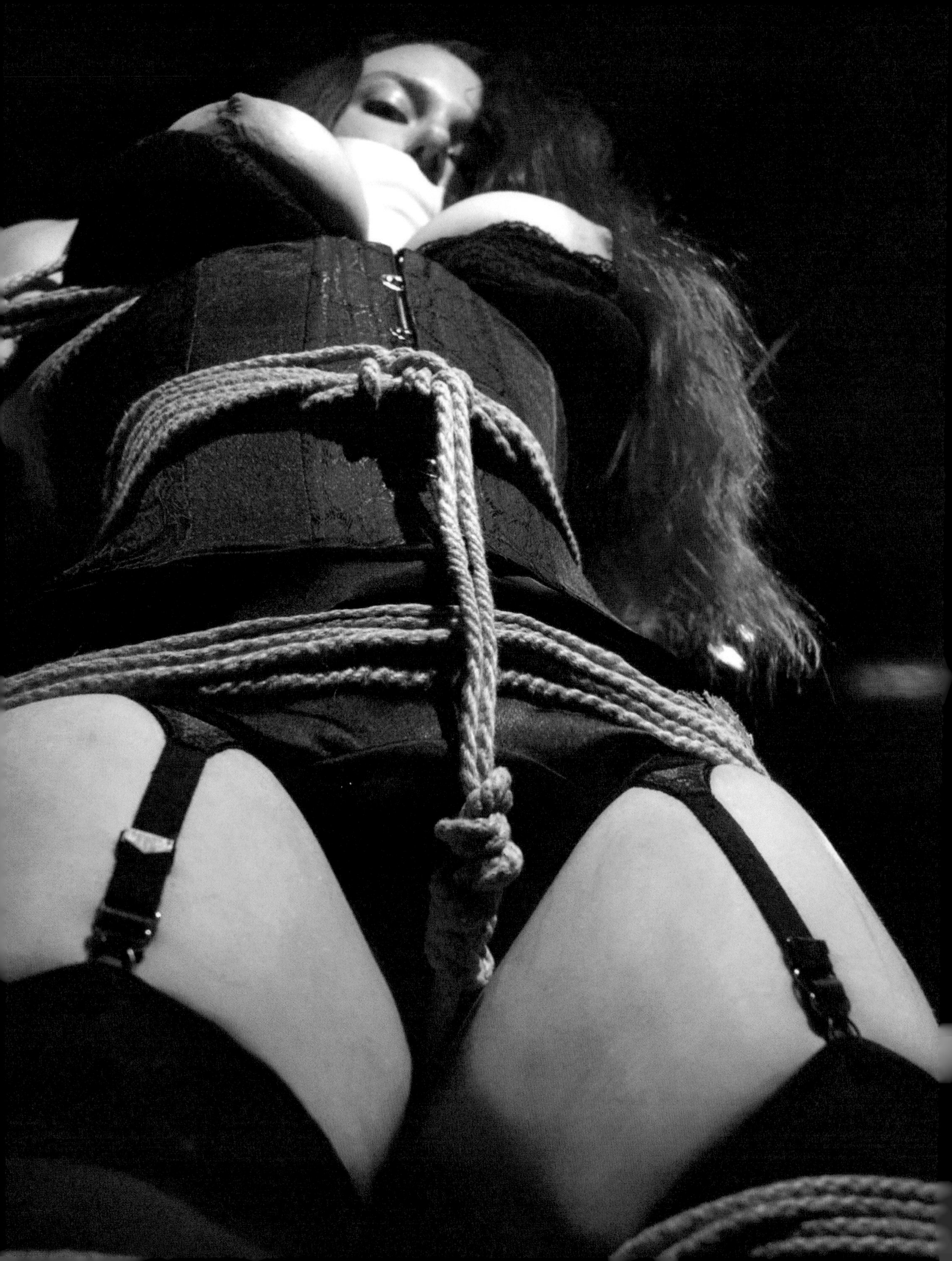

Chapter 6

For Curvy Rope Bottoms

Everywhere we turn, the message is the same: Thin is supposedly in. We get it on a macro level from ads, TV shows, movies, magazines, and more, and on a micro level via comments from family and friends, rejection by potential partners, that person disapprovingly eyeing our lunch. According to research firm Research and Markets, the global weight-loss and weight-management market was $148.1 *billion* in 2014 and is expected to reach $206.4 billion by 2019.[1] That's a lot of business that depends on our feeling bad about ourselves for not being thin.

A few more statistics for you:

- Anorexia has the highest mortality rate of any mental illness.[2]
- 50 percent of teenage girls and 30 percent of teenage boys in one study used unhealthy weight-control behaviors such as skipping meals, fasting, smoking cigarettes, vomiting, and taking laxatives to control their weight.[3]
- 46 percent of 9- to 11-year-olds in another study were sometimes, or very often, on diets, and 82 percent of their families were sometimes, or very often, on diets.[4] For more heartbreaking statistics on and help for eating disorders, visit http://www.eatingdisorderhope.com/information/statistics-studies.

This chapter is particularly close to my heart, because I've struggled with feeling bad about my weight and body shape for my entire life—and the most I've ever weighed was 135 pounds pregnant. In my 20s I exercised maniacally, often going to the gym twice a day, and would make myself throw up despite not overeating. I got down to 95 pounds and shopped for clothes in the children's department—a source of pride at the time. People kept telling me how amazing I looked, and I kept dieting to the extreme and making myself throw up. I was obsessed, unhealthy, and often miserable despite looking "fabulous."

> ***"Everyone looks beautiful in ropespace."***
> ***~ Dani_Red***

Even now, recognizing that at my thinnest I was my most unhappiest, I struggle every time I look in the mirror to not feel bad about my body, and subsequently myself. It's a struggle I usually lose. And I'm one of the "lucky" ones, because my disorder hasn't killed me.

As deviant as the rope world is, its public face often seems to share mainstream views about body image. Just look at FetLife's Kinky & Popular page, all the rope groups on Facebook, bondage photos published in magazines and books...more often than not, the rope bottoms are thin, young, very flexible women—in other words, *not representative* of the majority of rope bottoms, who have a wide range of body types, whose ages run the gamut, and who include men and transgender people.

This is not to judge thin, young, bendy women, by the way, who deserve to be who they are without being shamed or judged, just like everyone else. Nor is it to

Dani_Red. Bondage and photo by ModusVitae_SF

"I am short, fat, and much older than the beautiful girls on [FetLife's Kinky & Popular page].... Guess what? I can still be a rope bottom. Do I do the bendy stuff on K&P? Nope nope nope! But I can do what works for me. And it is hot!"

~ Kurious

say that every single rope top or photographer uses only young and thin females as rope bottoms. But what we're exposed to publicly—on social media, in professional bondage performances, even in many rope scenes at clubs and dungeons—is overwhelmingly focused on what appears to be a small minority of rope bottoms as a whole.

What we see all around us affects how we see ourselves, and hopefully this will help everyone see the fuller spectrum of beautiful rope bottoms in all their glory. As more than one person has said in different ways, everyone is beautiful in bondage. This book is one small effort that I hope will take root and grow until every rope bottom sees their beauty.

Let's hear what some beautiful curvy rope bottoms have to say.

Challenges

The No. 1 challenge for curvy rope bottoms seems to be a tie between dealing with self-image issues and finding a rope top. "There's definitely an internal anxiety I have about asking people to tie me, because I am afraid that they might make a face or reject me," JoyfulNoise says. Starberry cites "self-confidence and self-esteem issues," and Kori cites "my own insecurity and finding riggers willing to tie a larger rope bottom" as the biggest challenges. Gnethys says, "I've always been self-conscious about my image due to my weight, which has made me a bit shy when it comes to putting myself in positions where I would be looked at, and more vulnerable to negative messages."

The majority of photos we see on social media certainly don't help. "My biggest challenge has been my own perspective of my capabilities and my self-doubt," Sous says. "I struggle with insecurity, particularly when the majority of the photos I see of suspension bondage are women who look like [two well-known rope bottoms]. I am so much bigger than they are, so I convince myself that I am not as worthy of a rope bottom as they are." Starberry says, "It is intimidating to see a constant stream of images of rope bottoms who are superskinny and flexible and, well, I'm not."

WyldOrchid_soumi adds, "It has been very hard to feel less bendy than most bottoms I see on Fet. Emotionally, I often have felt inferior."

It's not just photos, either; curvy (and male and gender-nonconforming) folks are rarely seen bottoming for instructors in classes. "Most of the people in my country that do rope on an advanced level do it with supersuperthin and quite young girls," says a rope bottom outside the U.S. "The more advanced you go, the thinner they get it seems. So even though I know I can do it, I still feel insecure about it because the thinness is everywhere, while us curvy people are a minority." Here in the U.S., I've seen demo bottoms who are not superthin and young (including myself), but the majority do seem to fall within a limited weight and age range and be female.

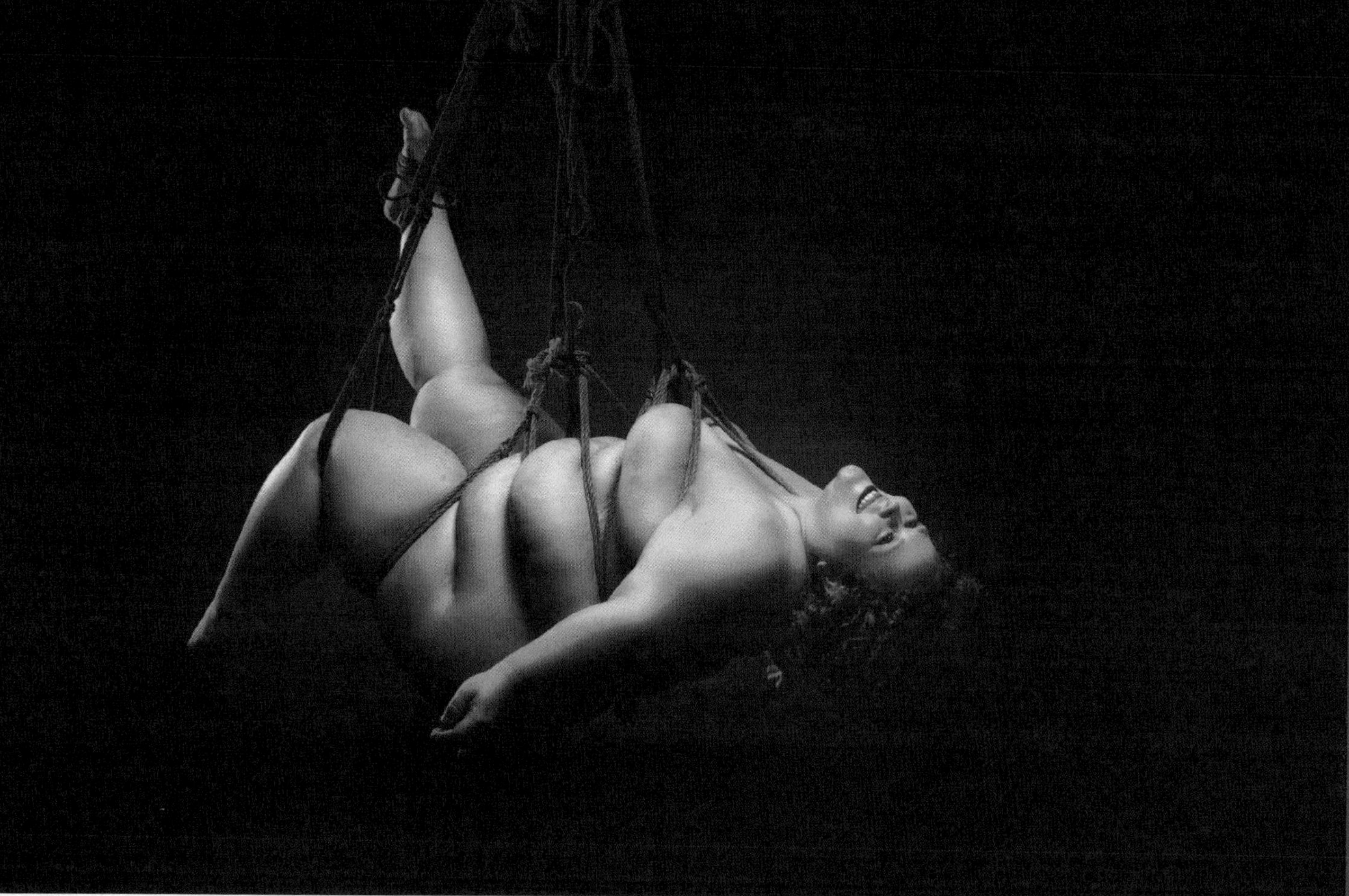

JoyfulNoise. Bondage and photo by The Silence

The Right to Choose

Before we go any further, it's worth pointing out that there are definitely those asshat rope tops and photographers who deliberately shame rope bottoms for their size, insist they *can't* be tied, or are otherwise insensitive or downright disrespectful in turning down a request to be tied. (If you need support for calling bullshit on those, see Shay Tiziano's article at the end of this chapter, along with all the photos of and writings by curvy bondage bottoms if you dig deeper than FetLife's Kinky & Popular page.)

And then there are those rope tops who aren't asshats but simply don't have the knowledge, skill, or desire to tie people beyond a limited range of body types. And those tops should not be shamed for that whether or not they have any intention of ever changing. Every top has the right to personal preferences—whether aesthetic, emotional, mental, or based on any other quality—the same way every bottom does, and the right to decide what is within their comfort zone. A rope bottom who shames a top who respectfully declines for any of the above reasons is being just as insensitive as the putzes in the first category. It may be a frustrating experience, but anger, blaming, and shaming are not justified here*

Frustrations and Misassumptions

So, back to finding a top. "There are just some people who will not tie people my size," Elsie says. "It can be extremely frustrating to drive an hour to an event and not get tied." Bri Burning offers this:

**One could argue that there are better responses than anger, blaming, and shaming in pretty much any situation. But that's a discussion for another book.*

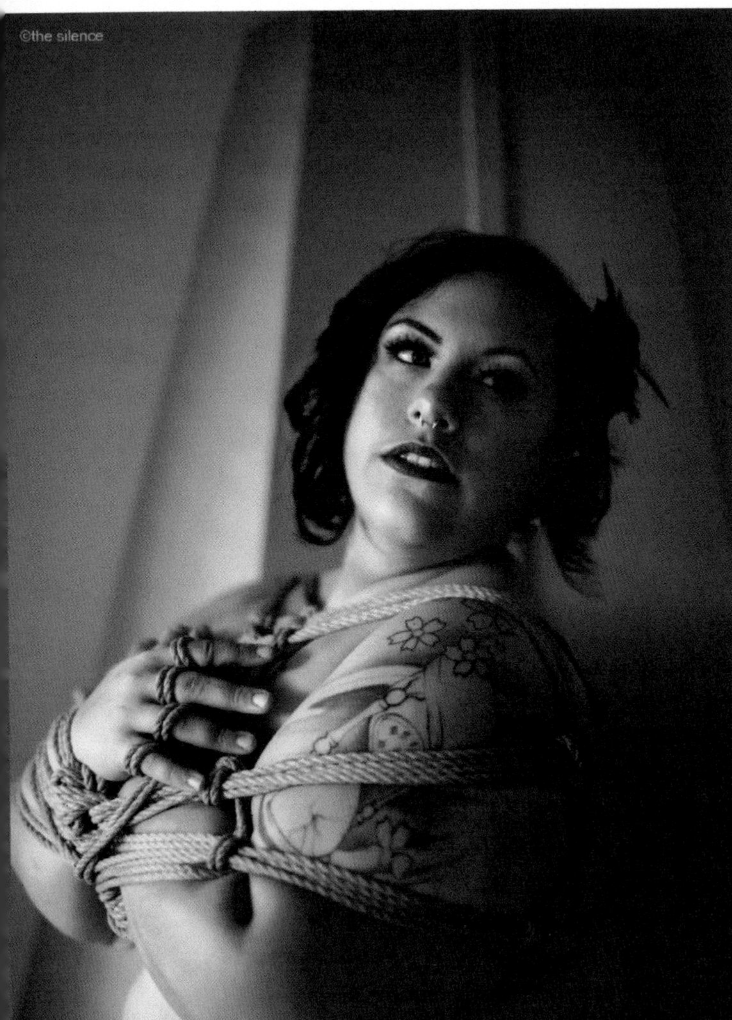

Bri Burning. Bondage and photo by The Silence

"The biggest challenge I've faced being a rope bottom is the doubt of tops—whether that be doubt in my body and what it can do, or insecurities in their own skills." That last part brings up another part of the challenge: incorrect assumptions about the limitations and capabilities of larger bodies. "I'm a very curvy woman who is extremely flexible," Bri continues. "[But] most people assume that I can't stay in stress positions for long or can't bend a certain way."

Let's be clear: Flexibility is *not* related to size. Curvy bottoms run the gamut from having very limited flexibility to having very high flexibility, the same way noncurvy rope bottoms do. (See Chapter 12 on ties for limited range of motion if you fall into the former category.) As Starberry says, "There may be some things I can't do, but those are my limitations and not necessarily due to weight."

Bottoms sometimes make assumptions about themselves that may or may not be true as well. "Flexibility started out to be the biggest issue in my mind. But it was only in my mind," Kurious says. "My rope top carefully makes sure there is not too much pressure on my joints. And as time has gone by, my flexibility has improved." Another rope bottom adds, "I think that if I approached one of the well-known rigger/photographers in my country, I would be refused as a model, but that's based on what I see them shooting and not on actually asking."

Figuring Out What Works

Some bottoms know from experience that specific parts of their body may need extra care. "Because I'm large-busted (I wear a 38M cup)," one rope bottom says, "if I'm not in a supportive bra, then chest harnesses and other breast ties are much more difficult and less aesthetically pleasing to me. There's a lot of flop to deal with, and heavy breasts on rope can get very uncomfortable." Usually I recommend trying to avoid underwire bras for suspensions involving chest harnesses, because rope pressure on the wire can add unbeneficial pain, but figure out what's right for you—if an underwire bra or any other type of support works best for you, go for it!

Similarly, certain tying positions may be out of the running. But as I've said elsewhere, no rope bottom that I know of doesn't have some kind of limitation.

Take fuoco, who performs at the top level and studies contortion. "I have very exposed nerves," she says, "and so I always tell play partners in negotiations that 'you can tie a perfect TK on me, but at some point I will have a nerve issue. It's not really a question of if but when.'" She makes sure that suspension sequences include positions in which the takate-kote is not bearing the weight of support, and that her rigger will be ready to transition her out of a TK as soon as it becomes an issue. So remember that not being able to hold certain positions or even do them at all is no reason to feel that you're not "good enough."

Along with learning about what works and doesn't work for your body, which applies to bottoms of all shapes and sizes, let's look at some other helpful suggestions from the community.

Helpful Ideas

Developing a positive self-image is a personal journey that's unique to every individual. But surrounding yourself with people, writings, and images that make you feel good about yourself, as opposed to things like most fashion magazines and FetLife's K&P page, is a good bet. "Do not read beauty magazines. They will only make you feel ugly." Wise words from *Chicago Tribune* columnist Mary Schmich (later lifted by Baz Luhrmann for his spoken-word song, and misattributed to Kurt Vonnegut). Similarly, read Hedwig's essay later in the chapter and take the concepts not just to heart but to put forth into the world. Anyone or anything that makes you feel bad about yourself is not worth your time and attention.

Focus on the good instead: "what you can do, and doing it well," as Starberry puts it.

> ***"Once I get in the air, all the self-doubt and self-criticism fall away and I lose myself in the joy of flying."***
>
> ***~ Sous***

Growing Awareness

"Physically I have been practicing yoga and meditation for the last three years," Bri says. "This has helped me understand my body further, what it can and cannot do. Mentally I continue to practice self-care and self-love daily. The insecurities that pop up have to do with my inner workings as a human that I have to take responsibility and action over."

WyldOrchid_soumi also recommends "meditation and body awareness—it is very important to be in tune with your own body. This really is for every bottom, but I feel for me that without that mindfulness, I would not have the mental fortitude to ever be naked in rope. You can't help but begin to love the body you have as you discover all the intricacies of how your body works."

Through meditation, you may also find yourself embracing the Hindu concept that your true self (*atman*) is completely distinct from the external body (and the mind too). Your real self is beyond all temporary designations like the body, age, gender, and race. It wasn't until I started meditating on the "inner beloved" who exists in all of us (Sally Kempton offers a guided meditation on this on Yogaglo.com) that I began to let go of my self-loathing and to realize that my true self is love, and that it has nothing to do with how big my thighs are.

The Value of Education

Finding a rope top who has good knowledge of tying curvy bodies, is creative in tying, and who is emotionally supportive is also key. "I truly think that having healthy relationships with my rope tops and building that trust is what helped me the most to accept my body type for what it was," Roxy says. "The first time I tried a rope suspension, I was really nervous that it wouldn't hold me or that the tie would hurt too much because I had extra weight on it. My rigger assured me he had suspended people of my body shape and bigger with no problems. It made me feel a lot better, and I ended up really enjoying the suspension."

Beautiful Words

"The first time I was tied in a karada, I cried. I cried because I felt fat and ugly. I cried because the rope was digging into my belly and I felt like my blubber was oozing out of the rope.

My top took a picture and showed it to me.

I was right. The rope was digging into my belly, and my fat was sticking out of the rope. I also saw the beauty in it. The rope was forcing my belly into diamond shapes and shaping it into ways that my top wanted to see." —thisgirl_m

"An educated top is your biggest ally," Kurious says. "Ask the questions...'Have you ever tied up a big [person]? What do you do differently with someone my size versus someone that is half my weight?...Will you be prepared to catch me if I am falling?'"

Consider having a spotter present too. More than once, a rigger has asked someone to help hold me up while getting me out of a suspension, and so now I evaluate a partner's ability to support my body weight if no one else will be around to step in if necessary.

If you just can't find an educated top, consider creating one! Do your own research and educate your partner. Learn together. "There are always workarounds to an uncomfortable tie," says WyldOrchid_soumi. "My top has added wraps or changed the point of the primary pull, and it has made all the difference. Also, a good wrap clearing or cleaning can make a huge difference when you have a lot of fleshiness under those wraps. Hurts like a bitch in the moment but is worth the extra minutes I can hold the tie."

If anyone says or implies that you're too big to be tied, that's a wonderful opportunity for a teaching moment. "I've done dozens of suspensions and been told by experienced tops that I was too heavy for that kind of play. I'm not and I love it!" Dani_Red says. Many other bottoms know the same thing. "Don't ever let anyone tell you that you're too big to be tied up. That's complete hogwash. I've been doing rope since my second kink event, and I've always been about the size I am now," JoyfulNoise says. "When it comes to something like suspension or complex,

WyldOrchid_soumi. Bondage by Bry1970.
Photo by D&R Photography

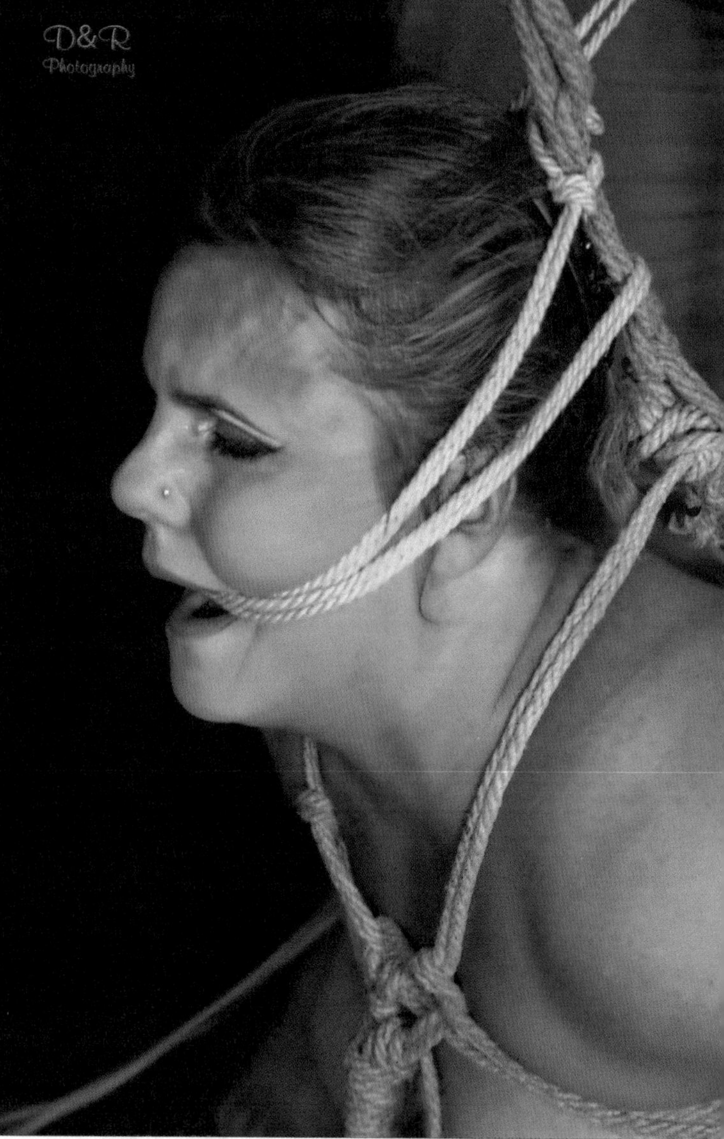

physically demanding ties, there may be some tops who aren't comfortable or don't possess the skill set to tie you. That doesn't mean it's impossible—it simply means you need to keep looking to find a rope top who has the skill set."

Boldly Go

And yes, we've already noted that finding tops can be an issue—as it can be for all bottoms. "Be brave, attend rope events, and get to know different riggers and bottoms," Kori recommends. "Ask the other bottoms for recommendations on who to tie you. If you get rejected, don't get angry or upset; there are plenty of people out there who like to tie all body types." Elsie adds, "Keep trying. There are people who will tie you; you just have to look a little harder."

Consider what signals you're sending about yourself too. "If you're not happy with yourself, you're not attractive," one rope bottom says. "There are enough people around that like curvy [people], or don't have much of a body-type preference. So when I started being a generally happy person and stopped feeling fat and ugly, I didn't have any problems with meeting nice people that wanted to have fun with me."

"I had to reshape my thinking completely," Starberry says. "I had to realize that society is trying to sell me something that I just don't want to buy anymore, and force myself to constantly remind myself that there is nothing wrong with me, at all. My body is exactly the way it is meant to be in this moment."

Kori adds, "I love myself, and I actually think that photos of me in rope are the only pictures where I look the way I see myself. I decided that if someone doesn't want to tie me because I'm fat, then it's their loss. I'm pretty fun to tie."

Find Your Tribe

Being part of a supportive community is invaluable. "Going to rope group has been huge for me...seeing other people with regular bodies and folds and rolls just enjoying the art, and being able to appreciate how others look (I am my own worst critic) and getting feedback from people who don't have

"I love myself and I actually think that photos of me in rope are the only pictures where I look the way I see myself."
~ Kori

any stake in my game, as it were," one rope bottom says. "It's done a lot to make me feel more comfortable." Don't have a local rope group, or the one that exists doesn't fit your needs? Make one of your own! Yes, you have the power and all the knowledge you need to do it right now—you can learn and grow together as you go; the important thing is finding like-minded people for mutual support.

For an online community, FetLife has two related BBW (big beautiful women) groups: One is BBW Rope Lovers (https://fetlife.com/groups/60427); and the other is BBW in Bondage (https://fetlife.com/groups/44239). If you are a big beautiful male or transgender person and can't find an online support group, consider starting one!

Tie One On

Learning how to tie and even self-suspend can be helpful as well. "Self-tying has helped me the most physically and mentally to rope bottom," thisgirl_m says. "I've gained knowledge about the technicalities of the ties that allows me to judge the safety of the ties I am in. I have learned my body's 'normal' in rope so I able to tell if something is causing me harm." Gnethys adds, "If someone tells you you're too fat to fly, nothing will shut them up faster than self-suspending in front of them."

Find Your Bliss

And remember that *you* get to define your rope experience. It's not about what other bottoms do in their own scenes or photos, or what they look like. "You don't need to do what you see others doing to be good at bottoming. You need to have a good time," says Dani_Red.

"You need to communicate and have confidence that you're sharing something beautiful with another human who is enjoying what they are doing to you.... It's about the energy you share with them." Starberry says. "I started trying rope without taking pictures and just feeling it. [Then] I allowed pictures, and for every negative thing I saw I gave myself two compliments. I am willing to try anything once and feel it for what it is before deciding I don't like it because of how it might look."

Bri adds, "When I first learned of rope, it was all about the aesthetics and looking a certain way. I stayed clear from that type of rope because I wanted connection, energy play, and pain.... The way rope can be taken off can send me into subspace. The smell of jute leaves me floaty. Rope is a different experience for every person.... Whatever body type, gender, or sexuality you happen to be, you can have these beautiful moments."

And Sous says, "Once I stopped worrying about whether or not my stomach fat was hanging down in a facedown suspension, or whether there was too much extra flesh bulging around my futomomo ties, I enjoyed all my bondage scenes so much more. One of my partners told me, 'Everyone looks sexy in rope,' and she is 100 percent correct."

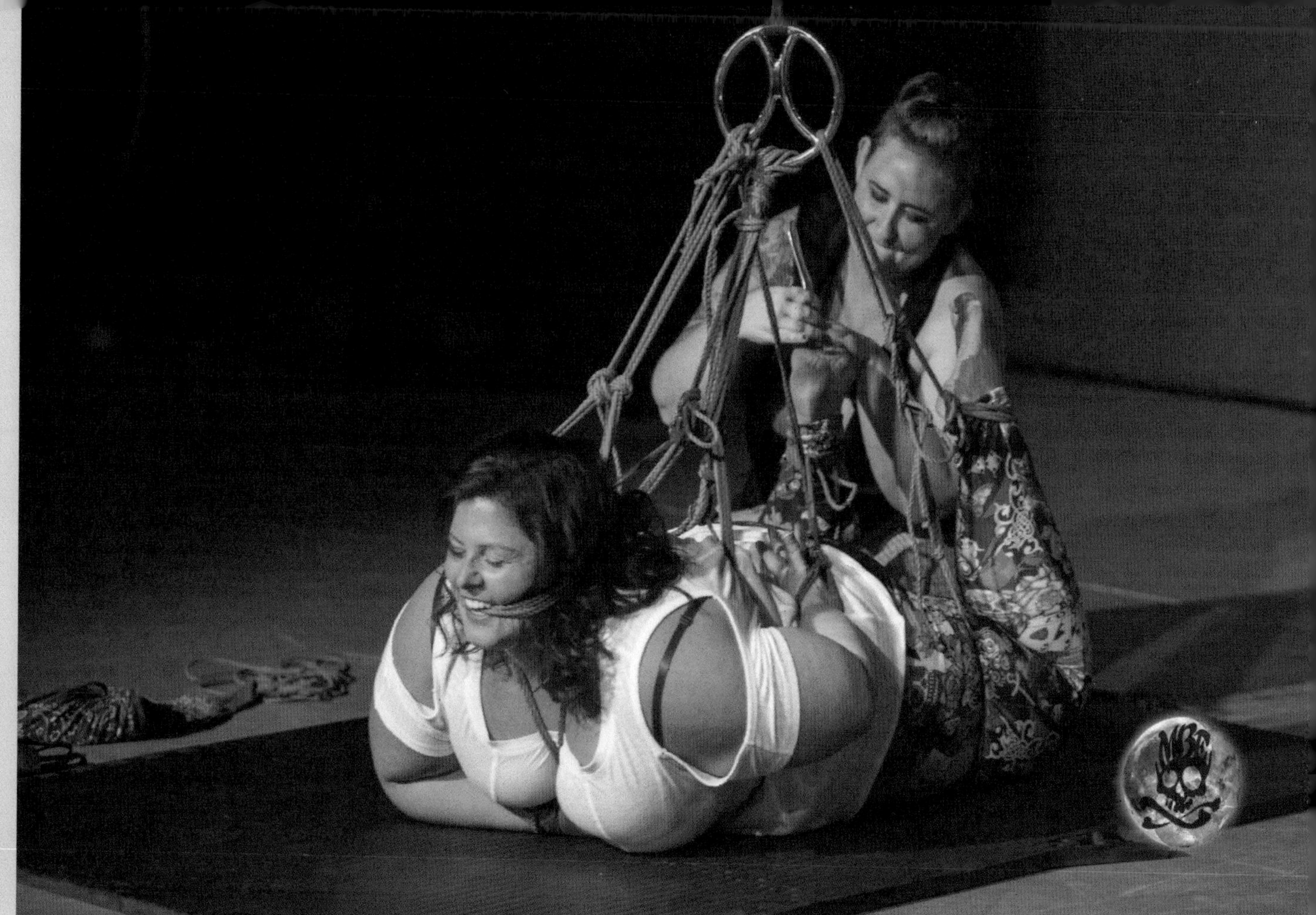

TheStuntDouble and RunningAemok. Bondage by RunningAemok. Photo by Taylor Roehr; www.rareglassphotography.com

Everyone looks sexy in rope. Everyone is beautiful in ropespace.

I can't repeat those truisms enough. Please consider sharing that message near and far. "So many people do bondage, of all shapes and sizes, and everyone deserves love and support for that," Starberry says. "We can be the change we want to see by putting ourselves out there—go to events, do private scenes, share your pictures, support everyone big, small, and in between. Rope is not just for small and delicate women—rope is for anyone and everyone who wants it. Go get it!"

Hedwig

Sharing the Journey

Hedwig is a rope bondage and sex educator, the cofounder of Hitchin' Bitches, and a feminist. Visit www.senseshibari.com to learn more.

If there is one thing I want you to know, it is this: Everything that you are is allowed to exist. Even if the world is telling you otherwise, that you need to be thinner, more flexible, stronger. Even if the photography you see, the pornography you see, the ties that are taught, the fitness forums, and the diet crazes are telling you otherwise. They are wrong. You exist in your form; you have a shape already. You are not a project to be improved upon or a problem to be solved.

I have struggled for a long time as someone who is not the flexible, tiny rope lover. Ropes initially helped me to find my way back to my body, to my sense of self, through a fog of dissociation and self-hatred. Through eating disorders and suffering. Ropes on my body have helped me to find where I am, and who I am, the boundaries of my body; both flesh and mind. Sadly, it has also brought new problems, because of some ideas in our rope world that keep on being circulated. Because we are a part of a world with structural inequalities that cast judgment and build hierarchies dependent on gender, sexual expression, ethnicity, physical dis/abilities, class, and so on. These structural inequalities bleed into our kink communities, and those who find themselves outside of the "normative" experience the consequences. Bodies are being seen as problems to be fixed, improved upon, but the problem is those who judge what does not adhere to cis-sexist, ableist, racist expectations. As a femme-identified individual, I know what it means to go through life having every curve inspected by society, media, culture, even family, and to internalize the fat hatred.

Here is how I try to fight this.

There are some images I do not accept and actively shut out from my life: the ones we all have been force-fed our whole lives. I actively avoid any culture that trash talks about any femme body, as well as any culture that preaches about exercise/"clean" living/diets only for the sake of looking thin or for the sake of "wellness," a culture that constantly measures and judges the body. Instead, I actively try to seek out counterexamples, the counterculture that has a stronger range of diversity both in images and in having more sound theories in regards to exercise and eating. Exercise can come from joy, not from the idea of transforming a body that is not "right" just as it is. The obsession about being healthy/fit can be as damaging as the obsession about being thin. If we don't give our bodies and our minds the care they need, they will have less energy to bring about the revolution.

I avoid the discourse about thin = healthy/strong character and fat = unhealthy/weak character. One thing all of us can do is to not comment on bodies at all, even if we think it is a compliment. Don't ask others if they have lost weight as a form of praise. Last time somebody asked that, I had been sick for six months and could hardly stand up. Weight loss is not automatically amazing, nor weight gain something negative. Do not assume. Be kind. That includes yourself; do not trash talk that amazing person who you are. It is surprisingly hard, because everything around us encourages us to do so.

A question that gets asked a lot is what one can do to become a better rope bottom. Most of the time the answer is to do yoga. That irks me. While yoga can indeed increase body awareness, flexibility, stamina, and body management, it is not going to do that for everyone. As someone who was completely disconnected and dissociative, I had to start much more simply. With walks. A chiropractor. Wrestling with partners in rope. Having an orgasm. After some time with those, I found myself trying out Pilates, and it was there that I realized what I needed: activities that made me less afraid to be in a body I had worked so hard to forget. Activities that made me be more present in my body and more aware of it in a nonjudgmental fashion. That made me able to scan, assess, and process where I was at. Start listening to what it was telling me, rather than focusing on what I felt it had to be. These activities have made it possible to be more present in ropes too, to scan, assess, process, and communicate.

Start wherever you are in your own body, and do something that encourages you to be more present and communicative. It can be so many things. A rope partner of mine does weightlifting. Another one punches a boxing bag. A third is an elite equestrian athlete. Today, I do Pilates and kettlebell-based exercise, and the reason I do the latter is because it is in a space that is LGBTQI-friendly and body-positive, no posters on the walls with motivational quotes or thin, tanned bodies. No huffing mus-

Hedwig and Osaka Dan. Bondage by Osaka Dan. Photo by Petra Sundberg; petrasundberg.se

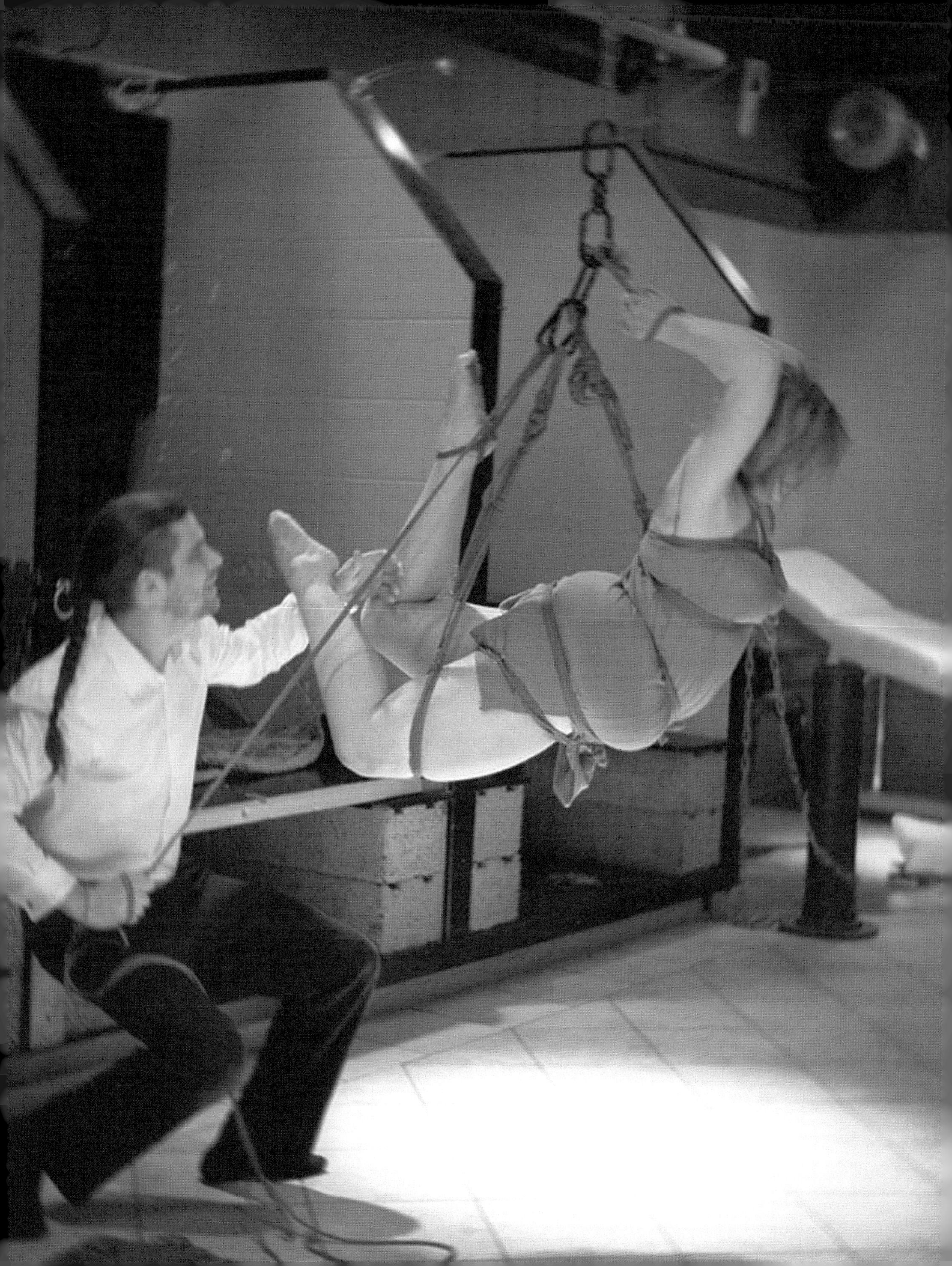

clemountains explaining what you are doing wrong. Instead I'm surrounded by queers, older people, those with injuries, of every shape and size. Instructors are from all walks of life and would never dream of verbally trying to push you to work harder or touching you for corrections unless you specifically ask for it. No silly expressions in the vein that an exercise will "burn off fat." Search for the places and the kinds of exercise that bring you happiness, not the ones that will make you feel worse.

Two years ago I decided to be open. I came out to my Pilates and kettlebell instructors about kink. About eating disorders. About injuries and weaknesses. I can go with my bruises and rope marks, but also my warped sense of self, and know that if something feels off, it's OK. I'm just working on all of those things I'm trying to reprogram.

I started to be much more open with those I tie with too. I started speaking with them about the emotional impact of how certain types of tying and rope make me feel heavy and ungraceful. Being open about this makes it a shared concern and will bring awareness to those who tie me, helping them treat me as the person I am instead of a figment of imagination. Furthermore, if they cannot accept and honor this trust, this is how I weed out those who are not worthy of my time. And if we can have these discussions about what makes us feel less worthy of love and rope and sexy times, then we can little by little change the entire culture that induces that shame.

Raise the bar. If companies make claims to be a part of the community, ask them to show the whole community, rather than thin, glossed-over, and edited versions of it. Regardless if it is a porn company or a venue in which you are supposed to feel safe in. Ask events to feature images and classes that reflect on the diversity, not just in regards to body shape but also in regards to ethnicity. Find that which speaks to you, that makes you feel as good as when the ropes are good. Change can happen. Change will happen. You have the right to ask for more. Demand more. More diversity. More respect. More visibility. Less fat shaming.

In rope, the awareness of where I am and who I am is so important. I find my strength, my fears, my boundaries, my lust, my voice. That is the starting point. Not the gym membership or the diet fads. The fault is never yours, though; the fight is not yours alone. It is a twisted world with structural inequality, that wants you to focus on you and yourself alone, to be so blinded that you won't fight against it.

Forgive yourself and keep on fighting for respect, kindness, and positive change. You are not a problem to be solved; everything that you are is allowed to exist.

BDSM Bullshit

Who Can Be Suspended?

by Shay Tiziano

Shay Tiziano is an ER nurse who has been teaching rope bondage for more than a decade. See her full bio in Chapter 11. A number of other awesome folks, including MietteRouge (a kinky MD), Guilty, and Frozen Meursault, also gave feedback on this article.

Let's start with an easy one—here's a statement I hope we all recognize as bullshit: "Only skinny people can be suspended!" With me so far? OK. Now, here's what I sometimes hear as a counter to that particular piece of bullshit: "Anyone of any body size can be suspended!" Unfortunately...also bullshit. It's a pit of snakes! Let's jump in!

Being larger-bodied does not exclude someone from being suspended. That said, I think making a general statement about anyone being able to be suspended is potentially dangerous, for two main reasons: rigger skill and health issues.

The first of these issues is rigger skill. A rigger is a person who also gets to have limits. Limits—they're not just for bottoms! Those limits may be knowledge-based ("I don't know how to suspend larger-bodied people") or preference-based ("I prefer to suspend only 100-pound bondage models"). Of course, stating one's own skills honestly is quite different from saying, "It simply cannot be done!" and having a personal preference is quite different from being a fat-shaming douchebag. There are unique

blissy and Rocket. Bondage by Rocket.
Photo by TwistedView

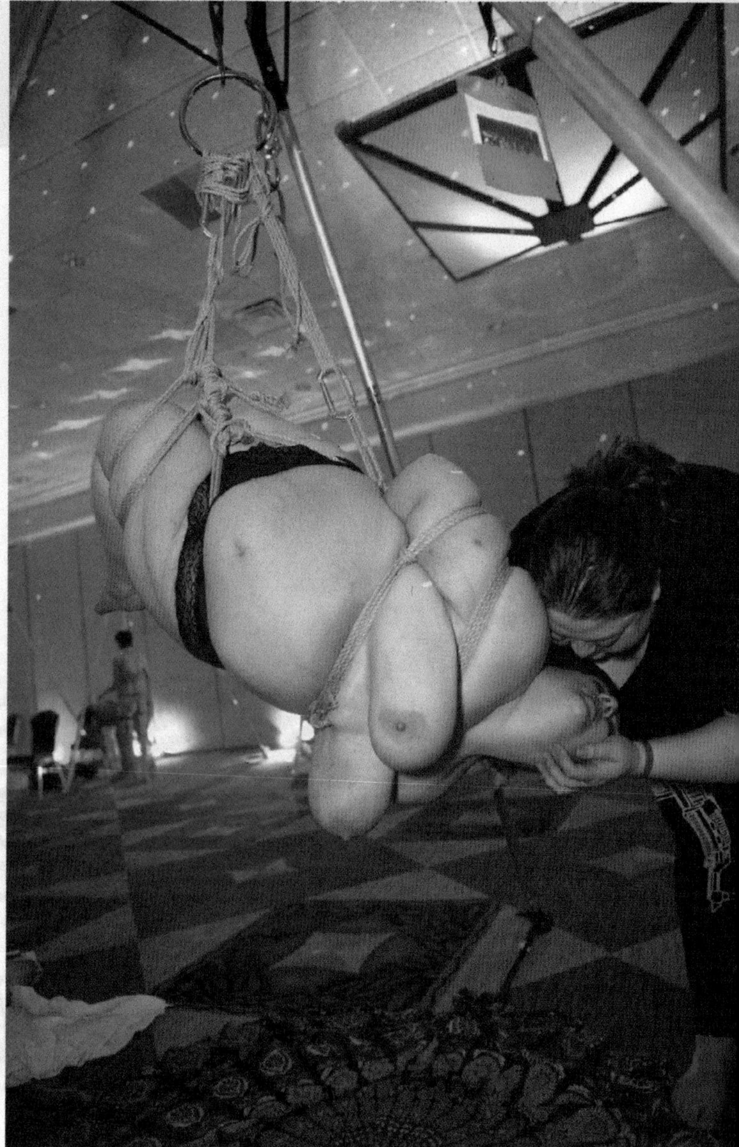

skills involved in suspending a larger-bodied person—not any rigger can or should suspend a bottom of any body shape. Some of that skill is relatively simple (generally, more wrapping turns are called for), but some is very specific and specialized.

There are safety concerns that extend to the rigger as well. If a larger-bodied suspension bottom needs to come down now, can the rigger partially support their weight while getting them down quickly and without injuring themselves? I think we can all intuit that this is more challenging with a 200-pound bottom than a 100-pound one. Having a spotter (another pair of hands to help should it be needed) and/or using an appropriate pulley system (which adds complexity and another potential point of failure) may be all that is required to mitigate this, but it's another area where additional expertise is required.

Moving on to the health aspect—being larger-sized doesn't exclude you from being suspended, but neither does being smaller-sized mean you can do all the suspensions! There are actually potentially increased risks at the other end of the weight spectrum. Most notably, very thin people are at higher risk for acute compression nerve injury.[5] With regards to assessing general health, fitness is a more important factor than weight: "Data from a 2009 study showed that low fitness is responsible for 16 percent to 17 percent of deaths in the United States, while obesity accounts for only 2 percent to 3 percent, once fitness is factored out."[6]

A focus on fitness is very relevant to rope, because here's something no one told me before I got suspended for the first time: Being suspended can be very strenuous! Dynamic sequences involving drops and position changes, or especially challenging suspensions (four wrapping turns around your ankle and up you go!) require a high level of fitness and body awareness. Which is not to imply that dynamic suspensions are more dangerous than static suspensions—in some cases they are safer, but often they do require more athletic ability. The best parallels I can think of are yoga or circus arts training (bar, hoop, silks). Are you healthy and fit enough, at whatever size, for those activities? You may need to build fitness before being able to partake in the most strenuous/dynamic suspensions.

The fitness needed and strain involved in being suspended are eminently scalable; it is not an all-or-nothing either-you-can-do-it-or-you-can't activity. If you want to do strenuous, dynamic suspensions (and there's no reason you have to; they're not everyone's kink), be realistic with your rigger and spend some time training. Rigging involves practice, skill, and training—a suspension bottom would be well served by developing or honing rope bottoming skills like core strength, balance, and body awareness!

Everything we do in kink (and, you know, life) has risks. Specific health conditions increase those risks, and at some point those risks outweigh the rewards of a given activity and we sit back and say, hmmm, maybe it's not such a good idea to do that. If you have frequent seizures, you aren't permitted to drive. If you are on blood thinners, your doctor will likely advise you not to go downhill skiing. Likewise, there's some kinky shit that you probably shouldn't do if you have certain health conditions. Someone with poorly controlled diabetes probably shouldn't bottom for bastinado (caning the feet), and someone on Coumadin (a potent blood thinner) shouldn't bottom for play piercing. This is simply about being rational regarding the risk-vs.-reward ratio of any given activity.

That said, here is a summary of conditions that at the very least require extra caution, awareness, and expertise (from both rigger and bottom) for suspension. In some cases these issues may make certain suspension positions particularly (and probably unacceptably) risky, or may mean someone shouldn't be suspended at all—these conditions all exist on a continuum, and evaluation needs to take into account the entire picture of a person's health and fitness, not just a single diagnosis.

• Conditions that cause significant neuropathy (nerve damage and impaired sensation), impaired circulation, or impaired lymphatic drainage require caution with any bondage, and in many cases may exclude the affected limb(s) from load-bearing bondage. Such conditions can include diabetes, lupus, stroke, mastectomy, lymph node removal, carpal tunnel syndrome, and Raynaud's disease.

• Serious respiratory issues (severe asthma, COPD, etc.)—these are especially a problem for chest-heavy ties and suspension positions like facedown or inversion.

• Heart issues (CHF, arrhythmias, valve abnormalities, etc.)

• Diabetes that is severe or poorly controlled—this causes increased risk of peripheral vascular disease, or poor blood flow to the legs, and peripheral neuropathy.[7] I think it is wise to avoid load-bearing lines on the lower extremities of someone who has peripheral vascular disease, and you may have to base this assessment on risk factors (diabetes, degree of diabetic control).

• Joint problems (this depends on the intended suspension, of course).

• Clotting abnormalities (hemophilia, taking Coumadin or other potent blood thinners, etc.)—I would not suspend anyone in this group, but others may have a different risk assessment.

• Aneurysms—cerebral aneurysms are a particular concern for inversion; aortic aneurysms are very high risk in general. Risk increases when combined with diabetes and/or obesity.

• Hernias

- Eye problems (conjunctivitis, glaucoma)—especially an issue for inversions
- Spinal injury
- Bone weakness (severe osteoporosis, osteogenesis imperfecta)
- Uncontrolled high blood pressure
- History of gastric bypass surgery—likely means the person should not do inversions. And be extremely careful of putting pressure on the abdomen with rope.
- Pregnancy
- Skin integrity issues (like long-term prednisone use)

This is not a comprehensive list! If you're comfortable being "out" to your doctor, asking them if you're healthy enough for suspension bondage is an excellent way to get a personal check. If you don't feel you can be out to your doctor, you might ask whether you are healthy enough for strenuous yoga and rock climbing, which have some parallels with suspension bondage.

Inversion requires special consideration, and there is actually quite a bit of literature specific to this topic—on the use of "inversion tables" to treat back pain and on the safety of various inverted yoga poses. A few things happen when you're inverted—for one, the weight of your abdomen (including organs and adipose tissue) presses up against your diaphragm, making it harder to breathe. Your intrathoracic pressure is increased (especially if you strain or hold your breath while inverted, which us perverts are known to do), as is your intracranial pressure. Blood pressure is increased.[8]

Common contraindications listed for inversion include high blood pressure, glaucoma or other eye problems, pregnancy, cardiovascular disease, diabetes (I would add that degree of diabetic control is the key here; some diabetic people can do inversion and some probably should not), and ear or sinus infection. As a side note, most articles on yoga inversion I researched also listed menstruation as a contraindication for inversion. The only reason I could find for this had to do with beliefs about chakra energy flow rather than anything I would consider a medical contraindication.

Suspension can be amazing, sexy, and fun—but it's also one of the riskier things we kinky perverts do. It's edge play and is not for everyone—top or bottom. I hope you can use this information to help you make a more accurate risk aware assessment... instead of believing bullshit.

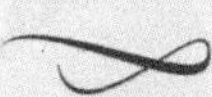

Notes

1. http://www.researchandmarkets.com/research/xvpflx/weight_loss_and

2. Sullivan, P. (1995). *American Journal of Psychiatry*, 152 (7): 1073-1074.

3. Neumark-Sztainer, D. (2005). *I'm, Like, SO Fat!* New York: The Guilford Press. p. 5.

4. Gustafson-Larson, A.M. and Terry, R.D. (1992). "Weight-Related Behaviors and Concerns of Fourth-Grade Children." *Journal of the American Dietetic Association*, 92 (7): 818-822.

5. Winfree, C.J. and Kline, D.G. (2005). "Intraoperative Positioning Nerve Injuries." *Surgical Neurology*, 63 (1): 5-18

6. http://www.nytimes.com/2016/05/08/opinion/sunday/why-you-cant-lose-weight-on-a-diet.html

7. Marso, S.P. and Hiatt, W.R. (2006) "Peripheral Arterial Disease in Patients With Diabetes." *Journal of the American College of Cardiology*, 47 (5): 921-929.

8. Haskvitz, E.M. and Hanten, W.P. (1986). "Blood Pressure Response to Inversion Traction," *Journal of Physical Therapy*, 66 (9): 1361-1364.

Chapter 7
For Male Rope Bottoms

Nobody's done an in-depth study focusing on men who love bondage (or of any other gender, for that matter), so we don't know the total number or percentage. In a survey of 1,516 people by researchers at the University of Quebec and the Philippe-Pinel Institute of Montreal, however, 46 percent of the men reported that they fantasized about being tied up in order to obtain sexual pleasure, and 53 percent reported fantasizing about being dominated sexually.[1] So it seems safe to guess that the relatively small percentage of photos we see of men in bondage on social media and elsewhere is a really bad indicator of the actual percentage of the male population who get tied up—or wish they did. It also seems pretty easy to guess why. Traditional cultural stereotypes of men's roles in many countries include a focus on emotional toughness, achievement, self-reliance, and being in control.[2] So it seems hard enough for most men to accept a desire to be in a submissive or bottoming role, let alone actually act on it, even in vanilla situations. Then add the idea of bottoming in a *kinky* way, and further add documenting that in public or semipublic places through photos...well, it seems like a Herculean leap for most men, doesn't it?

> ***"It's the fear of provoking ridicule or, worse, distaste in the girl I'm with."***
> ***~ Anonymous***

But we don't have to guess at the challenges and thoughts of men who love bondage, because here they'll tell us themselves.

Challenges

The biggest challenge male bottoms seem to face is finding tops. "Not many males want to tie men, and few females willing either," Hastingsbound says. Bound_Mnementh cites "finding riggers not only willing but capable and safe, able to not only rig but also keep me safe when I space out."

Body of Work

One layer of the challenge is that many people learn to tie on female bodies, and the male body is obviously different in key ways: "no boobs, no hips," as one bottom succinctly puts it—plus there's, you know, the cock. The presence of a cock can require different crotch ties or hip harnesses than someone has learned, and a person used to tying females may not know what to do with this body part even on a basic level—tie it gently? tie it roughly? ignore it completely?—and may shy away and stick with what's familiar. (Another instance where good communication can work wonders.)

Bodily differences may affect suspensions more than floor ties, but even in floor ties there can still be the challenge of tying a body that is bigger, heavier, or denser/more muscular. (By the way, I've noticed that more than one class has popped up on this very topic.) And adult males in general tend to be naturally less flexible than adult females,[3] so ties may need to be adjusted for that too. But of course that's a big generalization, and there are very bendy men and less bendy women and the whole gamut in between.

Luis Miguel Jiménez Villalba. Bondage by BrAxTeR. Photo by Tentesion

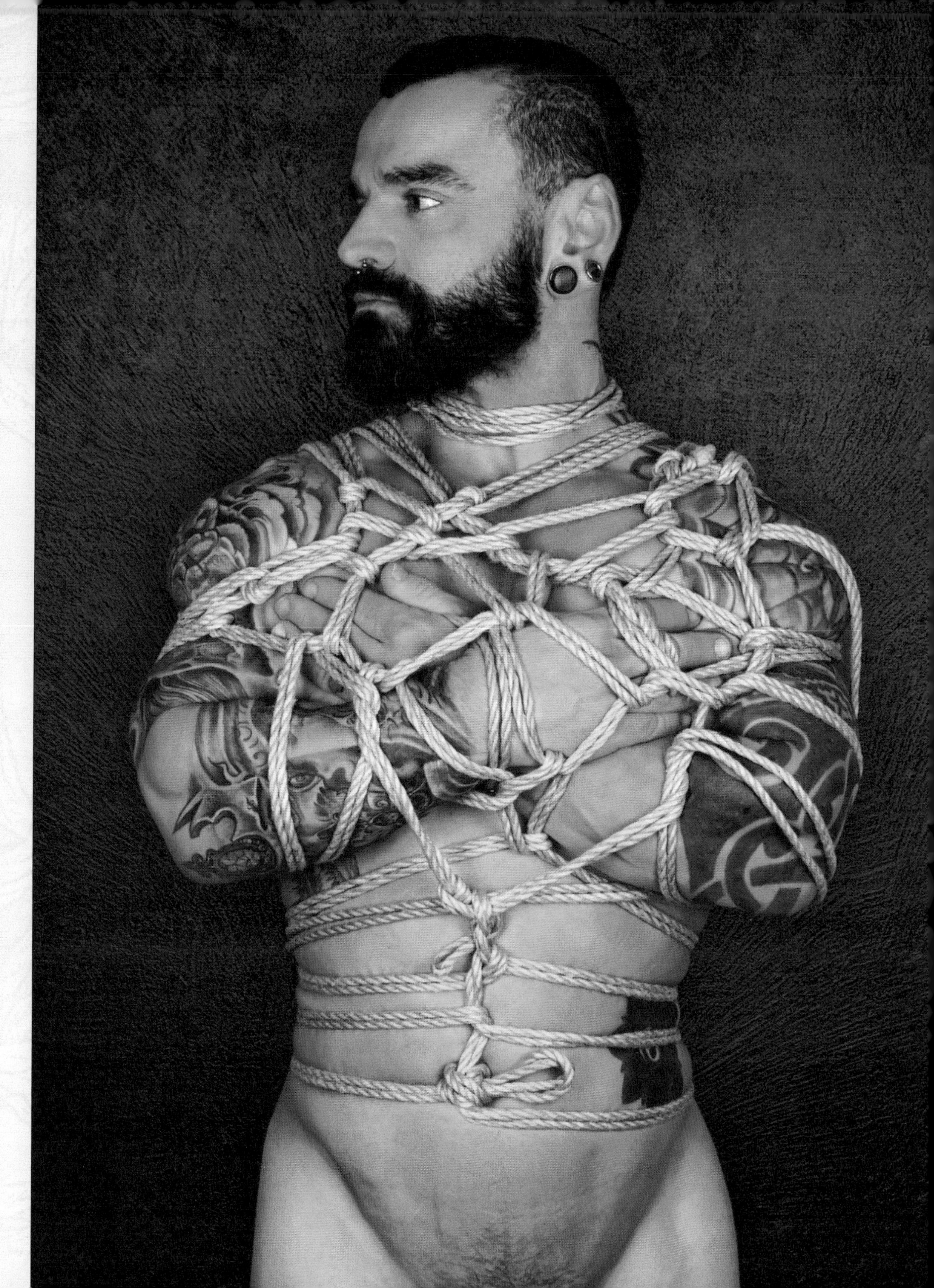

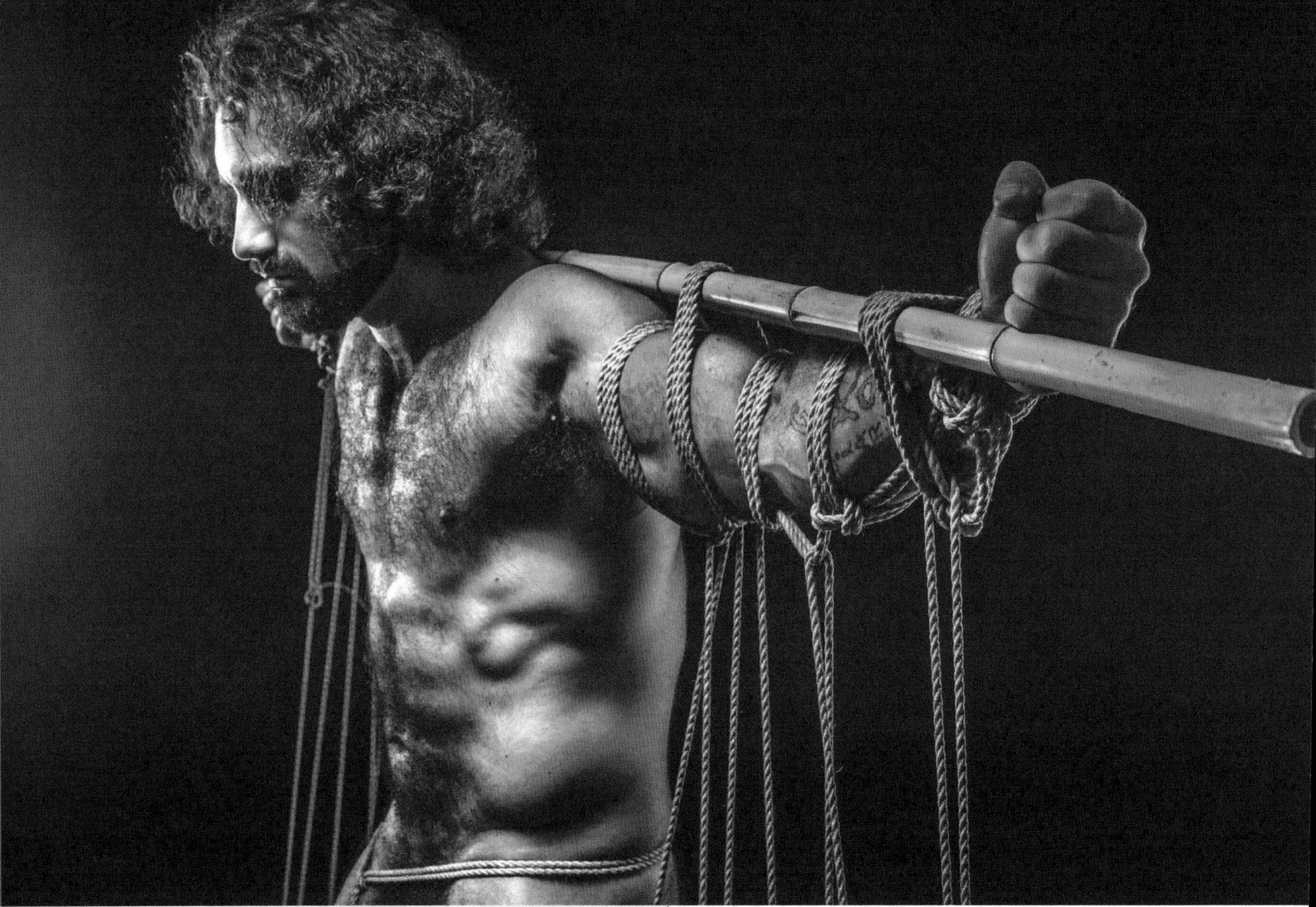

Christopher Ash. Bondage by MrMatt_PFM. Photo by Marshall Bradford; www.mbradfordphotography.com; http://mbradfordphotography.tumblr.com

Cracking the Cliché

Another layer is the stereotype of the male top and female bottom: "Female rope bottoms are presented as the default," Achilles says. This can be subtly pervasive or in-your-face. "The first time a friend took me to a peer rope event, one of the organizers asked for a volunteer and I offered myself," Gnethys says. "He ignored me, and instead made his partner (a lithe female) stand up and model for the demonstration (a simple single column tie on the wrist, where model skill or body shape wouldn't have been an issue). After that, my friend told me that riggers prefer to tie petite women, and that I shouldn't have volunteered. Foolishly, I believed her."

"[In the] early '90s, [I was told] I couldn't be a bunny, as I was a man. Only men could rig and only women could bottom," Bound_Mnementh adds.

As with other categories of rope bottoms, social media contributes to the stereotype. Female rope bottoms are "so ubiquitous that it was hard for me to fathom at first if it was even possible to apply these sorts of things—elaborate harnesses, complex predicament bondage, suspension—to a male-bodied person," Achilles says. "I couldn't find *any* examples of men in this context. After becoming more experienced and learning what to look for, I began to find representations of men bottoming, but I consider it a rare treasure."

Jessie Sparkles; www.jessiesparklesxxx.com.
Bondage by Tifereth. Photo by The Silence

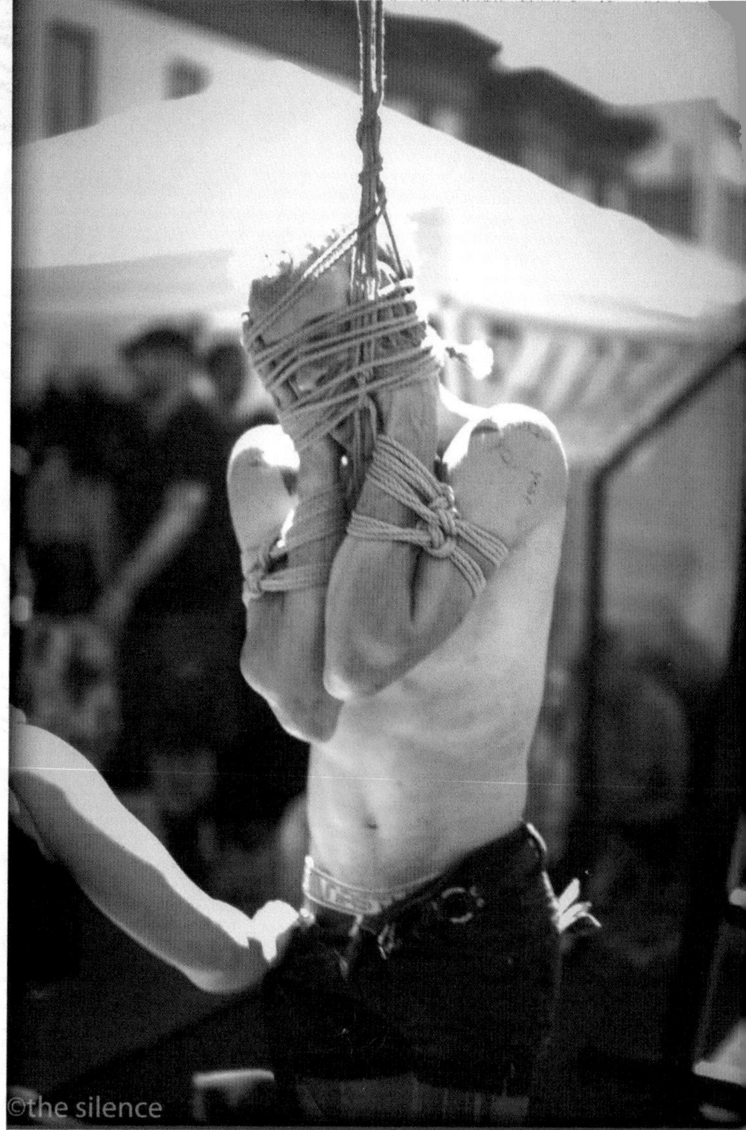

A Shallow Pool

Another layer is that the majority of the population is heterosexual. Estimates of the percentage of the gay, lesbian, and bisexual population range from about 1.2 percent (internationally) to 5.6 percent (in the U.S.),[4] and although it's safe to say a good number more just haven't reported being LGBTQ, the substantial majority is still clearly heterosexual. It's also clear just from being in the rope scene that the majority of rope tops and especially suspension riggers, at least the ones tying publicly, are heterosexual males. Since there's a smaller pool of both female and gay male rope tops to begin with, it can be tough for a man to find a rope partner regardless of sexual orientation.

Some female rope tops don't tie men, reducing the pool for heterosexual males even further. And if you're looking for an experience beyond just bottoming for someone in a class, workshop, or other nonsexual or nonsensual scene, it can be tougher yet.

"Although male rope tops are willing to tie other men, if your goal is to get sensual rope ties, then those are usually limited to female tops or very open-minded male tops," CuriouslySwitch says. Now of course some men can tie men just as sensuously as anyone else! But CuriouslySwitch's sentiment is shared by other (presumably heterosexual) males who responded to the survey.

"It was beyond ecstasy and peaceful all rolled into one. It is quite difficult to put it in words."
~ CuriouslySwitch

Fear of Flying

Then there's the challenge of overcoming personal feelings of embarassment or shame about being a male who loves bondage. While loving bondage doesn't necessarily mean someone is submissive, it does go against the cultural stereotypes regarding men mentioned earlier. One rope bottom describes it as "my own discomfort regarding the feeling that, as a male, I shouldn't allow myself to be put in a humiliating position.... It's the fear of provoking ridicule or, worse, distaste.."

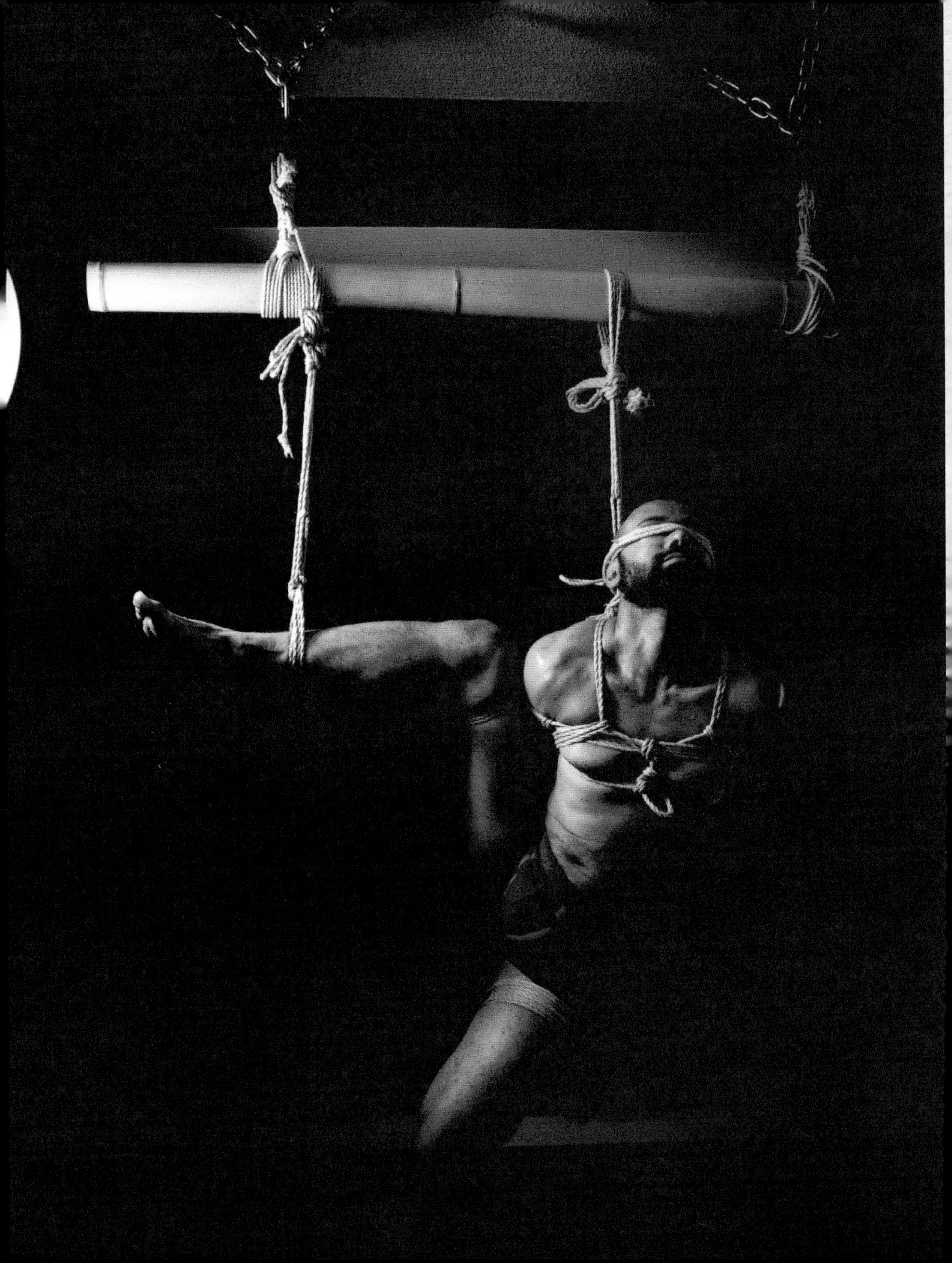

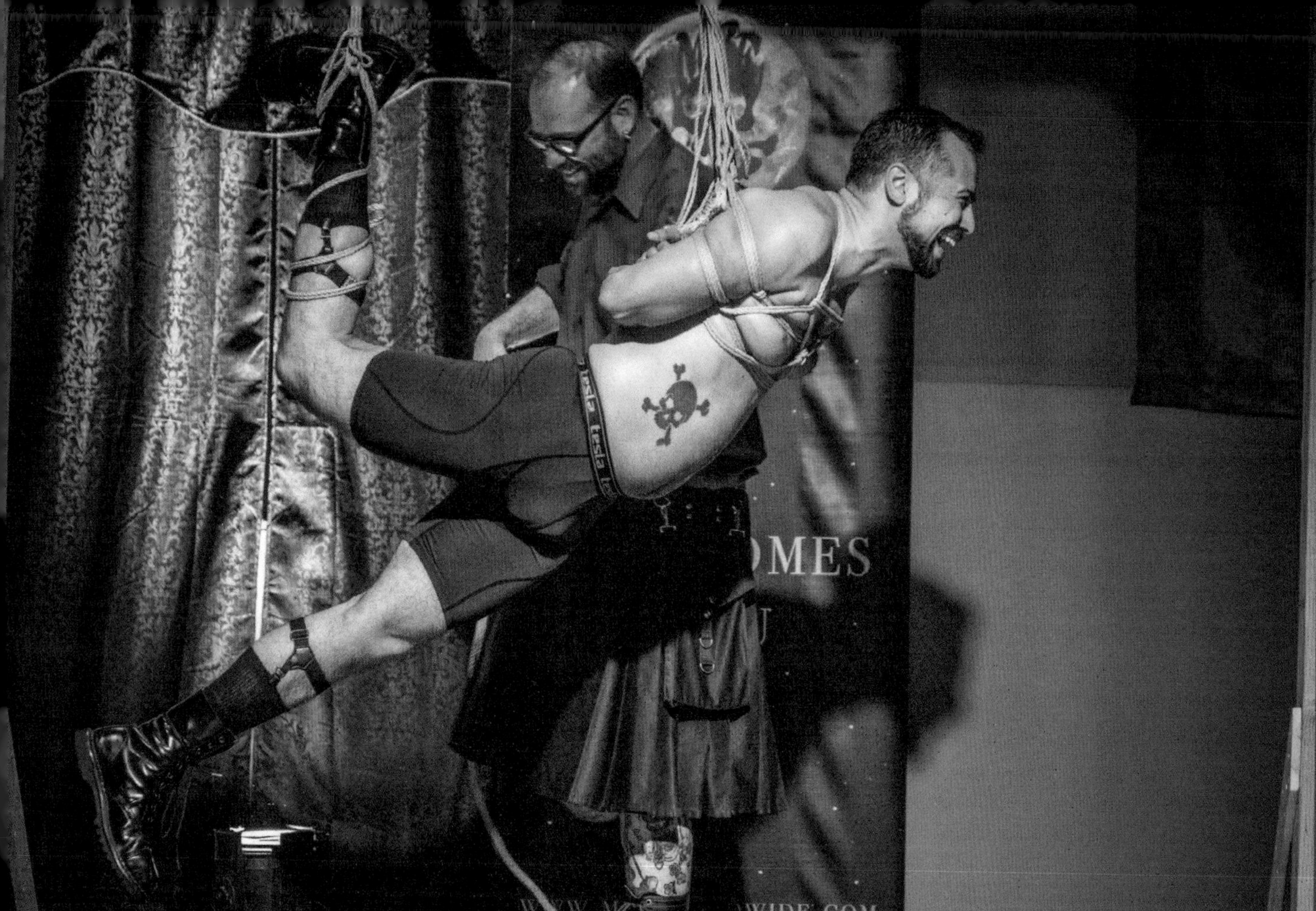

HeatHawk13 and MrKiltYou.
Bondage by MrKiltYou. Photo by iambic9

Even someone like Peter Acworth, who owns Kink.com—which has been producing videos for years for audiences including gay and heterosexual men who love bondage—says in his essay later on that he finds asking for bondage difficult, because "the role drilled into me was that I had to be in charge." Overcoming gender concepts imprinted on us in ways both overt and subtle since birth is no easy thing.

What's a man to do in the face of all of these challenges? Let's find out.

Helpful Ideas

As you can see from all the photos of men being tied in this book, it's not an impossible dream—it just might not be easy.

Get Your Group On

First, know that there are definitely female rope tops, and heteroflexible and heterosexual men who tie men. You might find female partners in the Hitchin' Bitches group on FetLife (https://fetlife.com/groups/47892), which at last count has more than 40 chapters worldwide. Founded by Hedwig, it's a group for rope tops that welcomes "all women who live full time as women and FTM, genderqueer and intersexed persons who feel that they still have links to women's communities."

CuriouslySwitch. Bondage and photo by NightWolfAJ

Being male, you can't join the group or go to most of the events. However, a proactive male rope bottom might check out the members of their local Hitchin' Bitches group and write a respectful note to someone they find appealing, asking if said appealing person might be looking for a prospective partner or even just someone to practice on. The Hitchin' Bitches group is specifically "not a cruising spot," so I'm gonna emphasize *respectful.*

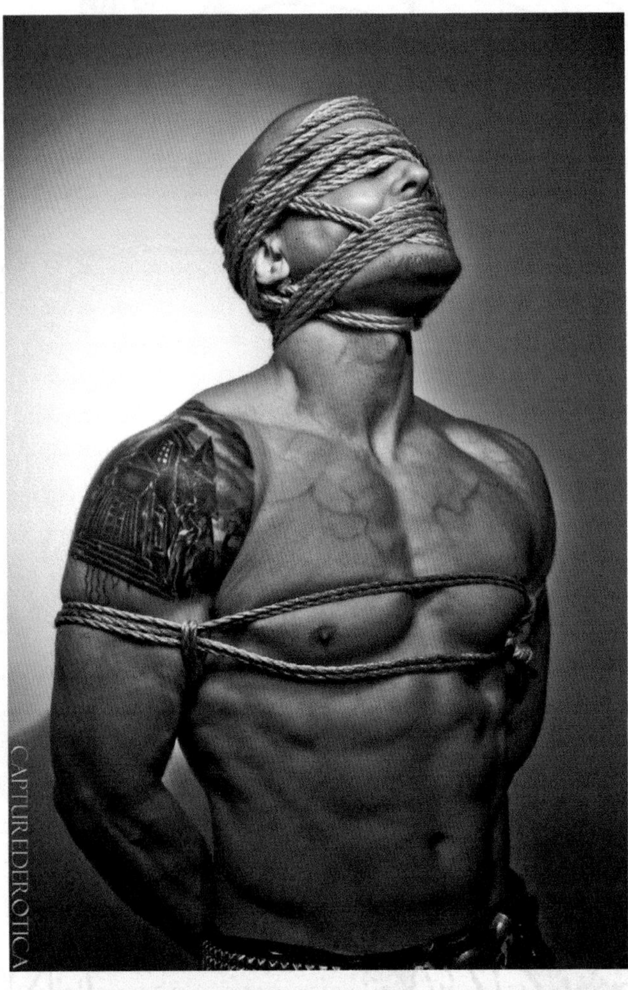

Anonymous. Bondage by Nikita. Photo by Captured Erotica; CapturedErotica.com

There are also two other relevant FetLife groups: One is Tying up Men (https://fetlife.com/groups/1144), which is for "women who like to dominate men through rope (or would like to) and for men who like to be dominated by being tied up"; the other is Men in Rope (https://fetlife.com/groups/117214), which has a sticky thread for male bottoms looking for riggers. Plus, you can perv the photos to see the names of the people tying all those men in rope. Maybe one of them lives near you.

Next, while we're on the subject of being proactive, why not consider helping someone learn to tie? Maybe all they need is a little encouragement and a willing partner. There are so many rope classes, books, and videos these days that you two could be getting your rope on together in no time.

Confidence Quest

Doing all the above things requires a bit of confidence, a word that came up in more than one survey response. "To this day I still need a lot of confidence with a person to offer to be tied by them," Gnethys says. Achilles recommends, "Take care of yourself! Get in shape, groom yourself, dress well. It does wonders for your confidence, and confidence looks damn good in rope."

Having confidence will help you toss aside those cultural norms that don't serve you, will help you reach out to potential partners, and will help you enjoy your scenes more when they do happen.

"Put whatever you may think of as cultural 'norms' aside," recommends one rope bottom. "This has nothing to do with your value, intellect, masculinity." Hear, hear!

Along with developing confidence goes being persistent—just the same as for rope bottoms in other categories. "Not everyone will want to play with you, but that happens to anyone," Gnethys says. "Don't let that discourage you; more people than you might think would love to tie you." Hastingsbound cites "bloody-mindedness" and determination as helping him, and recommends, "Don't give up trying to find someone."

Learning to tie can also put you on the radar of rope tops while helping you get to know your own body in rope and giving you a bit of a rope fix.

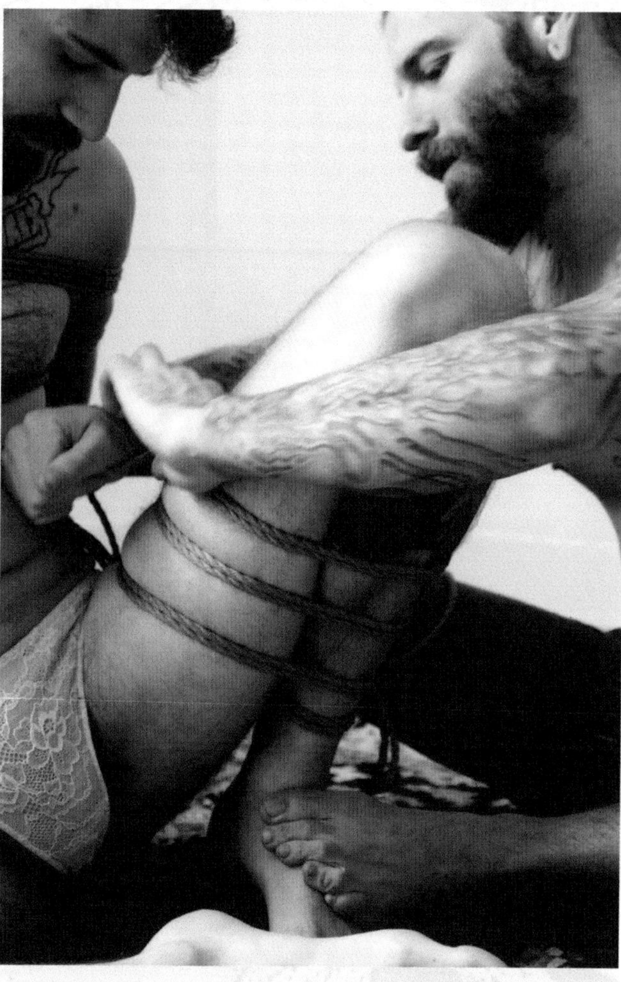

Bradley Cuttlefish and FredRx. Bondage by FredRx. Photo by Cam Damage

As for flexibility, remember that many ties don't require it (see Chapter 12 on ties for limited range of motion). But if you do want to improve flexibility, you probably already know that yoga or just general stretching can help. You may be outnumbered by females at your local yoga studio,[5] but so what? If you cared about being part of the herd, you wouldn't be doing bondage in the first place.

Toot Suite

Another bit of physical advice comes, not surprisingly, anonymously: "Try not to fart too much." Typical male stuff? Typical female stuff too, it turns out: A Salon.com article reports that according to gastroenterologist Michael D. Levitt, the "world's leading authority on flatulence," men expel an average of 38 ounces of gas per day, and women expel an average of 27 ounces per day.[6] And women's flatulence was actually found to have more sulphur gas and thus a more potent odor.[7]

Regardless of your gender, if flatulence is an issue for you (and you've ruled out dietary issues such as lactose intolerance), you can try Devrom, an over-the-counter medicine that neutralizes the odor; Beano, a dietary supplement that can help prevent gas in the first place; or UnderEase, airtight underwear that has a filter with a center layer of activated carbon. I haven't tried any of these personally, so read reviews and judge for yourself.

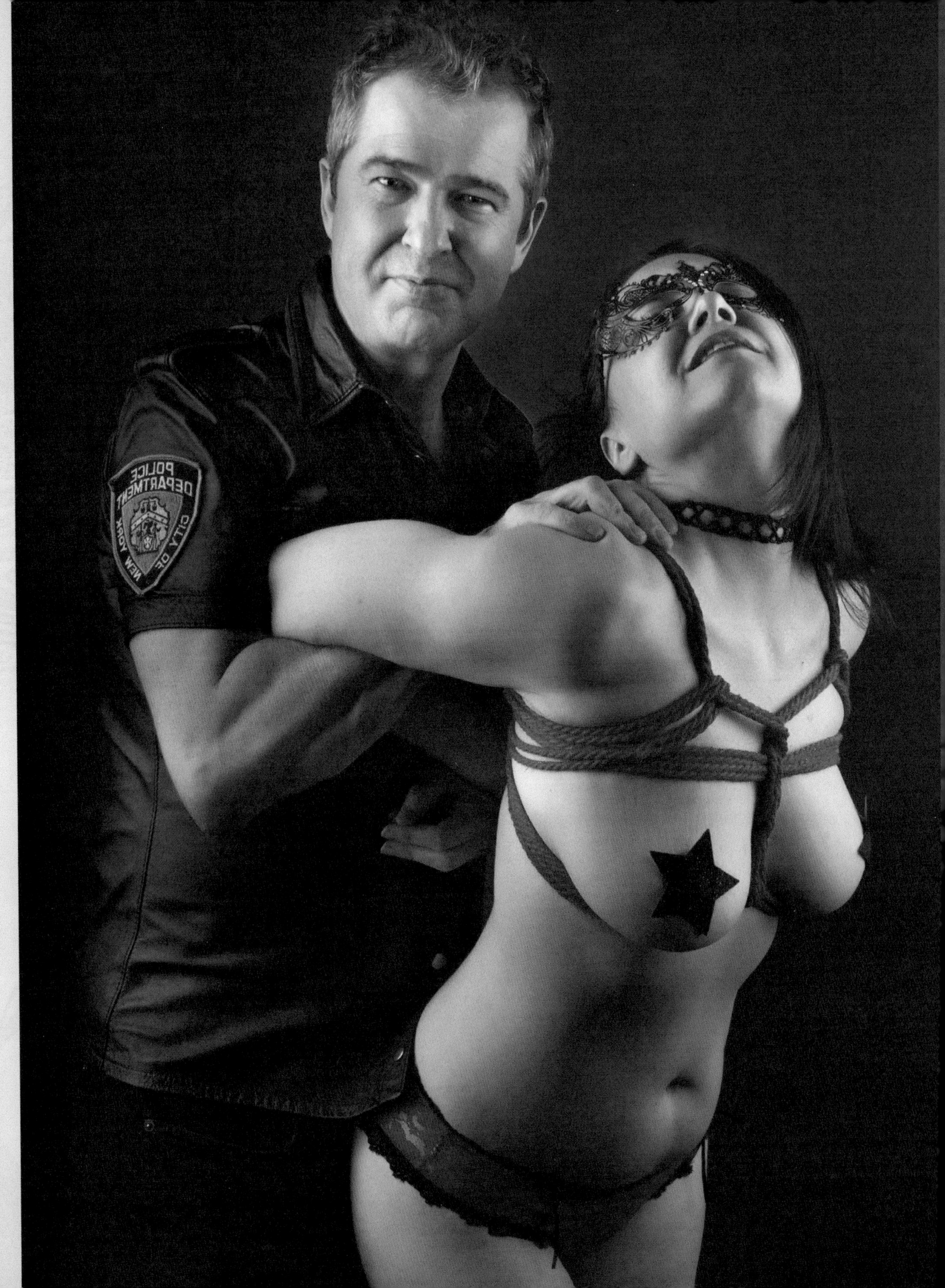
POLICE
DEPARTMENT
CITY OF
NEW YORK

Peter Acworth

Peter Acworth is the founder and owner of Kink.com.

I've been interested in bondage for as long as I can remember. I remember walking home from school, age 8 or 9, and seeing handcuffs in the window of an army store and being incredibly turned on by them. Initially the fantasies were purely about being tied up. Later on, around age 18, I would frequent seedy London sex shops and buy porn; those magazines were my first exposure to BDSM porn. They depicted women being tied up tightly, which I found very appealing, but to an extent I was also imagining myself being tied up.

During my first relationships I would bring bondage up and we would just sort of incompetently tie each other up, taking turns. I didn't know how to do it, and my partners didn't know how to do it either; we would just use rope and scarves, and later handcuffs.

I like the vulnerability and the loss of control in bondage. I like to be tied with my hands behind my back, very tight, and then fucked...it's a sexual thing for me. But I didn't really look for someone to tie me up because I was programmed for dating in a much more vanilla world. The role drilled into me was that I had to be in charge. It's potentially something quite difficult to ask for, certainly for me and maybe for most men, because we're led to believe that we should be in a leadership-type role.

I would describe myself as a switch, but I don't know if people see the rope that I do and just assume that I'm strictly a top. I think the challenge has also been finding a dominant woman who knows how to do it. I've fantasized about it a lot but it hasn't actually happened all that much.

We have a quite popular product line for submissive men on Kink.com, including Bound Gods. A lot of strong men are featured on those sites who want to get tied up and are perfectly OK with it, and I think that's a good thing. But I still find the idea of getting tied up myself somewhat challenging.

Peter Acworth and Evie Vane. Photo by Shoot That Klown; www.shootthatklown.com

"We cannot be that rare, can we?"
~ Achilles

So once you've got your confidence on, your support group in place, and your flatulence under control, is there anything else you might try? Achilles offers this beautiful insight:

"It's all a matter of doing everything you can to increase the chances of being in the right place at the right time, and being patient," he says. "What really helped me was when I came to the realization that there are people out there who want you, want to see you, feel you. Seeing the connection others have and understanding that you are just as capable of being wanted, needed, desired. Just because people or relationship dynamics that you identify with are hard to find, or less common, does not make them any less valid."

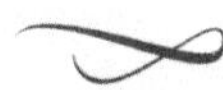

Notes

1. "What Exactly Is an Unusual Sexual Fantasy?" by Christian C. Joyal, PhD; Amélie Cossette, BSc; and Vanessa Lapierre, BSc; *The Journal of Sexual Medicine*, October 2014
2. http://www.psychologyofmen.org/male-gender-role/
3. http://www.livestrong.com/article/335439-range-of-motion-in-men-vs-women/
4. http://williamsinstitute.law.ucla.edu/wp-content/uploads/Gates-How-Many-People-LGBT-Apr-2011.pdf
5. http://www.yogajournal.com/article/men-balance/where-are-all-the-men/
6. http://www.salon.com/2000/02/24/farts/
7. http://www.ctvnews.ca/flatulence-expert-defines-normal-output-rate-1.269197

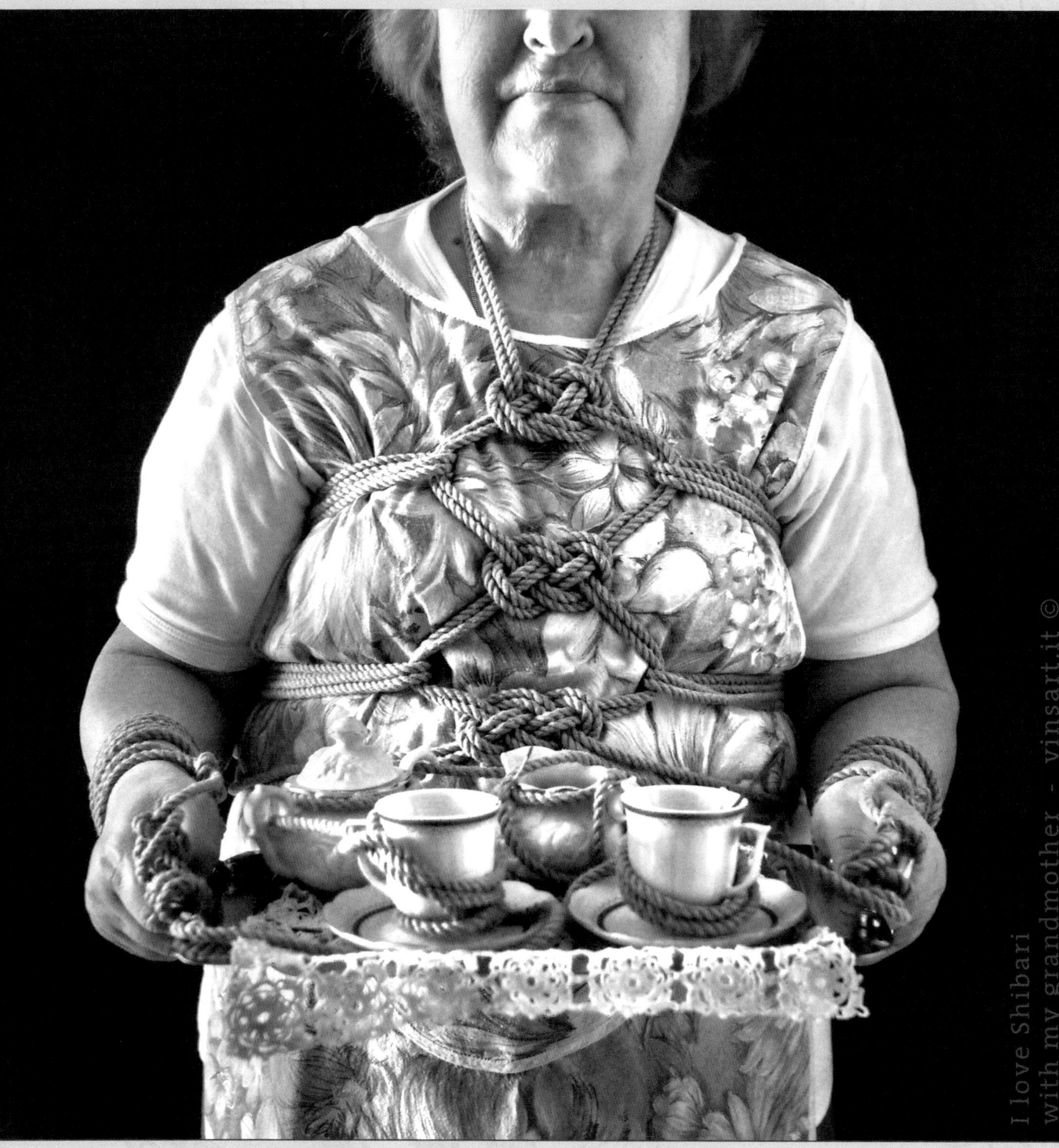

I love Shibari
with my grandmother - vinsart.it ©

Chapter 8

For Older Rope Bottoms

The American Academy of Orthopaedic Surgeons (AAOS) doesn't paint such a pretty picture about the effects of aging on the body. According to its website, muscles begin to shrink and lose mass as they age; the number and size of muscle fibers decrease; the water content of tendons (cord-like tissues that attach muscles to bones) decreases, making the tissues stiffer and less able to tolerate stress; and the heart muscle becomes less able to propel large quantities of blood quickly to the body, so we tire more quickly and take longer to recover. Our joint motion also becomes more restricted, and flexibility decreases with age because of changes in the tendons and ligaments.[1]

Sounds pretty bleak for older rope bottoms, huh? Let's put things in perspective.

At the **age of 86**, Katherine Pelton swam the 200-meter butterfly in 3 minutes, 1.14 seconds. The current women's world record for that distance is only about a minute less and was set by a *20-year-old*.[2]

At **age 99**, Teiichi Igarashi climbed to the top of Mt. Fuji, with a cane in one hand no less.[3] Oh yeah, and he did it again the following year, at **age 100**.[4]

Harriette Thompson, a two-time cancer survivor, finished her 16th marathon at **age 92**.[5]

I could go on. Visit www.50plusachievers.club for loads more inspiring accomplishments by folks over 50. But back to science. In *Aging Backwards*, Miranda Esmonde-White presents a chart of muscle mass remaining per decade. According to that chart, the muscle mass of a semisedentary person at age 50 is down to 80.5 percent, while that of a physically active person is still at *94 percent*.[6]

"At Shibaricon I had that 'one moment in time' where you absolutely know that being 26 or 56 just doesn't matter."

~ patrice, age 60

The AAOS says that "many of the changes in our musculoskeletal system result more from disuse than from simple aging.... Stretching is an excellent way to help maintain joint flexibility. Weight training can increase muscle mass and strength."[7] All those runners and swimmers and climbers and, yes, rope bottoms still using their bodies in amazing ways well into very advanced ages are living proof of staving off major musculoskeletal decline through physical activity. "Use it or lose it" is a mantra for a reason.

If you're interested in learning the latest info on aging from scientists (as opposed to, say, Suzanne Somers)—exactly what it does to our cells, what role genetics play, whether things like human growth hormone decrease the rate of decline, and so on—I highly recommend the surprisingly entertaining book *Spring Chicken*, by Bill Gifford. Sneak peek: One study cited in the book showed that exercise actually repaired the mitochondrial DNA in mice—"in short, it had reversed their aging."[8]

What does all of this have to do with rope bottoming? If you get tied up nonstrenuously and/or are blissfully unconcerned with what aging unexercised muscles

Grandmother. Bondage, concept, and photo by Vinsart; www.vinsart.it

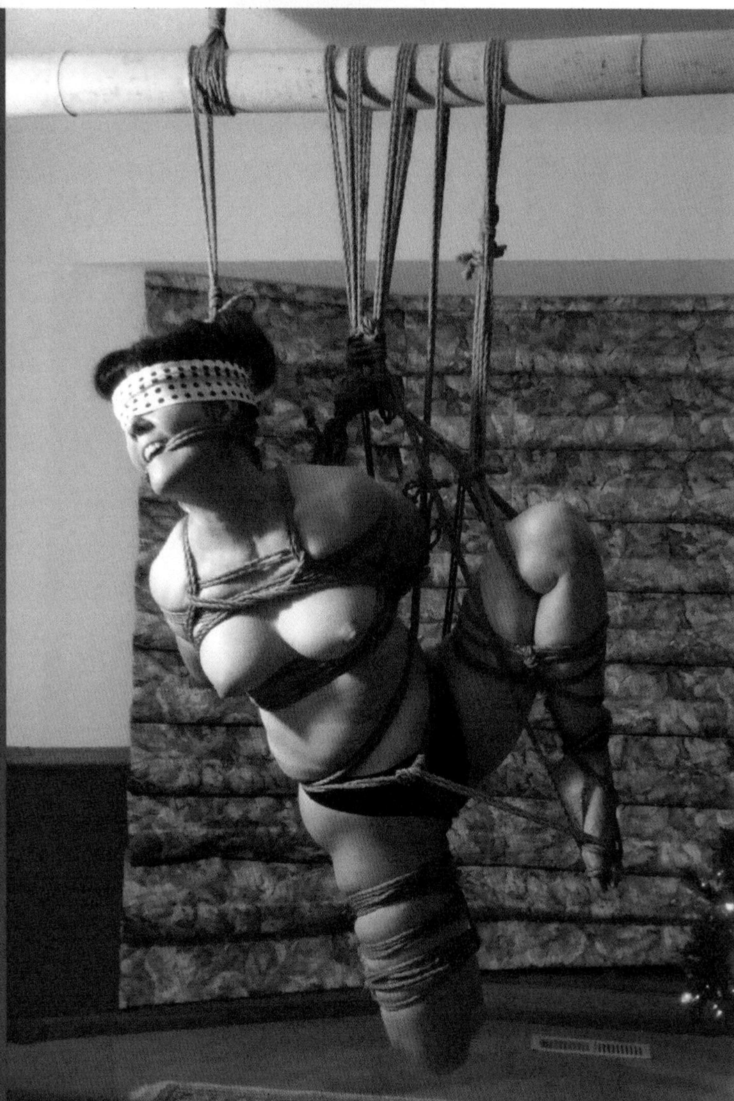

katabound, age 51. Bondage and photo by Katabind

should check with your doctor about any kind of potentially risky activity at any age, but even more so as you get older. You're old enough to know that already.

If, however, you want your body to work well and feel good into the advanced years, and/or you want to writhe and contort and have your body put into stressful positions—possibly including suspensions—then muscle mass, joint mobility, flexibility, tolerating stress, and so on are pretty important.

What Is "Older" Anyway?

If you ask any random adult what "old" is, they might say 70s or 80s, maybe 60s. But when I put out the call for older rope bottoms, without specifying an age range, more than one *40-something* rope bottom wrote in to say, "Well, I guess I qualify as old." As if rope bottoms are in the same category as pro athletes or supermodels, where the average career time span seems to end around the time crow's feet show up.

Bunk! Barring any prohibitive medical issues (or working around them), you can likely enjoy some form of rope even if you need a fire extinguisher to blow out your birthday candles. For example, Sarge started rope bottoming at age 65. And she says that after her second suspension, "I was flying afterward. I remember lying in bed that evening, believing I could accomplish anything."

The minimum age to be considered "older" for our purposes ended up being 40. Certainly not old, right? But many folks in the over-40 crowd are struggling with age-related issues, and we're all about inclusivity here.

"I think the older rope bottom, especially one with experience, can be a good rope partner because they know themselves better and are less likely to let a rigger injure them."
~ katabound, age 51

look and feel like, or you get tied up nonstrenuously and are not so blissfully unconcerned but wear a zentai suit and take a lot of pain relievers or something, maybe nothing. *Maybe* nothing, that is, because you

Evie Vane, age 47. Bondage and photo by Marcuslikesit; www.marcuslikesit.com

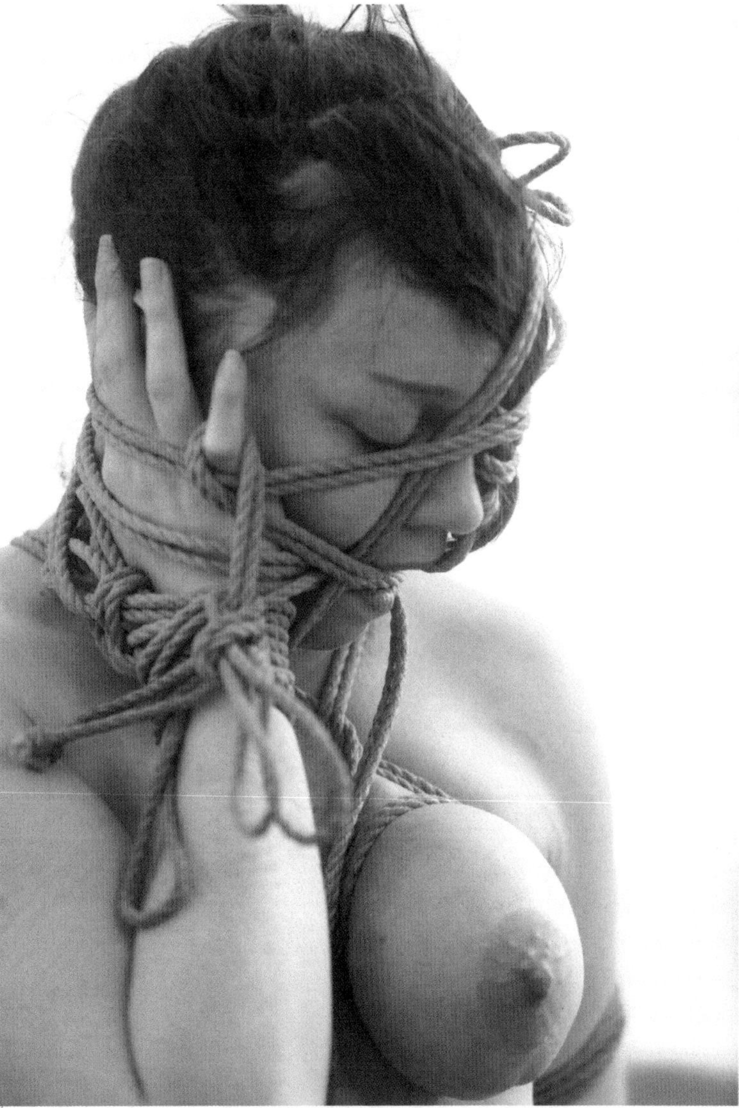

Challenges

It's no surprise, given the AAOS info above, that pretty much every 40-plus rope bottom who answered the survey mentioned physical issues.

Flex Time

The biggest challenge seems to be less flexibility, or having to work harder to develop or maintain it. It's worth pointing out here that some bottoms started working on flexibility after discovering rope, and are thus more flexible because of it! Still, flexibility clearly does not come as easily to the majority in the more advanced years.

"Loss of strength and flexibility [is a challenge]," says a 59-year-old rope bottom, adding, "Can't do the splits anymore." Lady_Hunny_Bunny (age 53), says, "Flexibility is the main issue. As we get older our body does stiffen up, and if you work a job where you sit all day, it is not hard to become extremely unfit." Lane (age 41) also cites "flexibility and working around previous injuries" as the biggest challenge. Lane added "non-rope-related" in parentheses after "injuries," but the longer you do rope bottoming, the more you may be at risk for rope-related injuries as well. Small amounts of damage that happen unnoticeably over time can add up to something very noticeable down the road. The more you get tied up, the more likely you are to eventually get some kind of damage even if you're well prepared and very careful. Unforeseen things happen.

Youth Orientation

Another challenge is the same as for many other types of rope bottoms highlighted in this book: "the ever-present 'thing' that riggers would prefer to tie the sexy, young 90-pounder...which I totally get but which really makes you feel like old news," as patrice (age 60) puts it. Not all riggers, of course, but it is indeed a "thing" for many rope tops. At first I thought it might be that the majority of rope tops are younger and that "like attracts like," but since there are lots of older folks, including *much* older folks, tying *quite* younger people, that theory went out the window faster than you can say, "Hogtie with a side of spanking, please."

So older rope bottoms may have to work harder to find partners, especially for suspensions and pickup play. And if you go to a club or party without a partner, you can end up feeling like the kid at recess whom no one wants on their dodgeball team.

Feeling inferior can, of course, be reinforced by social media. There's the emotional toll, as katabound puts it, "of seeing photos on FetLife of *much* younger models who are thinner, still uberflexible, and at the peak of their sexual attractiveness. On one level I'm quite thankful for what I can still do and am happy with my appearance—all my injuries, scars, and wrinkles are from a life well lived—but it's still difficult to keep my chin up when riggers continue sending out requests for young, flexible women only."

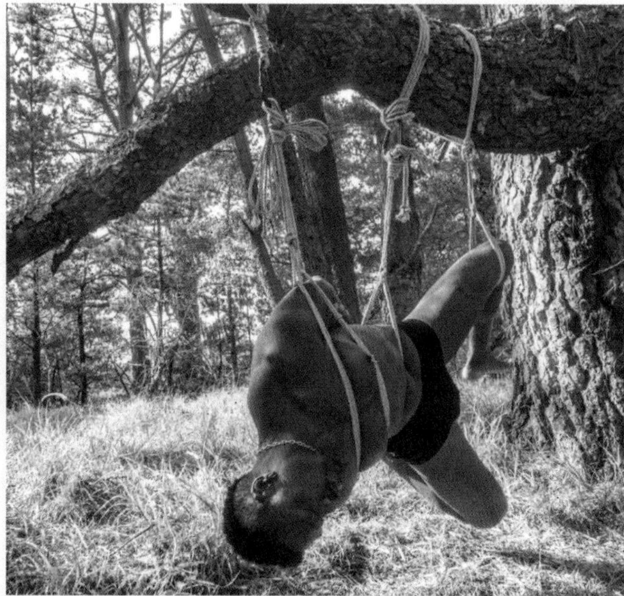

Jack HammerXL, age 50; jackhammer.xxx and interracialbondage.xxx. Bondage and photo by True Blue; miss_true_blue on Instagram

"Even though my body doesn't bend and flex the way it used to, I still don't feel that old; my mind is still very young and still wants to give everything a go—at least once LOL."

~ Lane, age 41

Time Goes By

Sometimes it's not finding a partner but finding the *time* for rope that's hard. "Real life and the reality of being a grown-up is one of the biggest challenges I have," patrice says. "Being able to get away to events and/or even practices." Fewer younger people have to deal with the same kinds of time constraints that older ones do, whether they stem from a demanding job (which by now may be a high-level one), a spouse/life partner who may or may not be kinky, children who depend on us (even harder if you're a single parent), our own parents who need taking care of, charitable activities...the responsbilities and involvements that can increase as we age can leave us with only a square or two on the calendar every month for rope time.

And when we do get tied up (whoo-hoo!), our bodies might take more time to heal. "Physically, I don't bounce back from injuries like I did in my 30s, or even my 40s, so I have to be much more mindful of the stresses on my body," says katabound. Sarge adds, "My body gets tired/achy more easily than in the past." Longer recovery time applies to rope burn and abrasion marks too. An abrasion on my skin that might once have taken a couple of weeks to disappear might now take months. Decades of sitting at a desk job in front of the computer takes a heavy toll on the body as well.

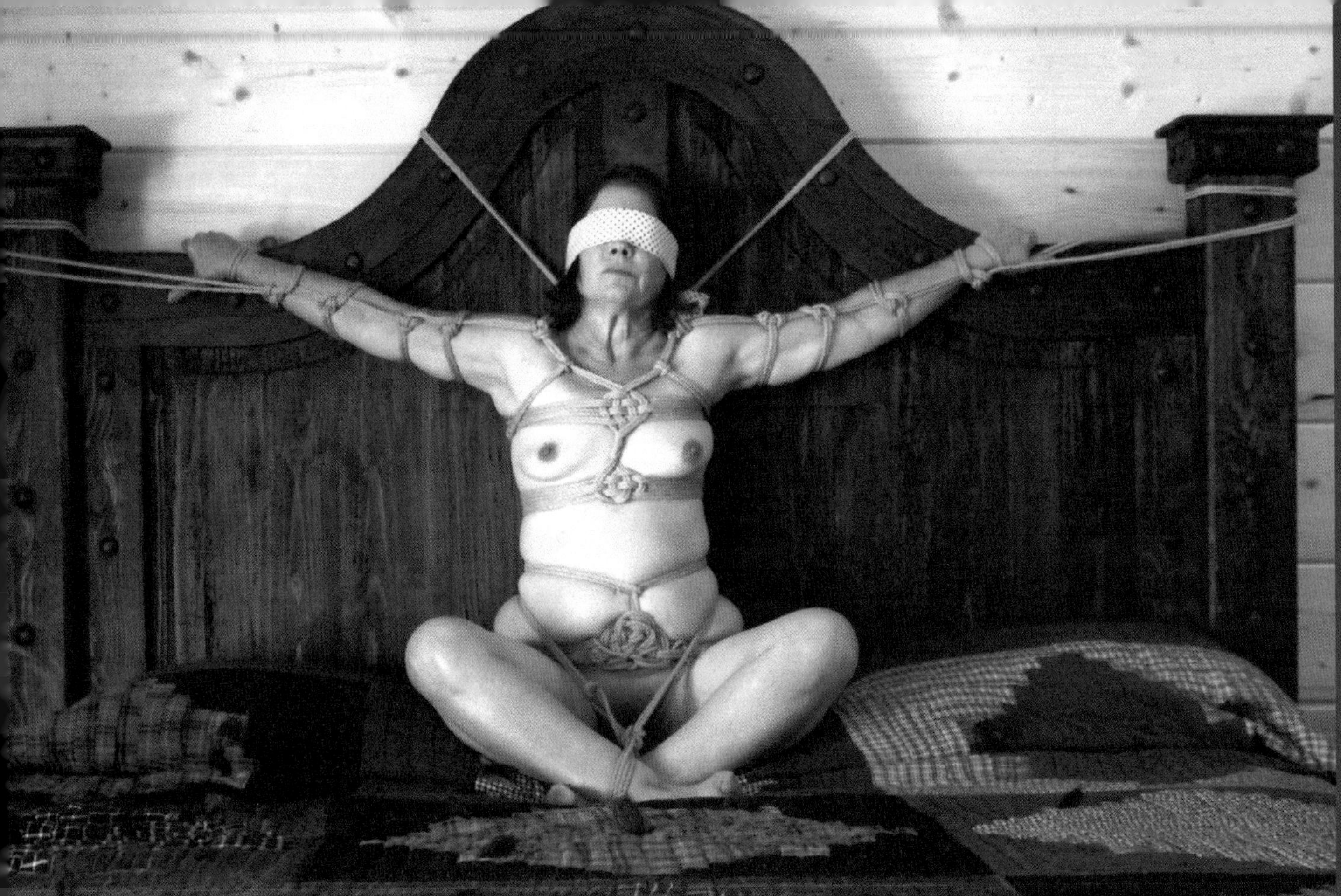

KnottySue, age 62. Bondage and photo by KnottyJames

Helpful Ideas

You don't get to this age without figuring out ways around, over, or through challenges, right? So let's look at some workarounds.

Body of Work

As you may have guessed from the first challenge mentioned above, doing yoga is highly recommended, as it helps the body stay flexible. It also helps cultivate mindfulness and self-awareness, and can improve balance, which otherwise can decline in the advanced years. Just make sure you have a good yoga teacher and learn the proper alignment and ways to use your muscles to support you in a stretch, because if you don't, it could actually cause issues that weren't there or make ones that you do have even worse. And keep in mind that many ties don't require flexibility at all (hello, head bondage!).

Overall, "stay in shape," patrice recommends. "Don't let it get you down [if there are times] when you don't have a regular partner. Keep moving!" The recommendation to maintain fitness is supported by a ton of major research. I would add here that you don't need to run on the treadmill until your legs burn or start lifting free weights like you're training for a bodybuilding competition. "Let's throw out the word *exercise* altogether and talk instead about how you are going to move your body joyously," writes Christiane Northrup, M.D., in *Goddesses Never Age*. She recommends things like dancing, swimming, and walking—but in ways that feel fun, that recall when we were children and did things just because they felt

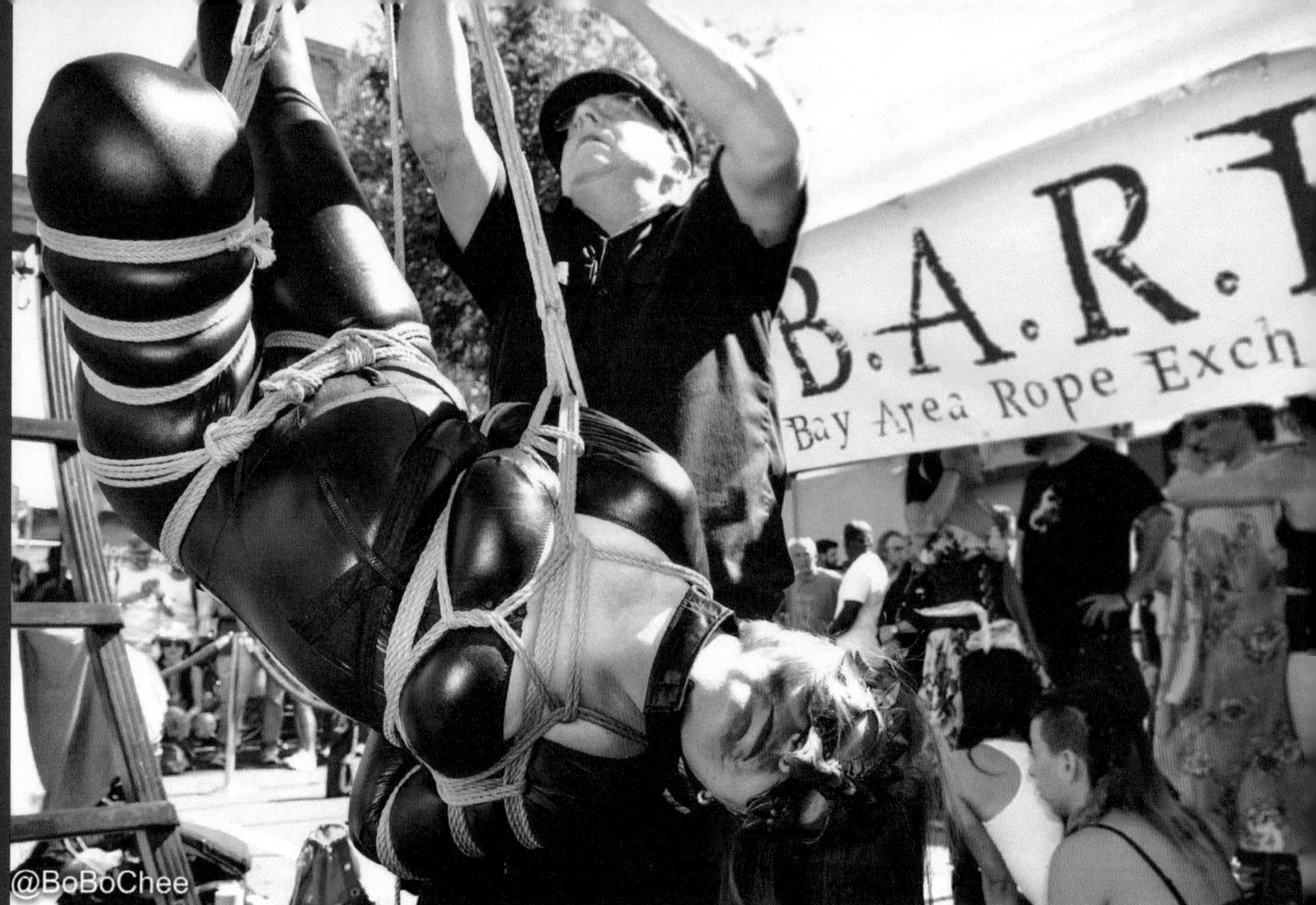

RopeGyver, age 65. Bondage by nawaji. Photo by BoBoChee

good. She says that if we don't enjoy the exercise, we'll eventually run out of willpower to do it.

Stretching before a scene is also especially important for older rope bottoms. Take your time with this—be gentle with your body. Warm it up first if possible, like with a nice brisk walk or a warm shower. After particularly intense scenes, I also like to take a warm bath with epsom salt, and to rub arnica gel anywhere the muscles are really sore. As for marks like abrasions and cuts, research has actually debunked and even advised against using vitamin E oil to treat cuts and many skin conditions, as it doesn't work[9] and can even cause contact dermatitis.[10] Check out some do's and don'ts for treating cuts and scrapes to reduce scarring, including things like covering the cut and massaging it gently with lotion, on Fitnessmagazine.com.[11]

Some rope bottoms take ibuprofen before an intense scene as well as after, to reduce both inflammation and pain. Taking *any* medication, even an over-the-counter one, however, is a personal choice and should not be taken lightly. Ibuprofen and other NSAIDs (nonsteroidal anti-inflammatories) can increase the risk of heart attack and stroke,[12] and common side effects include gastrointestinal issues[13]—among *many* others. I personally take curcumin with black pepper extract instead of ibuprofen; curcumin is the most active constituent of the spice turmeric and a natural anti-inflammatory.[14] But you should always do your own research and never take something just because it works for someone else.

Everyone should be aware of their medical issues and communicate them to their rope partner, and remember that aging can bring new issues, like high blood pressure or heart problems. If you're in denial about getting older—maybe you're still thinking your physical capabilities haven't changed much since your 20s and 30s, when you were a gym rat; maybe you've been putting off checkups and so on—it can cause trouble. It's always recommended to check with a medical professional before you do anything strenuous, and rope bondage is no exception.

"Physically, what helps the most is simply accepting my limitations," says RopeGyver (age 65). "By accepting where I am physically *today*, I am realistic about what my body is capable of. This helps me to keep within reasonable physical limits so that I have less chance of injury." She adds, "Pay attention to your body during your bottoming session and speak up about modifying ties when necessary." Good advice for rope bottoms of any age.

The Buddy System

On the mental side, having supporters—both in person and virtually—can be enormously beneficial. "I have an amazing dominate in my life," patrice says. "He never doubts my abilities to do whatever I want to do. He is always pushing me to be better. And I have some amazing contacts and friends who keep my head in the game even when I get totally discouraged."

If you don't have a regular partner for support, cultivating friendships in the rope bottoming community can be especially helpful. Maybe you even want to start a meetup for older rope bottoms in your area! And as much as we appreciate our bodies for all they've done for us throughout our lives, I recommend not spending too much time scrolling through tons of bondage photos on FetLife and Facebook. What we see all around us affects our self-perception, and older rope bottoms aren't well represented there despite being a sizable portion of the community.

"In all the years James and I have been together (since 1969), we have never experienced such a richness and closeness in our relationship as we have had with rope bondage."

~ KnottySue, age 62

Rope: The Fountain of Youth?

Research has proven that there are ways to stave off physical and cognitive decline even as the numbers on those birthday cards keep going up. And I believe that getting tied up is one of them!

"The brain craves novelty," says Vivian Diller, PhD, author of *Face It*. "To feel younger, you have to stimulate it with new associations and new things."[15] Sure, you could travel to Morocco or learn how to play the oboe. But you could also just keep doing rope. That new asymmetrical pose you've been processing, discovering the energy of the partner you just met for pickup play, learning something new about yourself in a tie you've done a dozen times...all of these are novel things that stimulate the brain.

"The healing power of touch also needs to be acknowledged as an antiaging medication," writes author Mireille Guiliano in *French Women Don't Get*

Morgana Muses

Morgana Muses is a feminist porn producer at Permission 4 Pleasure. To learn more, visit permission4pleasure.com.

Once upon a time, a girl was born in Sydney, Australia, to Slovenian parents. Her future was mapped out for her purely based on her gender. Her upbringing focused mainly on how a "good woman" should behave and appear in private and in public. She was taught that Prince Charming would come along; they'd marry, have children, and live happily ever after. Sex, sexuality, and all related pleasures were never discussed.

When the girl became a woman, she felt ashamed and at times angry because she didn't feel the expected and fervent desire to marry or have children. She was also enjoying the challenges and rewards of climbing the corporate ladder. More disturbing and conflicting for the woman was that she derived pleasure from pain, whether giving or receiving. The woman finally relented to the pressure from her parents (mainly her mother) and married at age 27.

The Prince Charming turned out to be a frog—a Catholic repressed frog with a 1950s attitude towards women and sex. When the woman suggested introducing kinky elements into their sex life, she was shut down immediately and told that she must be some sort of deviant. She never raised the subject again. Over the years she gave her parents two beautiful granddaughters. She became increasingly unhappy, emotionally and physically unfulfilled, which led to major depression.

At age 45 the woman asked the frog for a divorce, and at age 47 found the courage to begin her journey in exploring her sexuality and the pleasures that her body had yet to enjoy in her loveless and predominantly sexless marriage. She attended a weekend of workshops facilitated by a talented, amazing rigger and BDSM educator named Witcher.* Ropes, combat play, pressure points and knife play were all on the agenda. It was during this weekend that her love affair with rope and all things painful and pointy officially began.

Witcher enraptured the woman as he tied a model during a demonstration: the way he interacted with his model, the look of utter bliss on the model's face. The woman desperately wanted to be in the model's place, and when she was offered the opportunity to be

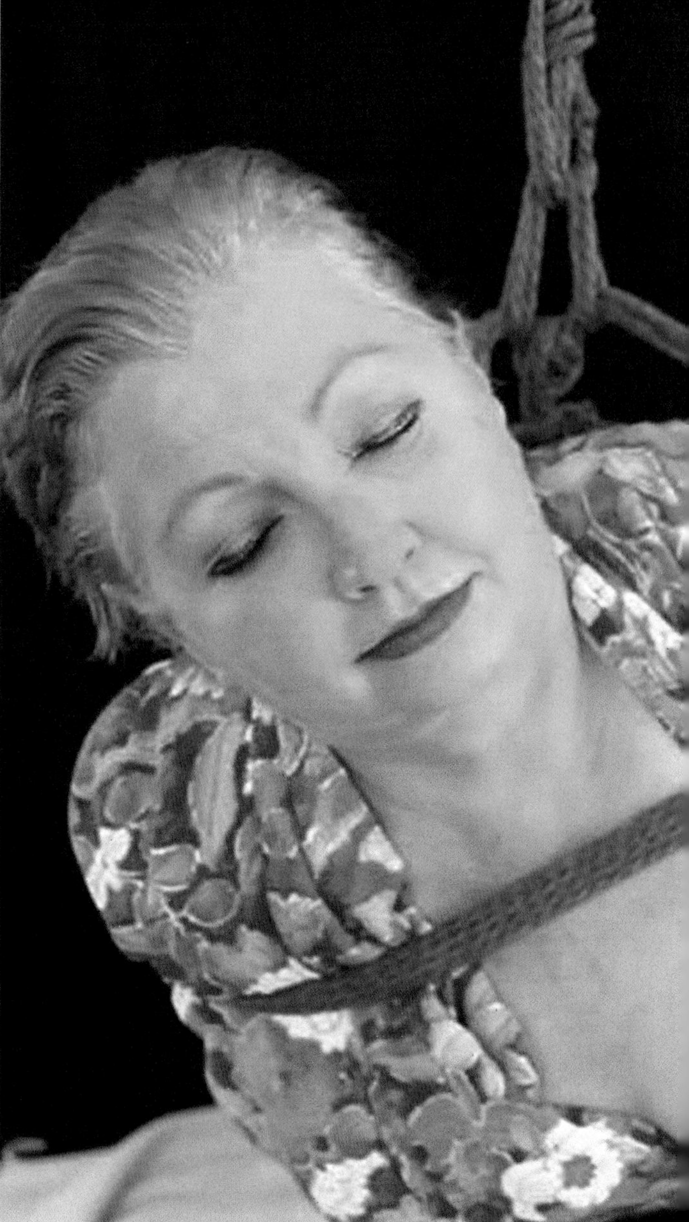

hogtied, any hesitations she felt just melted away by Witcher and his way with rope, leaving just an intoxicating adrenaline rush.

During this weekend, the woman also had her first experience being partially suspended, by a well-known Sydney dominatrix and rigger. Totally blissed out, the woman felt like she had just had some form of spiritual awakening. The rigger held her and whispered, "I think you're ripe for bondage!" And she was right!

That woman is me, Morgana Muses—feminist porn producer and explorer of all things BDSM- and kink-related. I no longer believe in fairy tales, but choose to make my own tales, openly and without shame, guilt, or fear of reprisal.

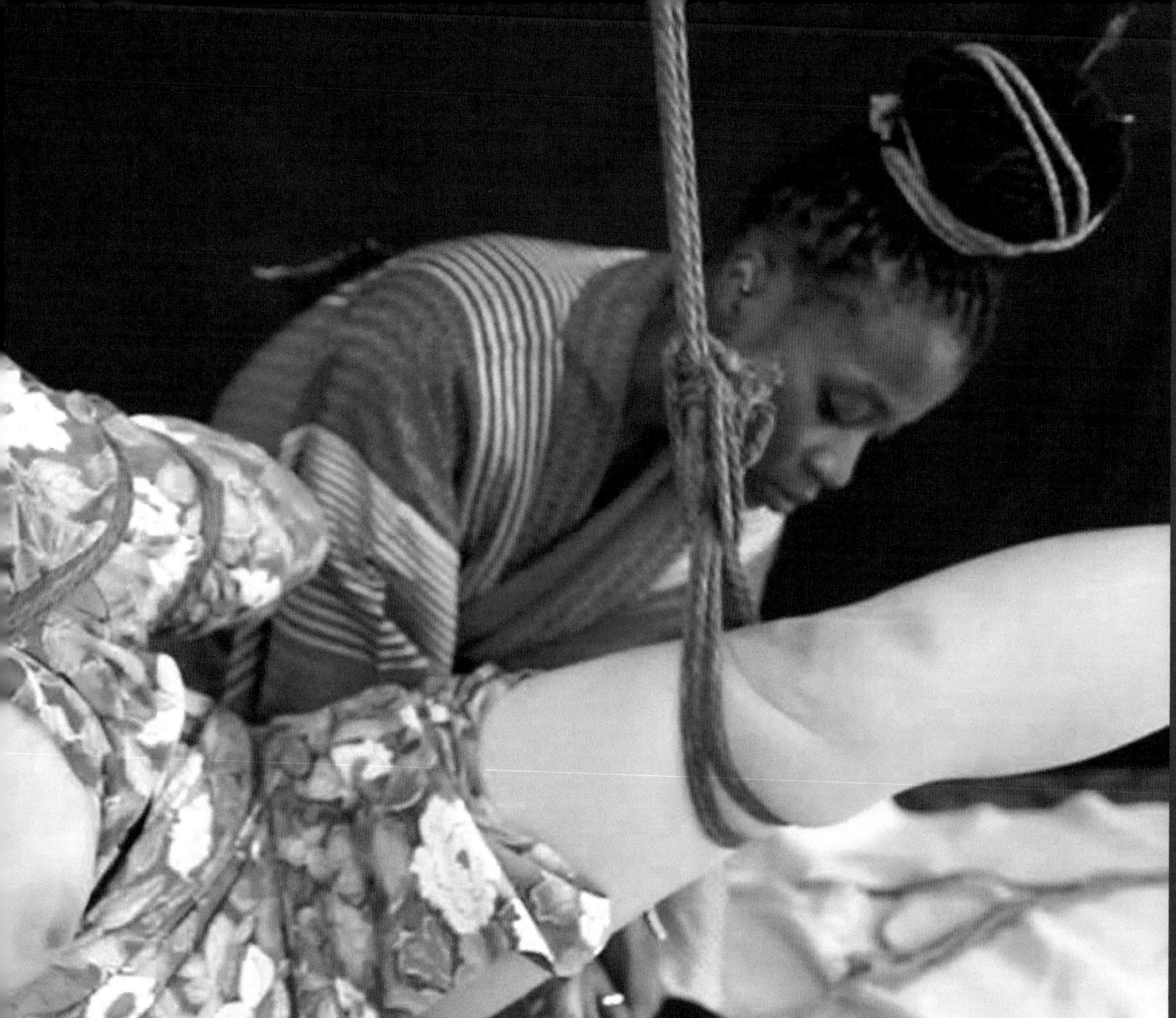

Being a "late bloomer" in my personal journey of discovery and producing porn, I found myself facing many classic stereotypes and taboos about sexuality, particularly for people aged 50-plus. I also discovered that many of these stereotypes spilled over into the rope world.

The mission in my life now is to bust as many age-related myths and show that there is no expiration date on our sexual pleasure and journey...and if that journey includes rope, I can assure you that you *can* teach an old dog new tricks. *Woof!*

*Name used with permission

Morgana Muses, age 51, and Caritia. Bondage by Caritia; www.caritia.com. Photo by Permission 4 Pleasure

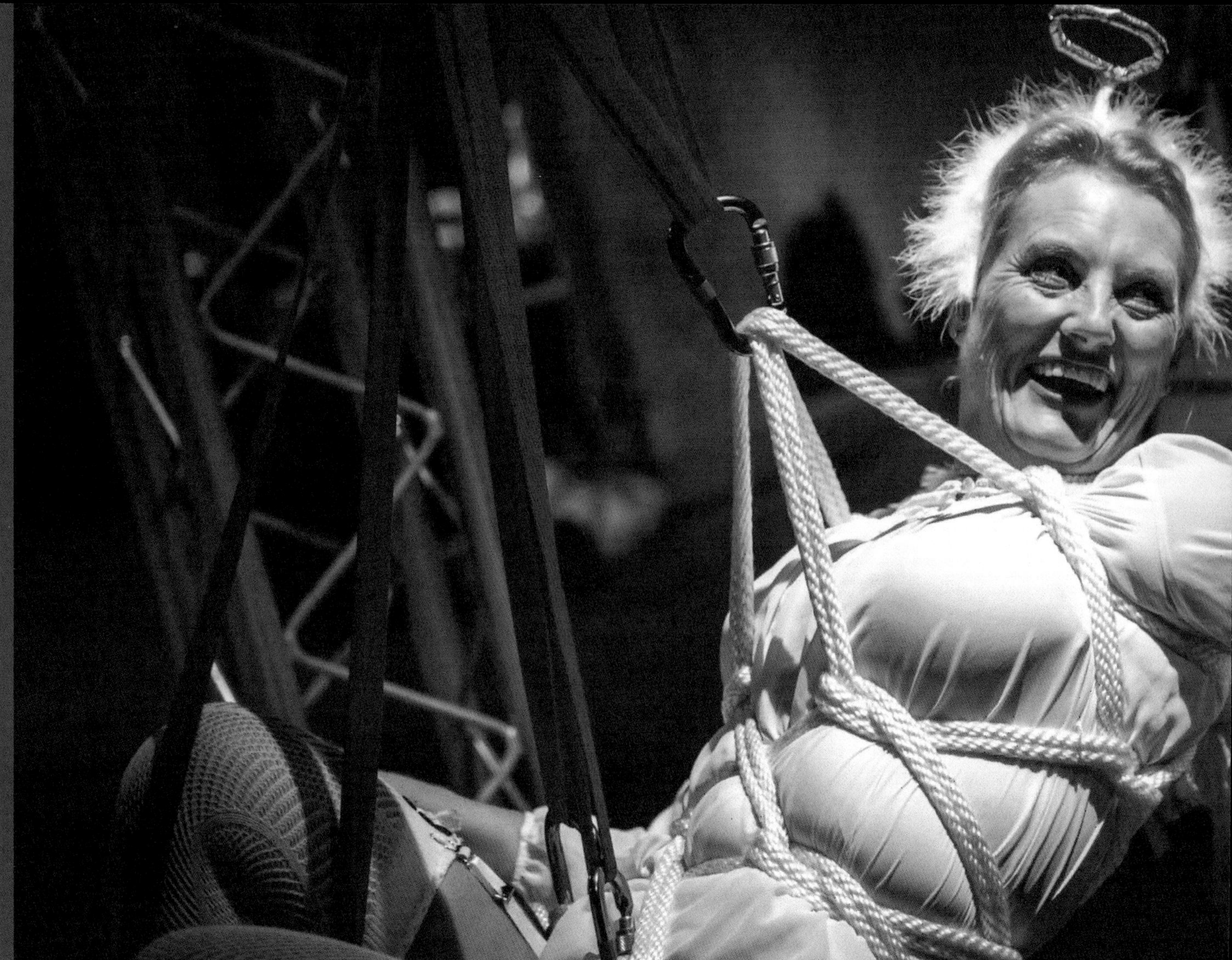

"Being in rope makes me feel alive."
~ RopeGyver, age 65

Facelifts. "Touches, caresses, and kisses during a day make a difference. All things tactile seem to." So write yourself that antiaging prescription by getting touched and caressed by a rope partner often!

Getting tied up is a physical practice aside from touch, usually involving more movement than just sitting around playing bingo. You may be engaging, stretching, or strengthening muscles you're not even aware of. And movement—or even just standing—is way better than sitting: In a study commissioned by the Cardiovascular Research Network, "inactive people who sat the most had double the risk of dying within three years than the active people who sat least."[16] Think of that the next time you're struggling on one leg in that predicament pose.

There's also the social factor. Research has shown that social disconnectedness and isolation can lead to depression, cognitive decline, and more, and that the risks may be particularly severe for older adults.[17] Being a ropester can be social in more ways than one: In addition to interacting with your partner(s), you can get your socializing fix with other rope lovers at munches, classes, Rope Bite meetups, parties, and

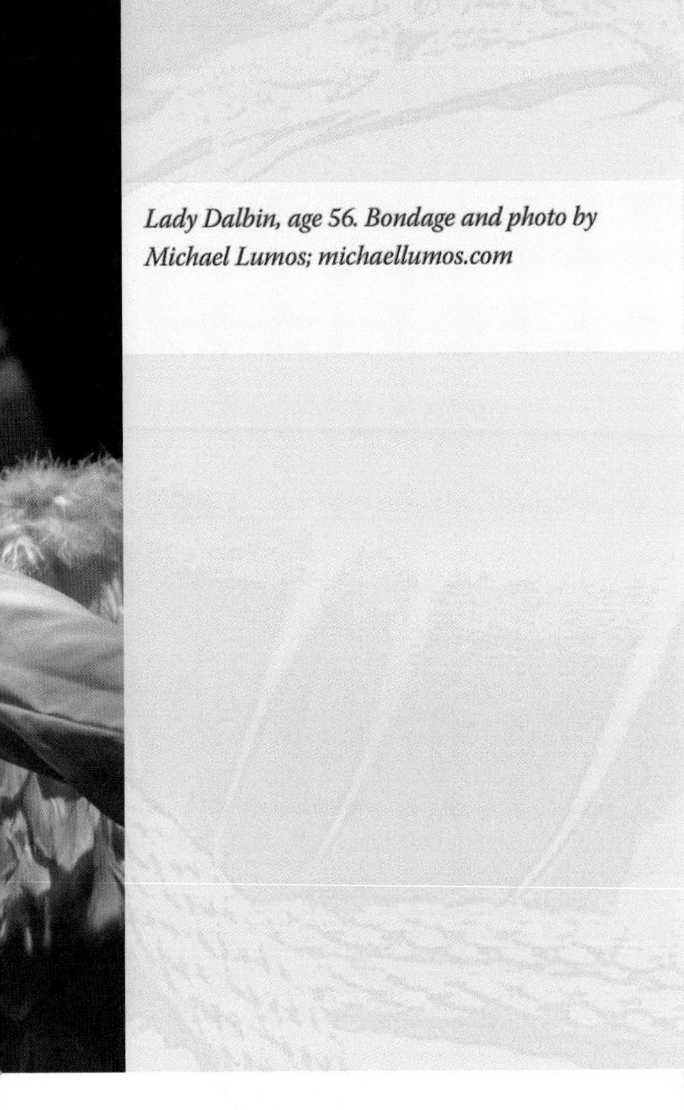

Lady Dalbin, age 56. Bondage and photo by Michael Lumos; michaellumos.com

conferences—and you won't have to rack your brain for something to talk about.

In *Goddesses Never Age*, Dr. Northrup talks about adopting an ageless attitude: "Getting older does not mean an inevitable decline in physical health or a slide into cultural irrelevance," she says. She believes that "the number-one thing you can do for your health is to live joyously." Rope certainly can help us live more joyously, feel more connected, and keep stimulating us and helping us grow in both physical ability and self-awareness.

Doesn't that sound like a recipe for living agelessly?

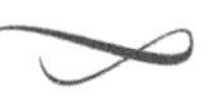

Notes

1. www.orthoinfoaaos.org/topic.cfm?topic=A00191
2. http://www.yourswimlog.com/200m-butterfly-world-record/
3. http://articles.latimes.com/1986-07-21/news/mn-26427_1_climbs-foot-fuji
4. http://articles.latimes.com/1987-08-03/news/mn-368_1_hoover-dam
5. http://www.cbsnews.com/news/oldest-woman-finish-marathon-92-year-old-harriette-thompson-ran-late-husband/
6. Esmonde-White, Miranda. *Aging Backwards: Reverse the Aging Process and Look 10 Years Younger in 30 Minutes a Day.* Harper Wave, 2014.
7. www.orthoinfoaaos.org
8. Gifford, Bill. *Spring Chicken: Stay Young Forever (or Die Trying).* Grand Central Publishing, 2015.
9. http://www.ncbi.nlm.nih.gov/pubmed/8221479
10. http://www.ncbi.nlm.nih.gov/pubmed/10417589
11. http://www.fitnessmagazine.com/beauty/skin-care/best-scar-treatments/
12. http://www.health.harvard.edu/blog/fda-strengthens-warning-that-nsaids-increase-heart-attack-and-stroke-risk-201507138138
13. http://www.drugs.com/pro/ibuprofen.html
14. http://www.drweil.com/drw/u/QAA400915/Curcumin-or-Turmeric.html
15. http://www.cnn.com/2011/HEALTH/07/19/defy.your.age/
16. "Stand up: Your life could depend on it." Sax Institute. http://www.eurekalert.org/pub_releases/2012-03/si-suy032612.php
17. http://www.ncbi.nlm.nih.gov/pmc/articles/PMC2756979/

Chapter 9

For Gender-Nonconforming Rope Bottoms

Probably everyone on the planet has some kind of body issue: too big, too small; too short, too tall; we wish we had a different nose or ass or shoe size. But those kinds of issues are fairly well understood by the majority. When your body doesn't match who you really are, or you otherwise have a gender identity that doesn't conform to society's expectations, it gets more complicated. And studies suggest that 0.3 percent of people in the U.S. feel strongly that their biological sex does not conform to their gender identity.[1] With the U.S. population at more than 323 million[2] as I write this, that means around *1 million Americans* are in that category. Yet gender nonconformity is still decidedly ***not*** well understood by the majority.

Language affects how we think, so let's start by defining some terms. These are courtesy of Erin Houdini, "rope mistress, anti-escape artist, and woman of trans experience." She created a short and sweet "trans glossary" and has kindly granted permission to reprint some definitions here. Erin's website has many more than the ones below; check 'em all out at www.erinhoudini.com/transgender-glossary.html.

Erin's site has a section on social etiquette too. Maybe you've avoided playing with or even just interacting socially with transgender ropesters for fear of saying or doing something wrong or unintentionally hurtful. Head over to that section to boost your confidence and comfort level!

For extensive coverage of the issues related to being transgender, as well as detailed explanations of related terms, I highly recommend Lee Harrington's book

Terms to Know

Gender: The sum of how one relates to themselves and others through their sexuality, personality, and physical body.

Gender identity: One's actual, internal sense of being male or female, neither of these, both, etc.

Trans: Prefix or adjective used as a simultaneous abbreviation of either "transgender" or "transsexual," derived from the Latin word meaning "across from" or "on the other side of." Because it avoids the political connotations of both those terms, many consider "trans" to be the most inclusive and useful umbrella term.

Transgender: Commonly used as an umbrella term for people whose gender identity differs from the sex or gender they were assigned at birth, and for those whose gender expression differs from what is culturally expected of them. Some people use "transgender" to describe their primary gender identity. The term "transgender" is not indicative of sexual orientation, hormonal makeup, physical anatomy, or how one is perceived in daily life.

Genderfluid: A nonbinary gender identity that indicates shifting between different genders, sexualities, presentations, etc. The term "bigender" is similarly used by those who feel they have both male and female sides to their personalities, such as cross-dressers.

Penny. Bondage by Naturalturn. Photo by The Silence

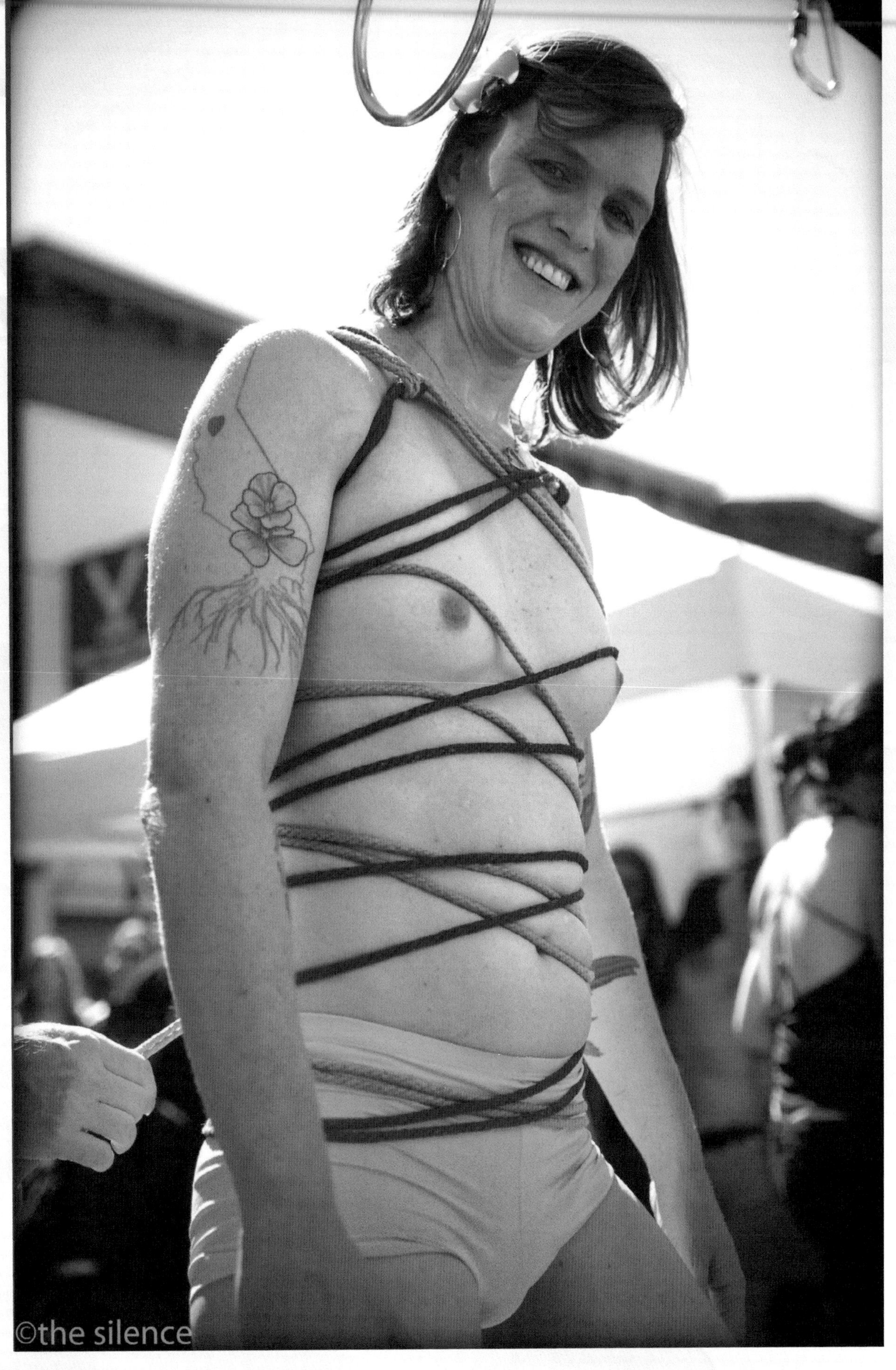
©the silence

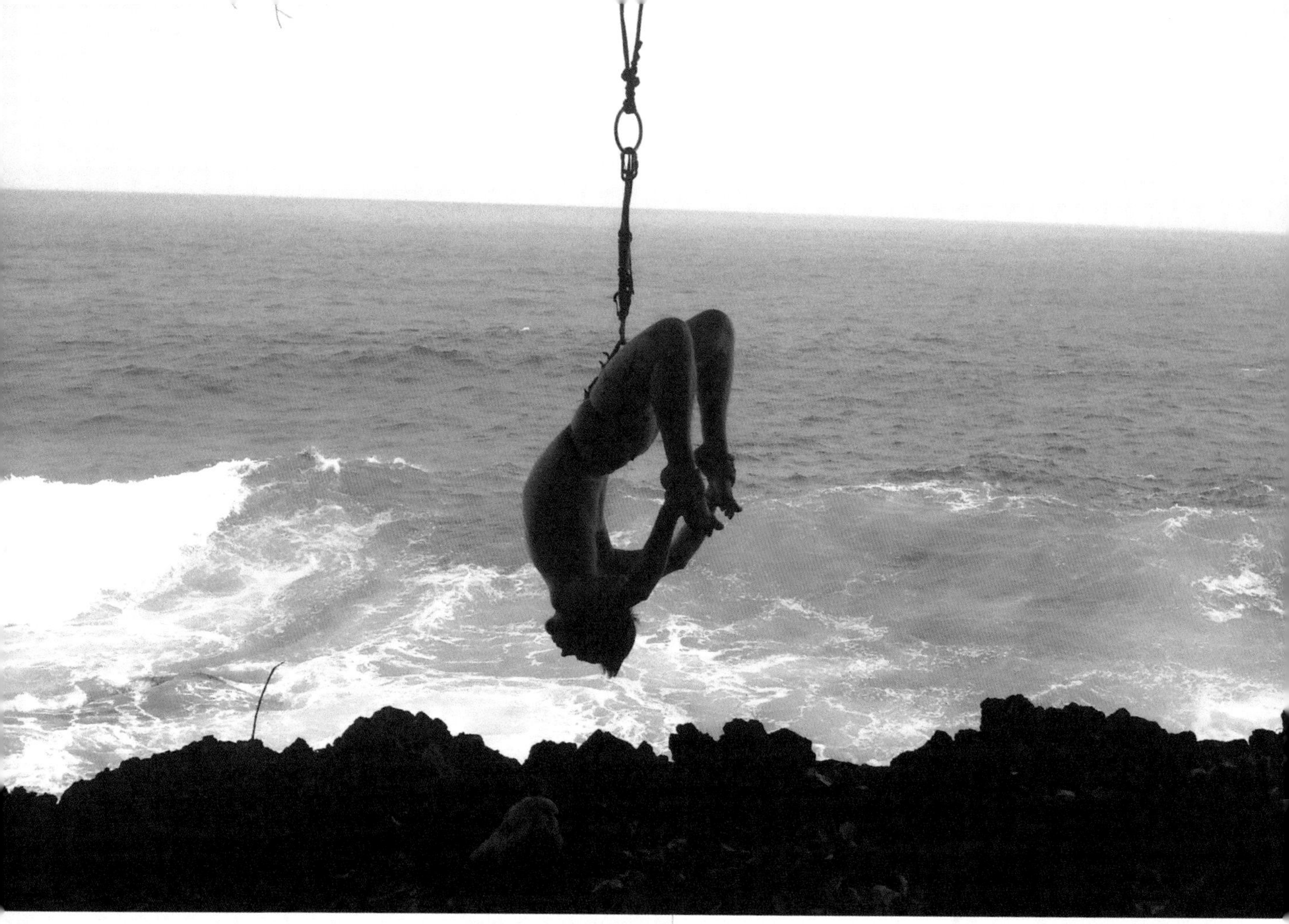

Lee Harrington in self-bondage.
Photo by AKButterfly

Traversing Gender. It's not just for transgender people but for everyone who cares about them. We are so lucky to have Lee in the rope community and as an invaluable consultant on this chapter, by the way! He is the author of eight books and the editor of or a contributor to 17 more, and has taught all over the world on spirituality and erotic authenticity. Lee has assembled a comprehensive collection of resources for transgender and gender-diverse people at http://www.traversinggender.com/ and you can find more about his work at http://www.PassionAndSoul.com.

Challenges

Being gender nonconforming in the rope community, as in life, can cause different issues for different people.

Finding Partners in Fun

One of the most common challenges seems to be finding a rope partner in the first place. "I've found that experienced tops aren't interested in topping me—whether it's because I'm fat, not especially flexible, not a masochist, or being a butch nonbinary trans, I don't know," writes Squirrel, who identifies as "agender, or nonbinary more generally." Nathaniel Flumen, "queer/nonconforming male," says of finding a partner, "It is a common difficulty.... The only two female rope tops of my area didn't want to tie my male form, and I couldn't find any male interested in males that was interested in tying me for nonsexual purposes." A gender-fluid male-assigned rope bottom says simply, "Not many people seem to be interested in tying men/transgenders."

Body Language

Being a female with external genitalia can be a challenge. "Many people only know me as female," says Jennifer Noble, who is trans and identifies as female, "and don't realize that I possess male anatomy at this point, so I have had several people freak out when finding out I was not born female. This has affected who I am able to partner with."

Others may more outwardly present as gender nonconforming, so there's no surprise involved. But that brings different issues, such as the potential for immediate bias or dismissiveness—people might not even try to get to know you beyond what they see.

Other challenges have to do with the body in rope. Some rope tops know how to tie only one kind of body structure, for instance, which can cause issues—especially in suspensions. One male-assigned rope bottom has found one of the biggest challenges to be "the fact that rope won't stay in place on my chest, as many ties seem to rely on the presence of breasts." A female who was born with a male body adds, "Ties around the hips may need to be a little tighter due to less curves." Some ties do assume a specific hip structure, when actually the rigger will need to feel out the individual hip.

A Time of Transition

If you're rope bottoming while transitioning, you and your top will be adjusting along the way. Surgeries and hormones can mean you might no longer have breasts to catch chest harnesses, for instance, or that you have breasts for the first time. Erin Houdini advises that rope shouldn't squeeze or put pressure on breast implants, by the way, so chest harnesses will need to be tied very carefully. Surgeries can also have unintended effects. "Chest surgery left me with a numbness under my arm," Lee says, "which changed the way the rope feels."

"When my partner and I are enjoying a rope scene together, our play transcends any sense of gender.... It is a pure emotional experience."
~ Snow, "male-bodied, gender-fluid"

Transitioning can mean shifts in body fat, changes in musculature, and different flexibility too, which may alter which ties and positions work for you. You may have scars or new hair or other things that take some getting used to. (Pro tip: If you're new to high heels, ask for some support while standing or walking while bound. Balancing when your arms are tied is hard even for longtime stiletto lovers! And if you're exploring makeup, consider avoiding body glitter and any makeup that could rub off on the rope—long-wear lipsticks are great for rope bottoming.)

Speaking of high heels, wardrobe malfunctions can happen: "I recently had a suspension scene where my genitalia slipped from beneath my panties where it had been tucked," Jennifer says. "I noticed a couple from the audience pointing, and the girl looked shocked." Experiences like this can be everything from a nonissue to traumatic, depending on the person.

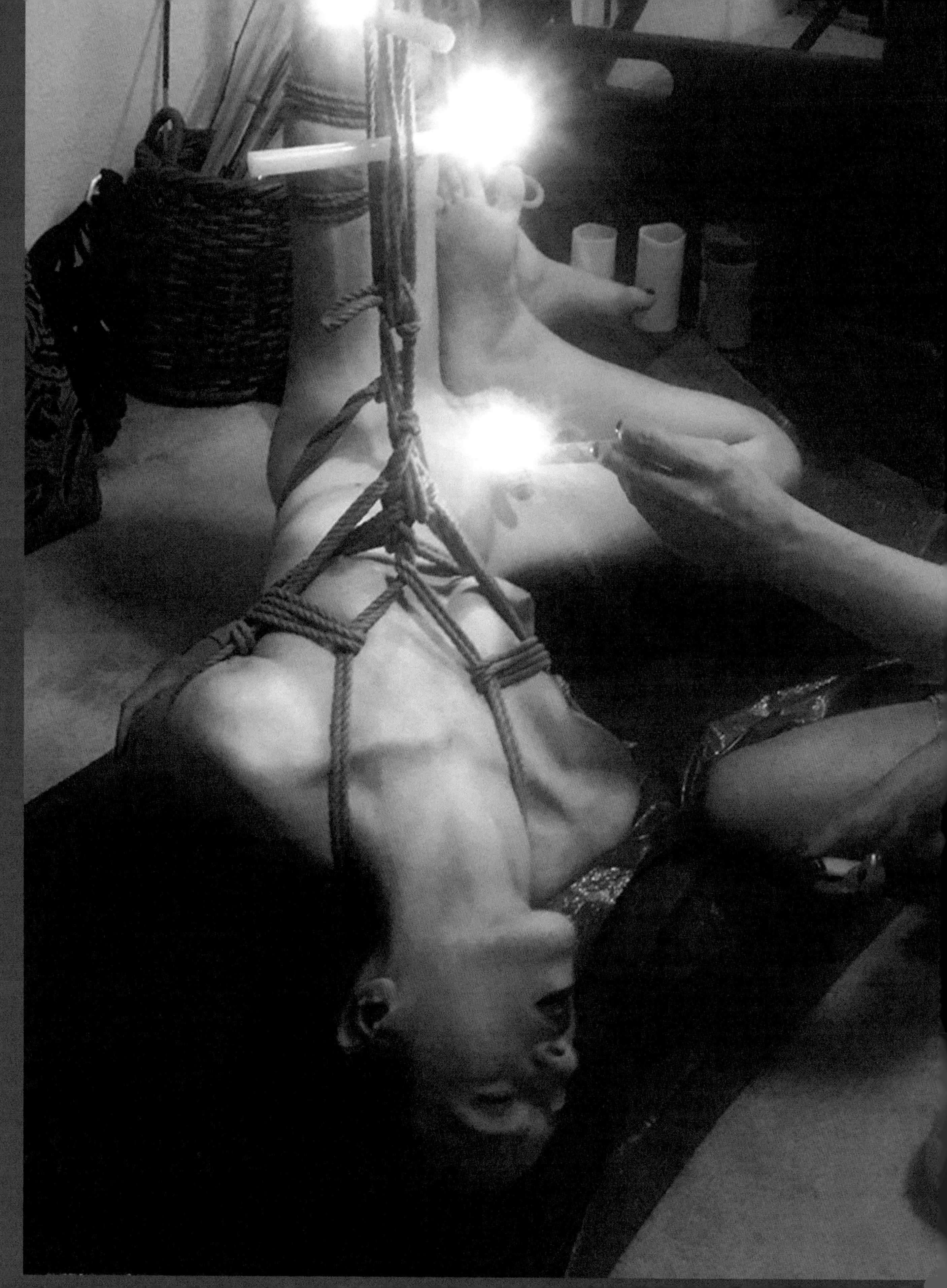

If you're not transitioning but your rope top is, you may need to readjust if they're getting used to tying with a different body, mindset, approach to rope, and so on.

Perception Is Not Reality

Sometimes rope tops shy away from tying male-assigned bodies based on perceptions that may or may not be accurate. "It's surprising how often people assume that male rope bottoms are not flexible," a male-assigned bottom says, "or are somehow less able to do challenging suspensions and partial suspensions. I love to do both!"

Or maybe it's the perception of the rope bottom that's initially skewed. "I had seen exclusively females in his ropes, which made me stupidly insecure," Nathaniel says about his first time tying with a well-known bondage instructor. And how did that end up? "He was highly focused on me and had an outstanding energy.... I adored every minute of it."

Working through feelings of insecurity can be enormously rewarding. "The largest challenge I've faced has been getting over my own issues with being undressed in front of people," says Jane J., who identifies as "female 90 percent of the time" but has "masculine and androgynous days." "While I was assured that being undressed was optional by the people that had tied me, I also knew that they preferred their bottoms naked to both make tying easier and to enhance the connection they were seeking. The larger obstacle was when it came to being tied in front of other people.... While I was incredibly nervous the first scene itself, I was fortunate enough to be a part of an incredibly positive community that has drowned me in praise afterwards and to this day."

Jane J. Bondage and photo by Knotty_Beth

"The only person that you should really be worrying about is your partner. If you and they are OK with who you are, then nobody else needs to matter."

~ Jennifer Noble,
"trans but I solely identify as female"

Helpful Ideas

While we're talking about community, if I had a dollar for every time I extolled its virtues for all rope bottoms...well, you know. You just can't underestimate how supportive, helpful, and resourceful other ropesters can be. "Being surrounded—on FetLife and in real life—by people who enjoy the idea of having male-bodied bottoms within the community sure was a game changer," Nathaniel says. "I felt appreciated and desired within the rope community. This support gave me enough confidence to keep believing and go forward."

So let's have a look at some of our awesome community's ideas.

Don't Assume the Position

"Don't let assumptions about limitations affect what you experience in rope!" advises Snow, who identifies as "male-bodied, gender-fluid." Nathaniel supports that point: "Always remember your sex/gender doesn't define your aptitudes.... Do not limit yourself to rope tops who clearly state an attraction that includes your sex/gender. People are not enclosed in their labels, and most people in the rope community are actually very open-minded and open to exploring different vibes with different individuals, at least at times."

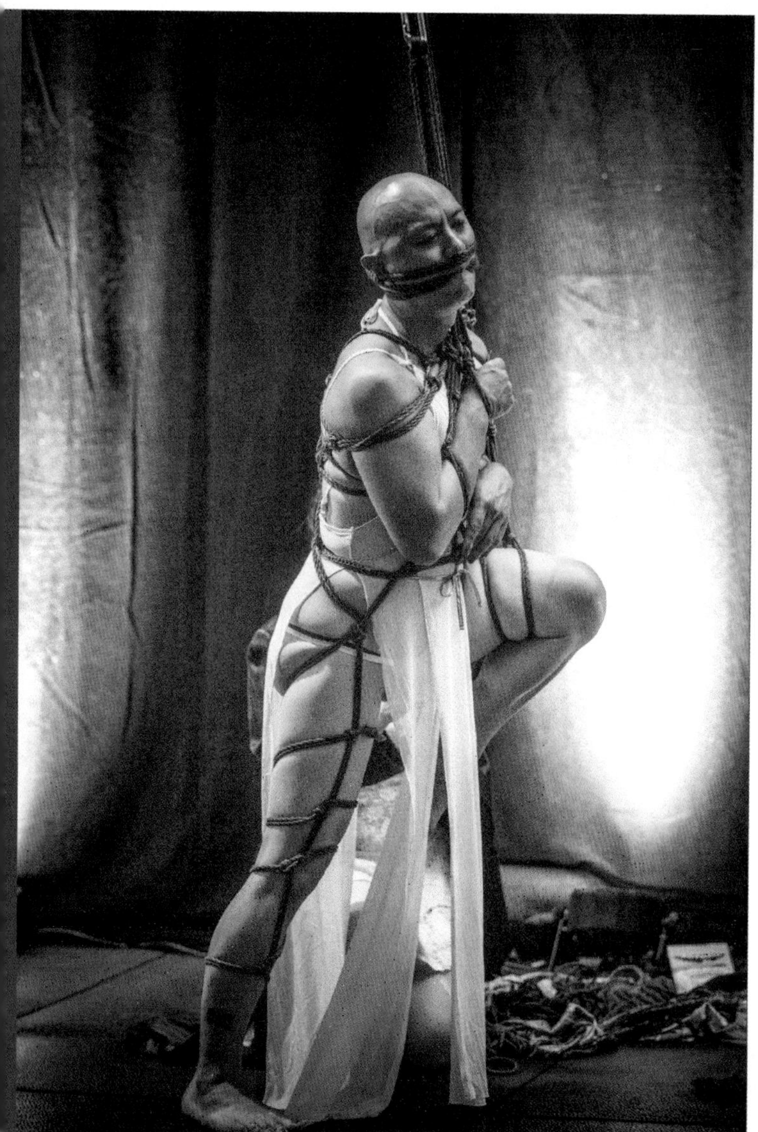

Obi Phoenix. Bondage by Ebi McKnotty; www.rope365.com. Photo by iambic9

Another trans rope bottom adds, "Confidence and being comfortable with who you are play a big part in moving along in many social situations, but I think it's especially important as a trans person to feel comfortable with yourself and what you're doing."

It Takes Two

If finding a rope top is a challenge, consider taking classes in tying others, and attending Rope Bites, rope munches, and other rope-related events. "Some people only do rope with a sexual attraction, but many also do it just to have a fun time, and gender or body type usually doesn't matter to those people," Jane says. You may or may not meet someone who's looking for a bottom at these events, but at the very least you'll gain a better understanding of rope and stay in touch with rope energy.

You can also try attending trans-oriented or trans-friendly events that aren't specifically rope-focused, like Queer Invasion or Dark Odyssey, Lee suggests. He adds that these events often have forums for hookup play online, and you can post a note there, along with attending classes and being available for random match-ups. See who plays with gender-diverse bodies, Lee recommends, as folks who play with diverse bodies (larger, smaller, male, and so on) are more likely to play with other gender-diverse bodies.

And keep in mind this golden nugget of wisdom from Obi Phoenix, whose descriptions include genderqueer, nonbinary, AMAB (assigned male at birth), and femme: "Being gender nonconforming, it's easy to encounter cis-male rope tops who will not tie you.... It might be disappointing, but then again, would you really want to send your one-of-a-kind parrot to a veterinarian who will not work with any other animals but cats?"

Uh, Wait, Actually It Takes Only One

The turning point for Nathaniel in finding partners was "learning self-bondage, attending classes as a self-tyer and an available bottom, and doing a bit of tying as well." That led to meeting some rope tops "who are still among my main rope partners three years later.... I actually stopped self-

Nathaniel Flumen and Osaka Dan. Bondage by Osaka Dan. Photo by PrometheusV

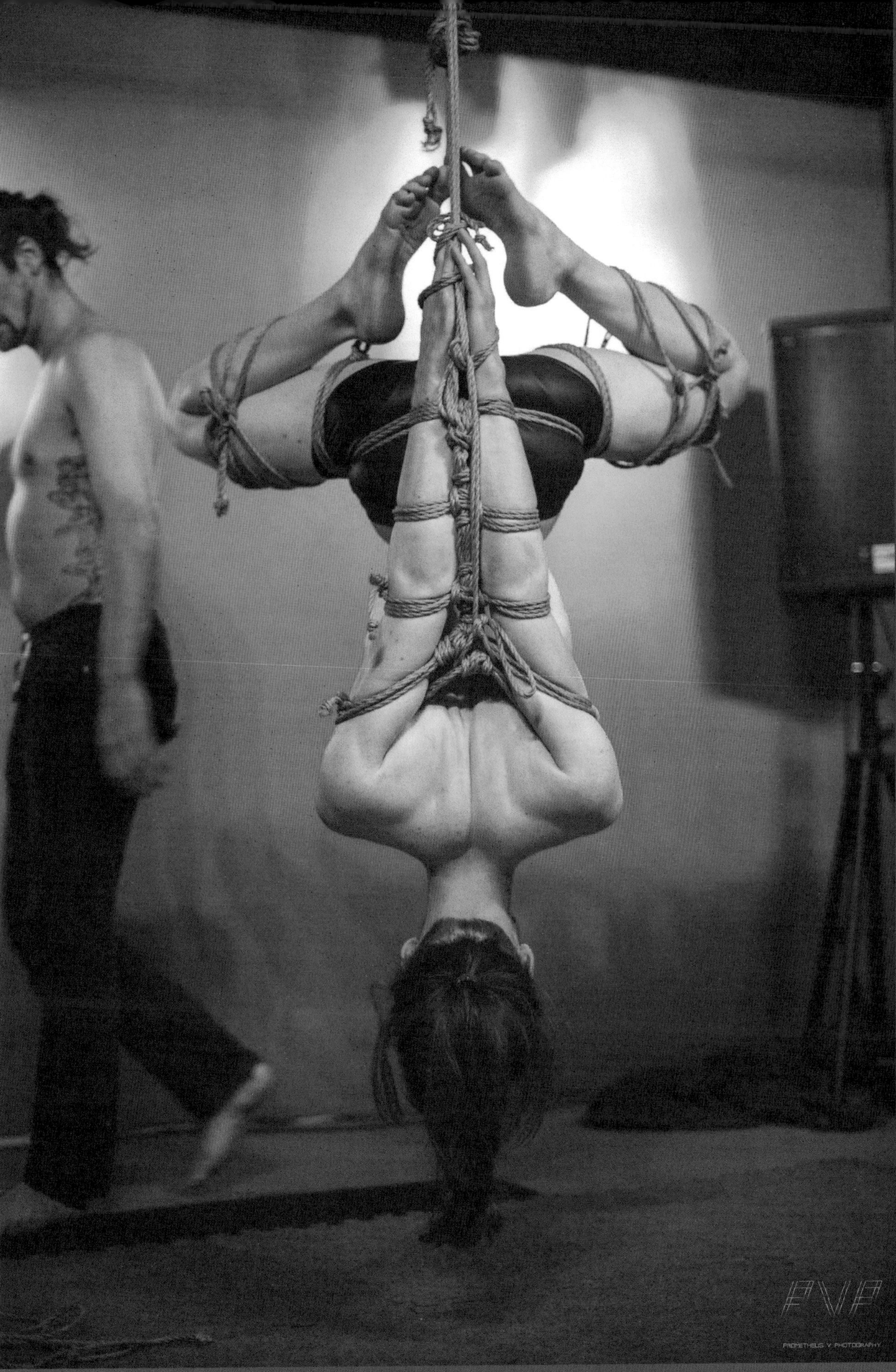
PVP
PROMETHEUS V PHOTOGRAPHY

"I do not recognize myself in any gendered concepts expressed in our modern society.... My crazy dream is to see a wide variety of rope bottoms regarding all possible aspects and not categorize them, seeing them as human beings in ropes."

~ Nathaniel Flumen,
"queer/nonconforming male"

tying and tying to concentrate only on bottoming." Jane also took the self-tying route: "Self-tying is something that a lot of people overlook....When I first started and even now, a lot of the work I did was on my self. It does lack the emotional side, but you can give yourself exactly what you want physically. It's like rope masturbation."

Some turn toward tying and stay there: "I've actually just kind of given up on rope bottoming," Squirrel says. "I started tying other people because others weren't interested in tying me, and I think I just got burnt out not getting my needs met to the point where I just don't want to do it anymore." If your journey in rope shifts course, consider it part of your evolution. You can always go back to rope bottoming later on if you want.

And remember that finding a rope partner, especially one you can connect with on a deeper level, can be a challenge for *everyone*. I hear it all the time, from people you might least expect. The more you put yourself out there—offering to bottom for people in classes, meeting ropesters at munches and Rope Bite and in the FetLife rope groups—the more likely you are to meet someone. As a person in our local rope bottoms meetup wisely said, in response to my lamenting about, yup, not being able to find a steady rope partner: "You're not going to find a dreamy rope partner sitting home alone dreaming about one." Putting yourself out there means opening yourself up to rejection. And while rejection might suck, not getting tied up can suck more.

For others, finding a partner hasn't been a major issue, and gender doesn't even necessarily play a role in rope scenes. Snow says of a strappado suspension that involved impact play: "The experience was very intense, and in the happy fog of subspace, I felt a strong connection with my partner. But in all of the emotions of that moment, I was not thinking of gender at all." One female-identifying rope bottom says, "I don't think I've faced anything specific challenge-wise with my gender or related.... I've played with a handful of people who had no idea of my trans status, without issue."

Major in Communications

When you do find a partner, communicating what language to use, along with where you do and do not like to be touched, can help you feel more comfortable and can help you trust your rope top more: "Communicate not just preferred pronouns," Erin advises, "but also preferred names for body parts, which parts of your body you want—or don't want—attention given to, which parts are completely off-limits, etc."

Touch is a personal and individual thing for everyone, so discuss preferences honestly and openly, especially regarding crotch rope and "the deeply personal choice of sharing genitals with someone," as Lee puts it. And know that those preferences may change from scene to scene. "I have days when genital or chest touching takes me out of ropespace," he says. Tell your partner what kind of touch is hot and sexy for you too, Lee adds—it's easy to focus on the no's, but telling folks what your yeses are is a great way to connect.

"Figure out what you need to stay in a bottom headspace," Squirrel recommends. "As in, what kind of touching, ties, language is liable to cause you dysphoria? What do you need to reaffirm who you are?" Squirrel says that learning "what areas on my body I wanted to have emphasized and which ones I didn't, and what kinds of ties would accomplish that" has greatly helped.

Other specifics to discuss with your partner might include tying over binders or compression shirts, along with wardrobe in general: "What clothing do you want to wear, whether for comfort, enforcing identity, or privacy?" Lee says.

He adds that trans people can also experience bodily dissociation, which may affect reporting safety issues. If this is the case for you, you may want to ask your rope top to check in more frequently during a scene.

Enjoy the Ride

In the end, your rope scene is between you and your partner(s) in the moment. Not the drunken jerk who wandered into the club off the street, not the uneducated person who said something unskilled and hurtful that morning, not previous partners or partners you wish you had. "I had to learn to let go and just enjoy the rope without wondering what others might be thinking," one rope bottom says. "As soon as I did, I was able to enjoy the rope much more."

"Keeping focused on staying in the moment and ignoring those who may see you outside of your partners," along with meditating, are a few things that have helped Jennifer the most.

Instead of being concerned with what other people might be thinking (which you might be wrong about anyway), let the rope work its magic in helping you connect with your partner, transcend the everyday, and celebrate your beauty and power like nothing else can.

As Erin says:

"Rope has always been a way for me to feel connected to my body even when my body wasn't physically configured properly and I felt very disconnected from it."

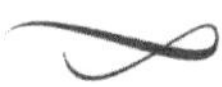

Notes

1. Russo, Francine. "Debate Is Growing About How to Meet the Urgent Needs of Transgender Kids," *Scientific American Mind*, Jan./Feb. 2016.
2. http://www.census.gov/popclock/

Chapter 10

For Rope Bottoms With Special Physical Conditions

I cried so many times working on this chapter—not just for the pain and suffering of all those who wrote in, but for their triumphs, their persistence, their empowerment in advocating for themselves in and out of rope. For many of these bottoms, rope has been much more than just a fun thing to do on a Friday night; it has given them relief, given them hope, and improved their lives.

"It's the only time I feel completely free; free from pain and free from stress."
~ Ashley B., who has severe pain involving the sciatic nerve

It's hard, if not impossible, to truly understand a particular condition if you haven't experienced it first-hand: Fibromyalgia, multiple sclerosis, amputation, systemic lupus, neuropathy, a brain tumor, chronic fatigue syndrome, degenerative disk disease, pulmonary fibrosis, ulcerative colitis…those are just some of the conditions people who responded to the survey are dealing with. Symptoms mentioned include searing pain, paralysis, seizures, depression, dizziness, sleep issues, digestive issues, extreme fatigue, stiffness, visual issues, nerve compression, hypersensitive senses, and slurred speech. Issues like these can make it hard just getting out of bed, let alone getting in rope.

As I'm not a medical professional, this chapter isn't intended to prescribe any course of action or remedy. It's to open the door and look at some of the conditions rope bottoms are dealing with, and *how* they deal—to increase our collective understanding and compassion in the rope community, and to show that whatever condition you're dealing with and whatever challenges you're facing, you're not alone.

Challenges

You've already seen a sampling above of physical symptoms some rope bottoms are dealing with. Depending on the specific condition, they may be mild to downright debilitating—and they can be accompanied by mental and emotional issues as well. Physical issues are at the heart of this chapter, so let's start there.

Physical Education

Fibromyalgia was the most commonly cited condition among rope bottoms who answered the survey questions. The National Fibromyalgia & Chronic Pain Association defines it as "a common and complex chronic pain disorder that causes widespread pain and tenderness to touch that may occur bodywide or migrate over the body."[1]

That description sounds so clinical, though. What does it actually feel like? "My pain-sensing nerves seem to get stuck in the 'on' position. This usually feels like constant burning in my muscles and joints, similar to the soreness from a hard workout," Lilah Rose says. Redfeline adds, "The senses of smell, taste, hearing, and touch can be hypersensitive; i.e., the sound is way too loud and people's perfume can be very overwhelming." Hikarin describes flare-ups as

Tarah Una. Bondage by MrMatt_PFM. Photo by Marshall Bradford; www.mbradfordphotography.com; http://mbradfordphotography.tumblr.com

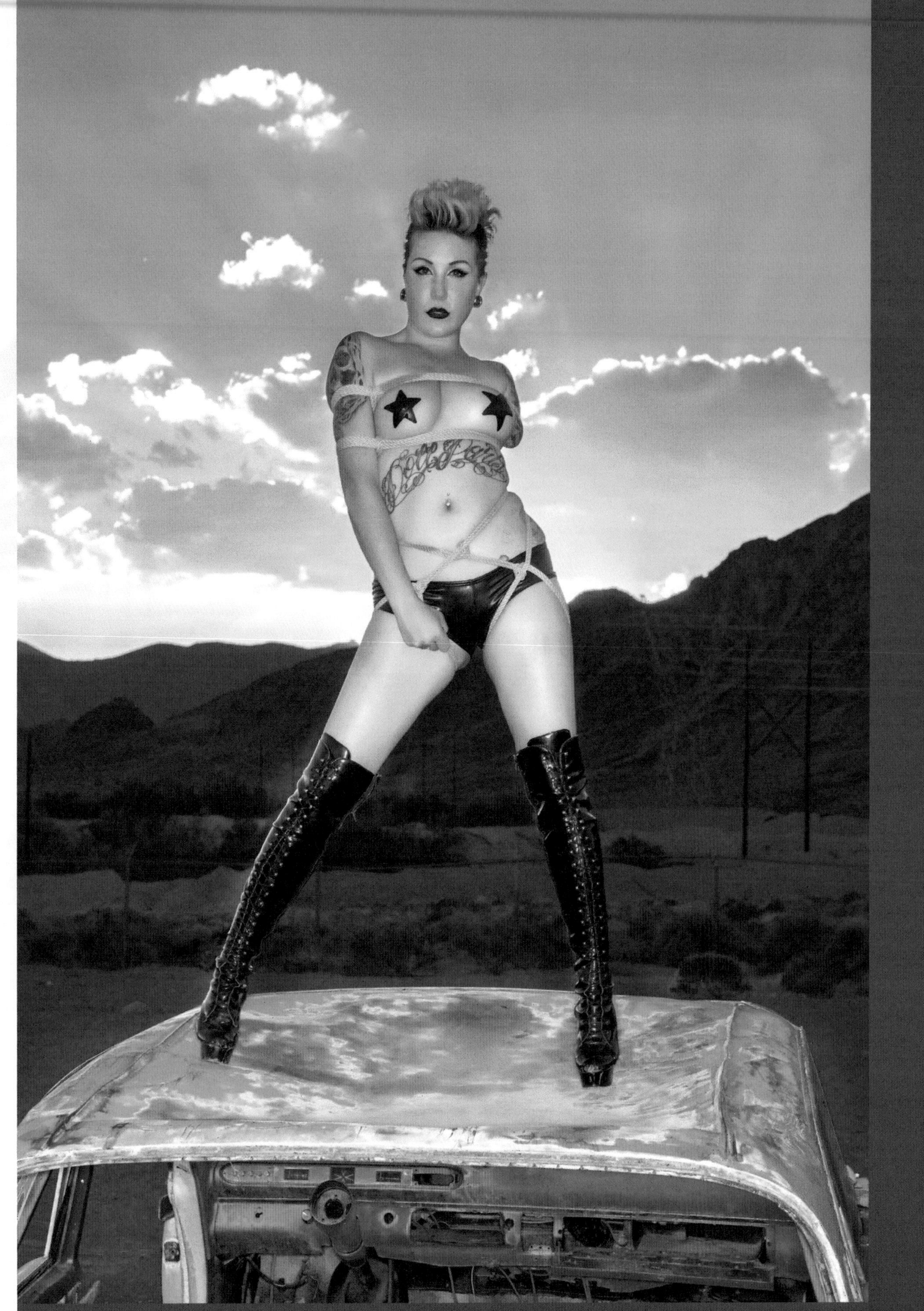

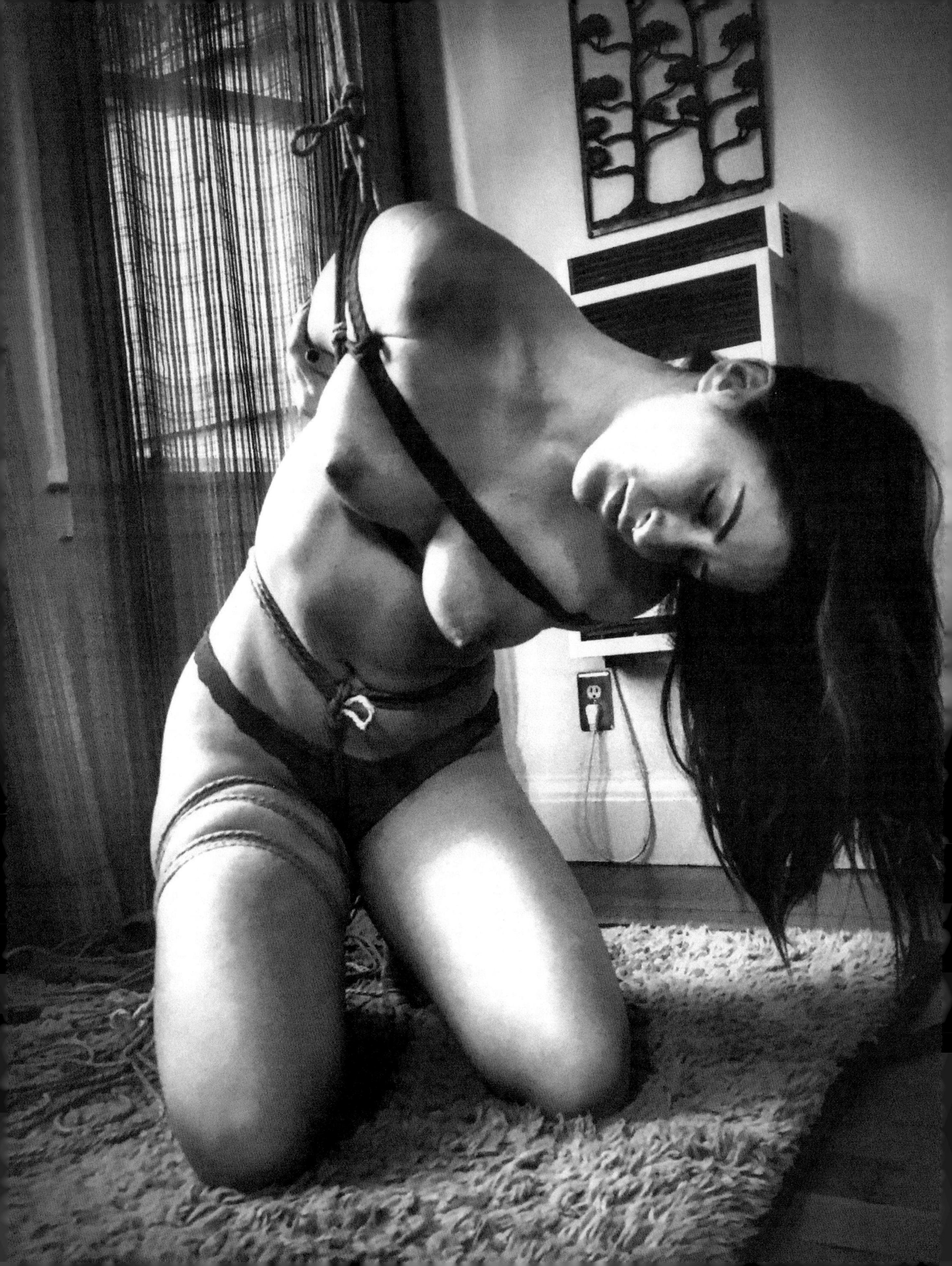

"like waking up with the flu, with my body feeling like it's on fire, pinned down by a large truck, and accompanied by a slow, foggy brain."

There is no cure for fibromyalgia, and the exact cause isn't understood. The pain can be excruciating. "There are times when I've been in too much pain or too ill to tie," says LucytheBrave. "I have had to cancel sessions and drop out of events. It's hard to say no to something I love that brings me so much joy."

It also can be hard to predict when the pain will be worse, and what will increase it, both in rope and out of it. "I have weird/random areas that may be hypersensitive depending on the day as well as significant joint pain—again varies based on the day and the weather. Finding ties/positions that I can tolerate has been somewhat challenging, especially just starting out," forgottendancer says. And it's not necessarily like you're home free once you find a tie that seems to work. "A tie that feels good one second may have to be untied and modified quickly," BioKim says.

Other rope bottoms have autoimmune disorders, which occur when the body's immune system attacks and destroys healthy cells by mistake. There are more than 80 types of these disorders.[2] As with fibromyalgia, there is no cure—treatment involves managing symptoms, and different kinds of autoimmune disorders involve different symptoms. "I have very little energy," says The Riss, who has Hashimoto's Thyroiditis, an autoimmune disorder that affects the thyroid. "In addition to fatigue, I'm more prone to—I kid you not—300 symptoms. I bruise and scar more easily than people without the disease, which means when the rope pinches my skin, that bruise is going to stick around for at least a week, and if it breaks the skin, that's a forever scar. I also have very stiff joints and muscles."

Then there's multiple sclerosis, an autoimmune disorder that affects the central nervous system. "When nerves short out, it causes symptoms like tremors, spasticity, pain, electrical shocks along the spine, foot drop, cognitive issues, and balance issues, to name a few," says kotori_kim, who has MS.

TheSuspendedDoll has relapsing-remitting multiple sclerosis, and says, "My biggest issue is the nerve pain. Constant tingling and decreased sensation I usually have in my hands."

Systemic lupis, which Lisa has, is another autoimmune disorder; it "causes joint inflammation and arthritis-like symptoms for me," she says. "Sometimes I'm in routine and daily pain. Other times I can be pain-free for months or years." Yet another disease is pulmonary fibrosis, which affects the lungs. "I now function with 39 percent of breathing capacity," says Blue, who has it, along with "poly arthritis, meaning chronic pain in the joints, and the hurting joint changing every day.... I deal with chronic pain on a daily basis."

The above disorders may be "silent" or "invisible," meaning you can't tell people have them just by looking. And "given the fact that my condition is not visible, it adds a certain level of difficulty for people to understand how much it takes a toll on me," says Blue.

Ulcerative colitis is another silent condition that comes with a host of symptoms. "I get tired super easily when I'm symptomatic," says His_anna, who has it. "My moods become very changeable.... I suddenly get hungry or suddenly get nauseous." Also dealing with ulcerative colitis is bubblerat, who says, "My large in-

The Riss. Bondage and photo by True Blue; miss_true_blue on Instagram

Lady_Hunny_Bunny

Lady_Hunny_Bunny has fibromyalgia and uses a wheelchair.

When I first entered the kink community, I was a walking, able-bodied person. I was shy and cautious. Everything was interesting and exciting. That all changed within six months, as I developed fibromyalgia. I went from fully walking to wheelchair-bound in a very short time.

Fibro is a cruel and unforgiving illness, and has many side illnesses. You can't be touched in any place it is without it causing you pain, and I have it on 100 percent of my body. The pain is mind-consuming. Your conversations rotate around your illness. Your life is one specialist visit after another as you try to find out what is wrong. You could get lost mentally.

I drowned at first. But as I started looking at ways to improve my quality of life, I returned to kink and what it could offer. I found that rope was a great way to allow me to meditate (by going into subspace), which helped to reduce my pain. I also found that orgasms reduced pain and increased my energy, and that flogging was the best deep muscle massage to my shoulders and back. It gave weeks of relief—not surprising when you realize all the endorphins you get.

I have an awesome partner who worked tirelessly to find ways to tie me without increasing my pain. For a long time we did not do suspensions, as there was no lower-body harness my skin could stand. I used to apologize for the inconvenience I was causing him, until he pointed out one day that I was really an asset to him by increasing his skills and toolbox of tricks. And I was happy, as I had rope on my skin and loved the euphoric feelings, not to mention the reduced pain levels.

My body is always changing. Weather affects how my body reacts—on rainy days I have high pain, sunny days not so high pain. My weight went up for a while due to edema swelling in my body, then as I got that under control my weight reduced again. When I thought about it, I realized he was getting a good deal because I was many different shapes and sizes to tie.

I also agreed that on my bad days we would find a substitute bunny for him. When we were going to classes, I would do as much as I could and then let the substitute bunny step in so he could continue. If the classes were over days, then I would attend but not bottom for him.

Our greatest challenge was how could I do a suspension? My partner suggested we use the wheelchair. OMG what dramas, LOL. First as you try to lift the chair in a suspension it folds up, so we had to work out a way to stop that. Then where can you attach the ropes without destroying the rope on the brake cables or having it move and change the axis of the lift? Figuring out the weight ratings on carabiners, rings, and ropes. Figuring out ways of preventing me from sliding out of the harness that attached me to the chair. It took six months of trying different ways of tying harnesses and attaching rope to the chair, talking to other riggers etc.

Finally we were ready, and on our first attempt I was able to stay up for five minutes. I had to come down because I had a corset on and a tab had bent into my stomach, causing nausea. I was wearing the corset for back support. I felt like I had failed when really I was suspended for five minutes, so it was not a fail but a success.

The second attempt I went with no corset and then rotated into suspension facedown. I was up for over 10 minutes. Awesome! I was flying and so happy. But our best was yet to come.

We were asked to perform at ARK (Amateur Rope Kaleidoscope), an event run twice a year for amateur rope performers by a lovely venue in Australia, where I live. Our performance had to last for 30 minutes. We took the wheelchair up in a suspension lift, then rotated it 360 degrees. I was suspended and flying, and not only that but I have done a suspension that few others have done!

Lady_Hunny_Bunny. Bondage by Fuggly and Chainwire. Photo by Georgia_63

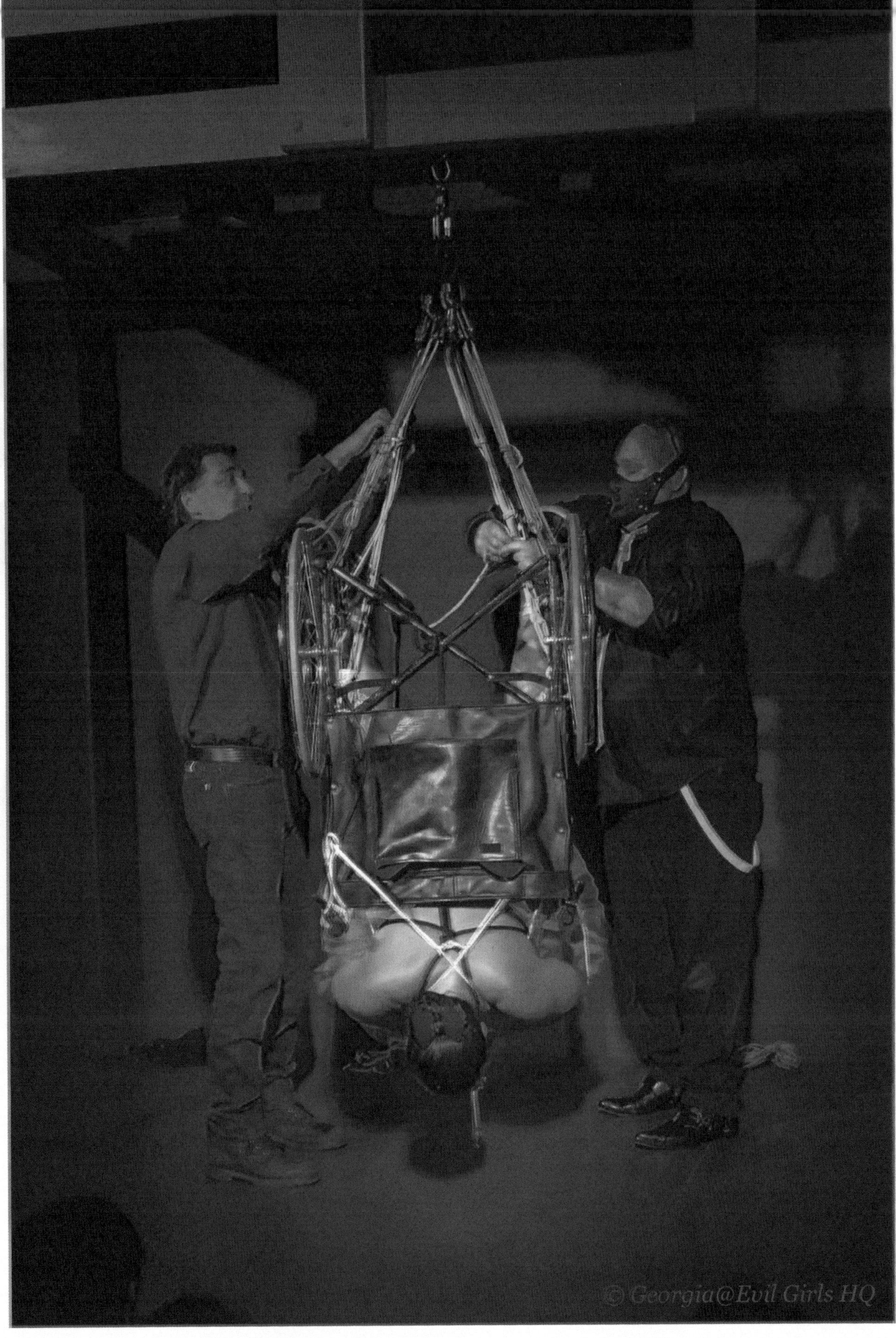
© Georgia@Evil Girls HQ

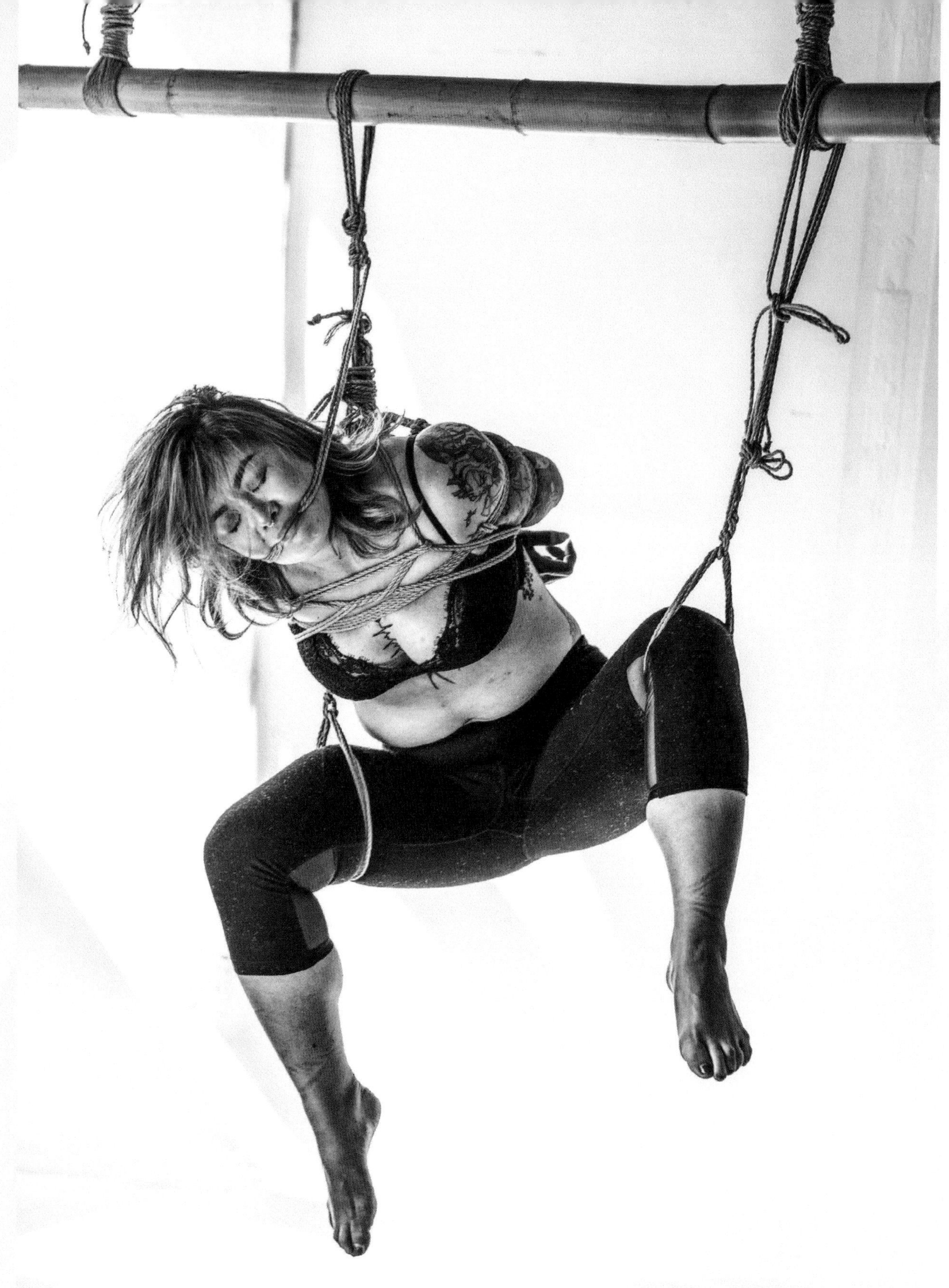

©the silence

testine is inflamed, has ulcers, and results in a lot of bowel problems—i.e., needing to go to the toilet very frequently and urgently, bleeding, and bloating."

Other silent conditions reported by rope bottoms include:

- Chronic fatigue syndrome (extreme tiredness that doesn't go away with rest)
- Glaucoma (increased pressure in the eyeball that causes vision loss)
- Cervical and lumbar degenerative disk disease (a damaged vertebral disk causes pain)
- Hypermobility, meaning the joints can move beyond the normal range of motion. This might actually seem like an asset in rope bottoming, but "my joints can bend in ways that are unsafe," FeistyTex says. "Before I started rope, I'd had frequent shoulder dislocations in my right shoulder and had shoulder stabilization surgery."
- Epilepsy (characterized by seizures)
- Knee reconstruction and a titanium plate near the hip joint. ("I opted to use hamstrings to reconstruct both of my torn ACLs," says nano_bites. "As a result, my leg muscles, especially my calves, are always tight.")

"Sometimes I wish I had more concrete issues that I could point to, e.g., a back issue, rather than having 'invisible' disabilities. I look strong and am flexible, and yet, my body often betrays me," LucytheBrave says.

Then there are less silent, or even readily apparent, physical conditions. Aubrey Metropulos, for example, has a leg amputated at the knee, and wears a prosthesis. Wheelchairs and blindness fall into this category

"I am not my medical conditions; I am me!" ~ RobinBoyHostage, who has a congenital heart condition and neuropathy

too—as does (at some point) pregnancy, which we will not be covering here. Getting tied while pregnant involves many possible risks even if you're not suspending; check out the article "Pregnancy and BDSM" on www.stefanosandshay.com to learn more.

Any type of condition may mean spending extra time preparing for a scene and/or less time in rope. "Before going to a class/event, I make sure I get a good night's sleep and a nap, then I take an epsom salt bath for least 30 minutes," says Redfeline. "I make sure I take all my inflammatory supplements and my medications to control pain.... I also go through my stretching exercise."

And having a disorder may make it harder to figure out your body's responses in rope, to differentiate between issues caused by a particular tie and issues caused by the disorder. The SuspendedDoll says, about the constant tingling and decreased sensation mentioned earlier, "This is a residual symptom I have all the time, which makes it very hard to tell the difference between actual nerve issues from rope and my regular dysfunctional sensation." And EveningRopes comments, "My body reacts differently to tying than other bodies, so I have little external information with which to compare my experience."

Mental Patience

Physical symptoms are only part of the picture. Mental and emotional issues can, of course, go hand in hand with chronic pain and other physical issues.

nano_bites. Bondage and photo by The Silence

Fibromyalgia "is accompanied by literally hundreds of other conditions, including sleep and cognitive disturbances, digestive issues, anxiety, and depression," BioKim says. "This disorder can and does do a number on our self-esteem," says Redfeline, also about fibromyalgia, but of course that applies to other disorders too.

"When I have to tap out of anything I could do before, I get frustrated," kotori_kim says. "Learning to overcome the tendency to beat myself up over things out of my control was difficult, and it's an ongoing learning process." Lisa echoes that: "It can be hugely frustrating to go from 100 percent able to nearly disabled," she says.

That transition can happen gradually or quickly, and it can be hard to judge what is right for your body on any given day. "I hit my wall almost before I knew it was coming," Lilah Rose says of a particular suspension. "I wasn't collected enough to 'red'; I just burst out, 'Down-down-down-down-down'.... I was devastated. I've dealt with severe mental health issues my whole life, and all I could think was now my body was failing me too. One of the most meaningful and enjoyable things in my life was being taken away, and I didn't know why or how to fix what was going wrong. The loss of something I took pride in, that helped define me and gave me such pleasure made enduring the pain and exhaustion that much more difficult to deal with."

"Mentally I'm still struggling a little, but I'm working on accepting that my body has changed and I can't expect it to perform the way it used to," Lilah Rose says.

Even if a tie feels right for your body, you can flash back to times when it wasn't, or to times outside of rope that were scary or even traumatic. "Twelve years ago, I was partially paralyzed and could not feel my hands or anything below my waist. Because I associate numbness with these frightening memories, I have experienced panic in rope before when I start to lose feeling in my hands," TheSuspendedDoll says. "I have been lucky to tie with knowledgeable, loving partners who have helped me work through this trigger, and now I do quite well keeping my panic in check."

Other bottoms with disorders or other conditions also shared that they are dealing with worry, anxiety, nervousness, stress, and depression. And while we will not be discussing mental illnesses specifically in this book (that could be a book of its own!), BDSM educator Naiia shares her story later on of how both mental and physical issues affected her relationship with her partner and with rope, and describes the realization that made all the difference.

Crowd Control

In addition to all the inner challenges to deal with, other people can contribute to negative feelings. Leaf-in-the-wind, who has epilepsy, says that responses of bystanders "range from pity to openly and aggressively berating me. Quote: 'How irresponsible of you to do suspensions with a condition such as yours!'"

Finding a top can be challenging as well. There's "the social stigma of having a medical condition. I've found it increasingly difficult to find a top to play with," says RobinBoyHostage, who has a congenital heart condition and neuropathy. Alexis, who has fibromyalgia, adds, "The fact that [rope bondage] has caused pain has discomforted my partner to the point that the frequency of rigging has gone down."

Then there's the point for some, like those with amputations, that we've covered in other chapters: "A lot of tops seem to not want to stray from the standard body type," Aubrey Metropulos says.

For others, finding a partner is less of a challenge. "One of my biggest fears was disclosing the disease to potential partners. I didn't believe that anyone would want to tie me," says kotori_kim. "I was wrong. The few people I felt brave enough to share with and ask to tie with were receptive."

A top may also have preconceived notions that may affect your scene. Some tops "would treat me like I am made of glass, therefore not pushing my limits—with consent of course—and making decisions for me, thinking for me, and not letting me follow my own path," Blue says.

When you add up all the challenges, you might wonder how tying ever happens at all, or why anyone with a painful disorder would even want to delve into an activity that can and does cause pain itself. Let's find out.

Helpful Ideas

Anyone who deals with chronic pain, struggles with a changing body and sense of self, and faces stigma, misperceptions, and even peripheralization on a regular basis without giving up can tell you a thing or two about persistence and resourcefulness. *Every* rope bottom can benefit from the ideas here!

Care, Care Everywhere

Self-kindess, physically and mentally, seems to be key. "Be compassionate with yourself," says EveningRopes. Lilah Rose says the most important thing is to "not get discouraged or be hard on yourself." And The Riss offers this: "Take care of yourself above anything else.... You're doing the best you can on any given day. Even if the bulk of that effort was washing your hair, you did it. Good job. Be kind to yourself."

"The passion outpaces the limitation."
~ kotori_kim, who has multiple sclerosis

For some, self-kindness includes managing stress. "I try to keep my stress levels low right before, during, and after" a tying session, says Hikarin. "Take care of yourself the day before and the day of classes/events," Redfeline says. "Reduce the stress as much as you can. Hot baths or showers and wholesome food go a long way."

Self-care might include physical therapy. "I have had a lot of success with lowering the threshold of constant pain and regaining strength by doing regular physical therapy, especially aquatic therapy," Lilah Rose says. It might also include yoga, and for reasons other than just flexibility. "I do a lot of yoga, which keeps me limber and flexible," LucytheBrave says. "[It] also helps me with body awareness—what is stiff or sore." Lisa also believes in yoga, saying it "has helped me physically more than anything. Not just that yoga has improved my joints, although it has, but it's improved my body awareness. I'm more able to gauge what I can and cannot do, and where problems might pop up."

Remember that no single discipline works for everyone, however. "Find something you love that works for your body," recommends EveningRopes. "For me, it's aerial and active stretch classes to prevent hypermobility injuries. For a good friend of mine, that's been barre, while yoga is an absolute no for her body. For others, swimming works well." Nano_bites uses a dense foam roller, which is great even if you don't have a special condition!

"Bondage has been incredibly empowering. It is empowering to know I can handle enormous pain and to have a choice in the pain I am experiencing."

~ EveningRopes, who has an autoimmune disease

Find Your Bliss

EveningRopes' advice about finding what works for *your* body was shared by many, in terms of both self-care and being in rope. "Develop exquisite knowledge of your body and your needs!" recommends LucytheBrave. Kotori_kim agrees: "Work with the issues instead of fighting against them; much greater things are possible that way."

You may find that entire categories of ties aren't right for you. "I can't do inversions, because my eyes can be affected. The eyestrain could be so high that I go blind," says Hiroshima Alarcon Blanco, who has glaucoma. "[Also], I can't recieve pressure on my upper part of the body, over the breast. For example, a simple TK."

There's no reason to think of yourself as lacking if you can't do a particular tie or even a group of ties—remember that limitations and issues of some kind or another are common among all rope bottoms! "Don't compete with anyone else and don't compete with yourself," Lisa advises. "Today's body and today's rope are what they are. It's not a failure if you can't fly." The Riss shares that sentiment: "Comparison is the thief of joy, and you'll never feel good about yourself or your life if you continue to see yourself as lacking."

"Mentally, remembering that it's OK to have boundaries and to have things I can't do because of my illness" helps forgottendancer. "I am not a bad rope bottom for not being able to do everything someone able-bodied could, and I am not a bad bottom for being unable to do all the things all the time." Hear, hear! And if you do find yourself falling into the comparison trap, you may find "The One Thing That Will Make You a Super Rope Bottom" in Chapter 1 helpful.

Finding what works can involve thinking creatively about clothing as well as the ties themselves. "I wear knee-high boots to protect my shin and an underbust [corset] to protect my skin during suspension,"

Making It Work

"My husband was disabled with cancer for over a year. He was in a wheelchair for six months and had to relearn to walk. Chemo left him with nerve damage in his hands and feet and with damage to his lungs. Tom has been tying since the '70s and is hugely skilled. Then suddenly our roles were reversed, and I was in better shape than he was. In skiing, they use the term 'adaptive' to describe differently abled ski techniques. We began doing Adaptive Rope. He could sit in a swivel chair and I put my leg up. Futo! We worked together in ways that were even more satisfying than more traditional styles of topping and bottoming and found ways to make things work.

Suddenly being the 'able' one felt strange, and I realized that it never bothered him when I couldn't do things. He loved tying me in whatever ways were available. I love being tied by him however he manages it."

~ Lisa, who has systemic lupus

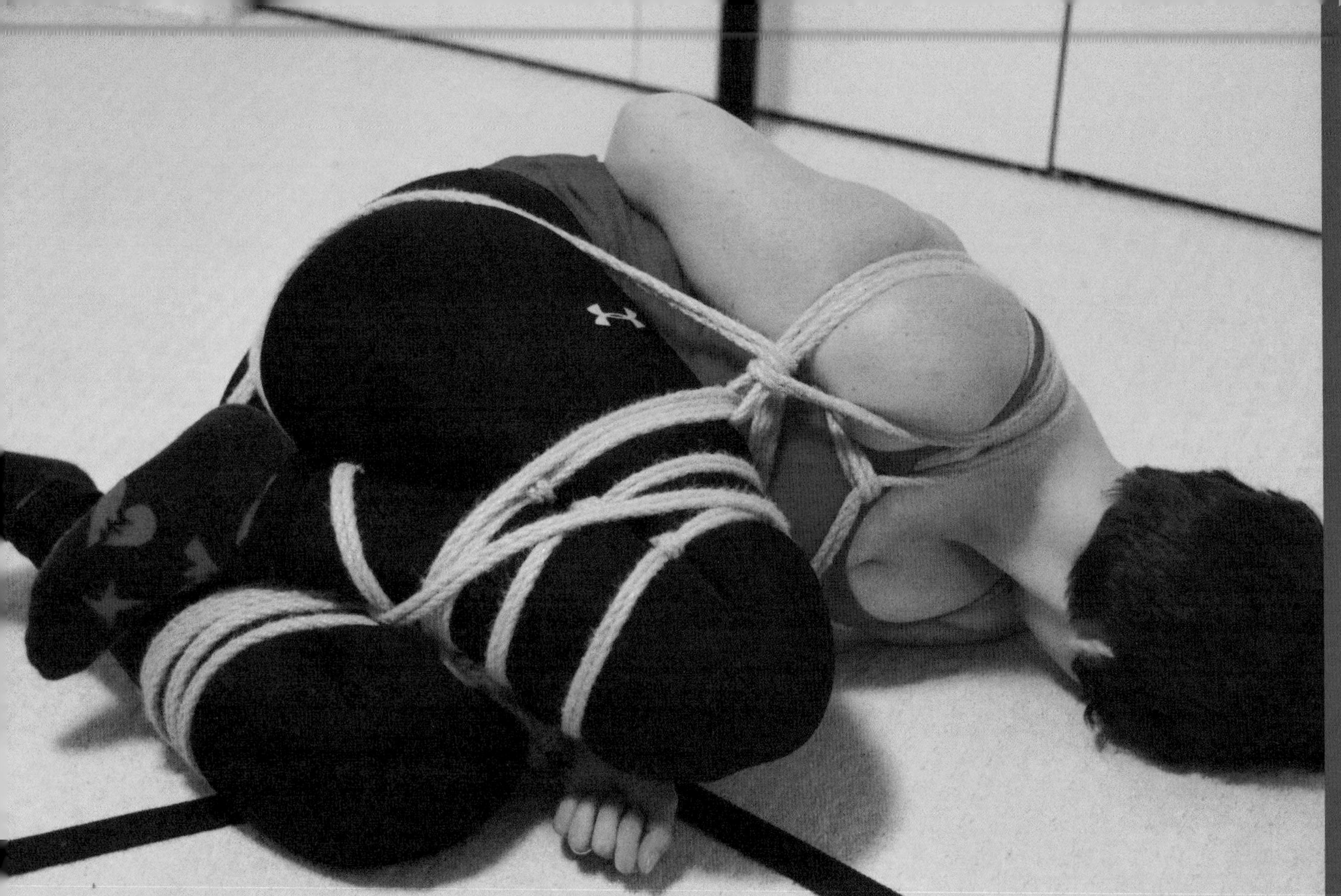

TheSuspendedDoll. Bondage and photo by a_dan

Redfeline says. And FeistyTex adds, "For a long time I had a difficult time staying in a TK, and especially had problems with the TK bearing any weight in suspensions. Strappados and bunny ears ties would often cause my shoulder to ache as well, so it took a lot of creativity on the part of my riggers to come up with ties where my right hand stayed in front of my body." Remember that you can ask for "lab time," with either a regular partner or someone else in a trade-type deal.

Self-tying can be a valuable tool in discovering what works too. "Learning to tie myself has been a fun and useful way to determine how my body behaves in rope, and I highly recommend it," BioKim says. "I've been able to experiment with different types of rope, ties, tensions, etc., and that's given me some valuable knowledge in my journey." Alexis says, "Self-ties have helped me the most, because I can modify these and then show my partner how I did them and help him understand what works for me."

Figuring out how your body responds to environmental factors is another piece of the puzzle. "Cold causes my body to lock up," says EveningRopes. "If I play outdoors, I have to be very careful that it's late enough in the day for sun exposure not to cause sun-related blistering and warm enough not to trigger a flare-up." Other environmental factors to consider include heat, light, noise, perfume/cologne or other smells, and amount of elbow room.

"I am different, and people that I do rope with acknowledge that and help me celebrate it."
~ Blue, who has pulmonary fibrosis and poly arthritis

Sharing Is Caring

Learning about how your body responds to rope is only part of the story—it behooves you to let your partner in on it, along with info about your condition. This includes how to handle any medical emergencies or symptoms that may occur. "Rope bondage is a partnership between two or more people. Clear communication and listening skills are very important, especially with health issues," Redfeline says. "*The rigger needs to know!*" leaf-in-the-wind emphasizes.

"Communicate with your top about what's going on with you that day. Make sure they understand how your condition interacts for you, and make sure they know where not to put rope and where it is more comfortable," recommends forgottendancer.

"Be honest and [don't] be afraid to speak up," advises Redfeline. "Don't be afraid to keep asking questions [about] how other people handle certain situations." Does your partner need to transition you extra slowly? Avoid tying over certain areas? Are certain positions a no-go? These are basic points to ponder. Do they know what to do if you pass out, have a seizure, need insulin, need an emergency bathroom break? Discussing these things may be more difficult, but you're putting yourself at greater risk if you don't.

And besides, every rope bottom has something to discuss with their top to reduce risk, whether it's a tricky shoulder, a position that triggers them, their preferred type of TK...why should there be a stigma attached to discussion points just because they're related to a medical condition (or a mental one, for that matter)? Thank you to the bottoms in a discussion group at NARIX recently for stridently making that point! And, as Aubrey Metropulos says, "the more comfortable you are with yourself, the more comfortable everyone else is with you."

Speaking of risk, consider what you are comfortable risking. In the short term, would you be OK with perhaps more pain, fatigue, or moodiness than usual the day after a rope scene? In the long term, how about permanent marks, nerve damage, or deterioration of your condition? It's important to share this information honestly with your partner too, because they may not be comfortable with the same risks as you.

"I have no way of being certain that I will be aware of a sensory nerve issue caused by rope, so sensory nerve damage is a risk I am comfortable taking," says TheSuspendedDoll. "However, it might not be a risk my top considers worth taking, so I make absolutely sure they know how things work with me."

Go Team!

Tying with a supportive partner—someone you're on the same page with, who is willing and skilled enough to come up with possibly creative ties—can make a big difference in your experience. "A good rigger can modify appropriately and appreciates the information," EveningRopes says. "It can be a way to figure out who the good riggers are as well."

What kinds of partners are right for you is a highly individual decision. "I no longer tie with people who want a submissive, more 'passive' bottom," Lisa says. "The rope tops I play with are happy to get feedback in

Hikarin. Bondage and photo by FreemanForever

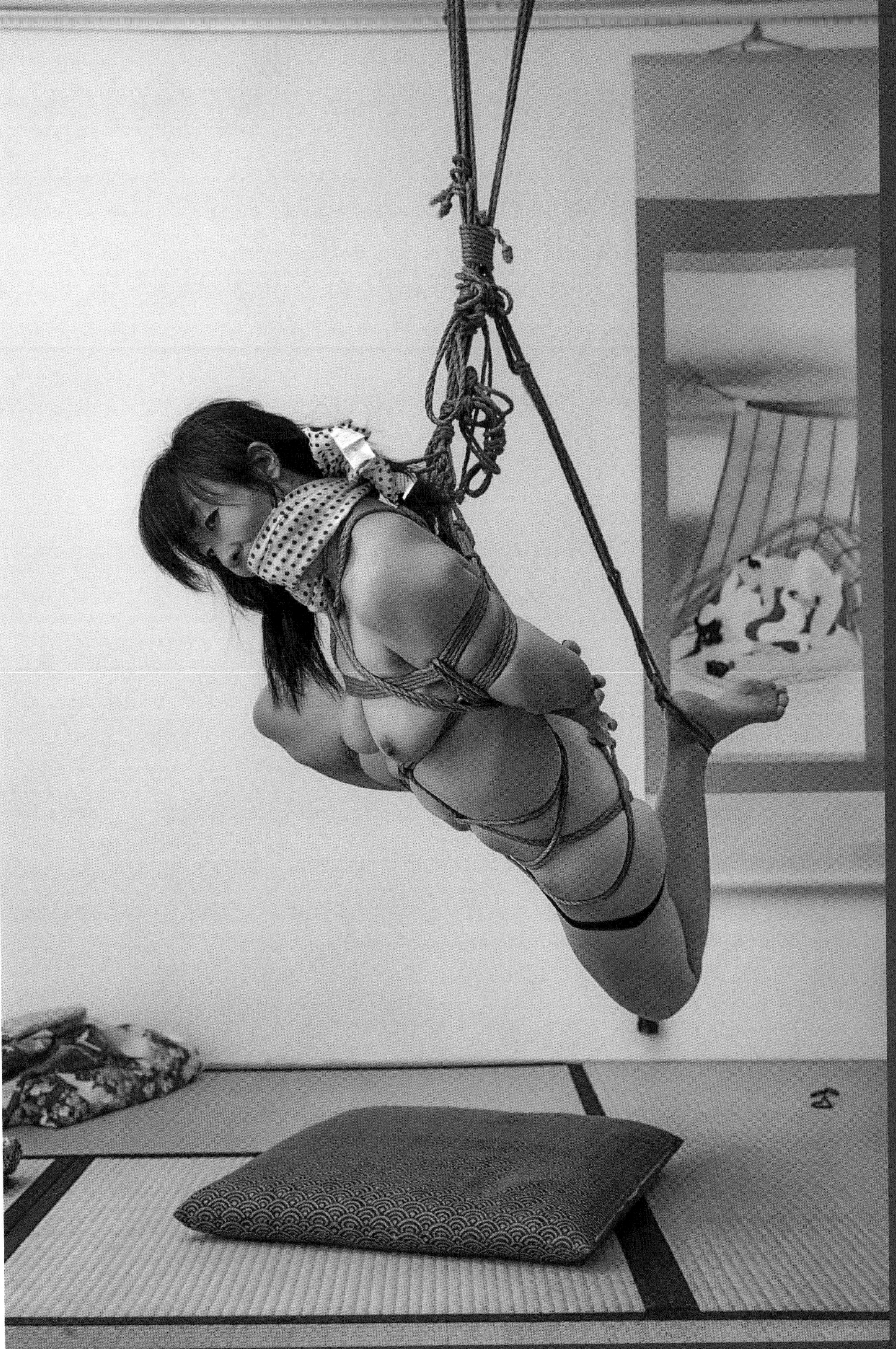

scene and to treat the scene as a partnership. If I'm expected to follow, I feel pressured to ignore my physical needs so as not to ruin the mood for my partner."

"I found that I don't do well with super-sadistic traditional kinbaku-loving riggers; they tend to go too far," Hikarin says. "I do enjoy receiving pain from someone who is willing to read me carefully."

"Being with my Sir, who is also my rigger, is a great comfort," bubblerat shares, "because he understands and listens to me, is always checking that I'm OK, and doesn't get annoyed if I ask to avoid certain areas/ties depending on what my body is feeling."

The benefits of a good partnership can go beyond just a single scene. "Having a regular rope top has helped me push myself further than before," nano_bites says. "Playing with someone that already knows where my sweet spots are and how far he can push me has helped me grow as a rope bottom."

Beyond your tying partner, who else could you have on your team to support you—physically, emotionally, mentally? "I'm fortunate to have many friends that like to snuggle with me after a class or scene," Redfeline says. "This helps me to relax and recharge." Alexis advises, "Find a community of people who understand you." As you may have figured out from previous chapters, I could go on and on about the benefits of community, so we'll leave it at that. FetLife groups include Kink and Disability; Fibromyalgia and Kink; Fibromyalgia (and other immune disorders) and Kink; Lupus and the Lifestyle; Blind Kink; and BDSMers in Wheelchairs and those who love them.

How about having a kink-aware medical professional on your team too? "Talk to your doctors about rope bondage as it relates to your condition," FeistyTex recommends. "Particularly try to find a physiotherapist who is supportive about helping you figure out how to modify ties, and can give you exercises to build up strength to compensate." EveningRopes shares that approach: "Be honest with your doctors. They might be less surprised than you'd think."

"Knowledge is power," kotori_kim says. "I immediately told my neurologist about my lifestyle—though at the time I was on a long and difficult break from it—and discussed how it might eventually change things. He told me to live my life. To stay active. That doing so would likely keep me going a lot longer. I strongly advocate finding a doctor people feel comfortable discussing their lifestyle with."

Whether you have just one person on your team or a whole slew of supporters, the important thing is to "embrace what you can do and align yourself with people who will help you do that," as kotori_kim puts it.

Pack Your Bags

A well-stocked rope bottoming bag is helpful for all rope bottoms, but may be especially important for those with physical issues. Water, snacks, and a lightweight blanket are great inclusions for starters. "Mine includes exercise balls for rolling, multiple layers of clothing (leg warmers, zip-up sweater), pain meds, candied ginger, Bio-Oil, Icy Hot," says LucytheBrave. Lady_Hunny_Bunny notes that a head support can be useful.

Consider what will help make you the most comfortable—a fluffy throw or cushy mat? Your own super-soft silk rope? A small pillow? Also bring along what will keep you safe, like medications, insulin, and an EpiPen. And don't forget any fun "extras," like a vibrator, a blindfold, and sex toys. Some bottoms also include arnica (in gel, cream, or tablet form) in their bags.

Persistence Pays Off

If you've read Chapter 1, you already know one of my favorite mottoes: "Patience. Persistence. Resilience." And it definitely applies here as an overarching principle. "Keep going," Alexis says. "Don't let one failure keep you from doing what you love. If it makes you feel beautiful, or complete, then keep going until you find things that work for you."

Even small efforts count. As kotori_kim says, "Whatever you accomplish is greater than choosing to abandon your goals because you think you can't." And TheSuspendedDoll offers this: "I think it is very important...to not get discouraged by what we can't do, and instead focus on being creative and enjoying the things we can do!"

But Know When to Say When

Having said that, there are times when *not* persisting is the right thing to do. "Know when to push yourself, and know when to focus on health. There's always time to play when you're feeling good, or at least not overly rubbish," His_anna says.

"I had to stop going to my weekly bondage night because the lack of sleep would mess me up for about five days after," recalls The Riss. "If rope bottoming is not your main source of income, do not let it wreck the balance you struggle to maintain in your life."

Sometimes it's hard to know when to say when. "The greatest challenge has been trying to make sure that I don't push too far in a session," Hikarin says. "The reason is not because of being in pain that day, but for the next day or afterwards." Keeping a log can help: Write down everything involved in the tying experience, including preparation, sleep, food eaten, and aftercare along with the types of ties, and then describe how you felt immediately afterward and in the days following. You may notice patterns over time and can adjust accordingly, which may mean canceling, postponing, or changing the rope session you had planned.

"Energy management is key for me," Blue says. "I need to know exactly in what condition my body is that day. Sometimes [I'll] cancel a session [or] change a full suspension into a partial and/or floorwork."

Bonus Benefits

You might think someone suffering from chronic pain or other physical issues would avoid activities that, you know, cause pain or other physical issues. But more than one rope bottom responding to the survey said rope bondage *makes things better.*

"Rope often helps to decrease my pain," says LucytheBrave. "Maybe it is the endorphins that are released afterwards, maybe it is the compression, maybe an inversion helps with back pain."

"What has helped me most in being a rope bottom is the relief I receive from pain while I am bound," says Ashley B., who has severe pain involving the sciatic nerve. Describing one particular scene, Ashley B. says: "Once I was unwrapped, I realized I was still pain-free and stress-free. The stress didn't return for three days."

Please talk with your doctor, however, if you want to try rope bondage for pain relief! You may have a completely different response; you may even make your condition worse. Here's a cautionary tale from BioKim, regarding a suspension: "I really felt amazing, though I was up for maybe five minutes at the most. The rest of the night was a mix of endorphins and suspicion about why I was feeling so surprisingly pain-free. I really should have enjoyed that time more! Long story short, the next three or four days were sheer hell and I could barely walk."

Interestingly, some bottoms report crossover benefits for overall health. "Pursuing healthy habits in food, exercise, and sleep has been amazing for both the MS and the rope bottoming," TheSuspendedDoll says. "I have lost over a hundred pounds and built up enough muscle to do things I never thought I could do when I first started bottoming for rope." Leaf-in-the-wind has also discovered extra benefits: "I'm more physically fit than ever, [which] I attribute to rope bottoming. It gives me motivation to keep up my physiotherapy, gives me courage to undertake other operations (knee surgery), and generally gives me purpose in life!"

Of course, only you can decide whether rope bottoming helps or hurts your condition and your life. But hopefully reading about the experiences here and the insight of all those who've been there has been only beneficial! Here's one last wonderful bit that I hope resonates with you as much as it does me, from Lilah Rose:

"Remember why you are doing rope, what it is you love, why it fulfills you. Remember that no one else is living your experience, and avoid making false comparisons. Allow yourself to enjoy what you can do, celebrate when you can do more, and be forgiving to yourself when you can't do as much."

Notes

1. http://www.fmcpaware.org/aboutfibromyalgia
2. https://medlineplus.gov/ency/article/000816.htm

Sharing the Journey

Naiia

Naiia is a BDSM educator; learn about her classes and events at www.naiiabound.com.

At the age of 38, I entered the public kink scene. It was so wonderful to feel fully and openly myself for the first time. I especially enjoyed bottoming to rope and learning to "fly" on the floor and in the air. I couldn't get enough and wanted to be inverted and spinning whenever I had the chance. I was at the top of my game and was able to demo bottom for my then play partner for his rope classes. I felt amazing in his rope and like I could do anything.

Fast-forward to age 43, with my now partner and I struggling to make our relationship work and him finally saying that I needed more help than he could provide. I was sure he was looking for a reason to leave, and then he said this: "No, I am looking for a reason to stay."

What happened next was a series of things that changed not only how I could play but my entire relationship with rope. I was diagnosed with dysthymia, a mild, long-term form of depression. Also severe depressive episodes, anxiety disorder, and premenstrual dysphoric disorder (PMDD)—all of which over the last two years I have learned to live with and treat.

But the medication lowered my pain tolerance, I gained weight—between 50 and 60 pounds—and I couldn't "fly" in the air anymore. The elevation in weight and the decrease in my pain tolerance made suspension too difficult for me. I felt like a failure and that I was letting my partners down. Why would anyone want to play with me? My anchor partner and I had been heavily into rough body play, and I wasn't able to do much of that anymore either. That first year of getting better mentally while my body betrayed me was intense. I started to talk to people and ask for help (something I am not good at), and found that I was not alone.

Depression lies. It is that simple. It tells us that we are worthless, useless, and a burden. Depression was ultimately the root cause of my weight gain and drop in pain tolerance. My partner had to tell me repeatedly that doing "those things"—the suspension bondage, the rough body play—were not the reasons he loved me. It took some time, but I realized that the stigma of mental illness, the fact that I needed the medication, my insecurity about my weight gain and ability to endure painful rope were what was holding me back. I learned that part of my healing and learning to love rope again required me to talk openly and publicly about my journey. I rediscovered my love of floorwork and "flying" (the ability to reach what some people call "ropespace," or an endorphin rush) on the ground.

I am also learning to tie for the first time and have found a passion for that as well. I have been doing a "one rope" technique and some rope dance. These things have helped me reconnect to my partner(s) through rope. They have given me the ability to feel strong and in control of my body again. Every time I learn something new I feel pride and a sense of moving forward.

The medication caused physical side effects, but along with therapy it gave me a chance to be and feel happy. It gave me a chance to fall in love with bondage again. It gave me a chance to discover new things about rope that I loved. I wouldn't change being able to feel those things for anything in the world. Not that every day is good, but I always know that there is a good chance the next day will be brighter.

Remember that playing in a way you love is possible—you just have to find it on your terms and not compare yourself to everyone else. For me, realizing this made all the difference between feeling inadequate and unfulfilled in my play, and rediscovering my passion and love of it.

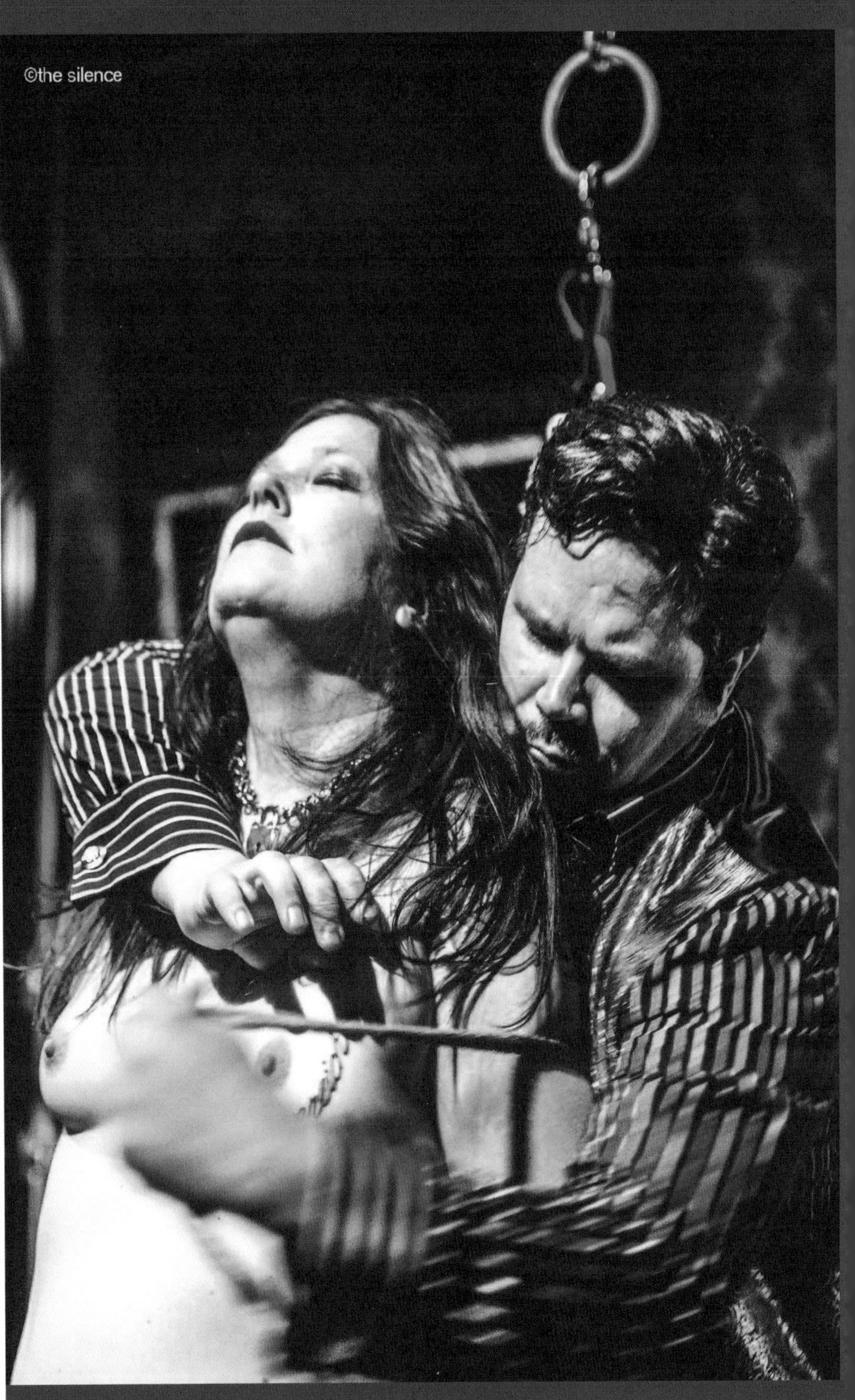

photo by The Silence

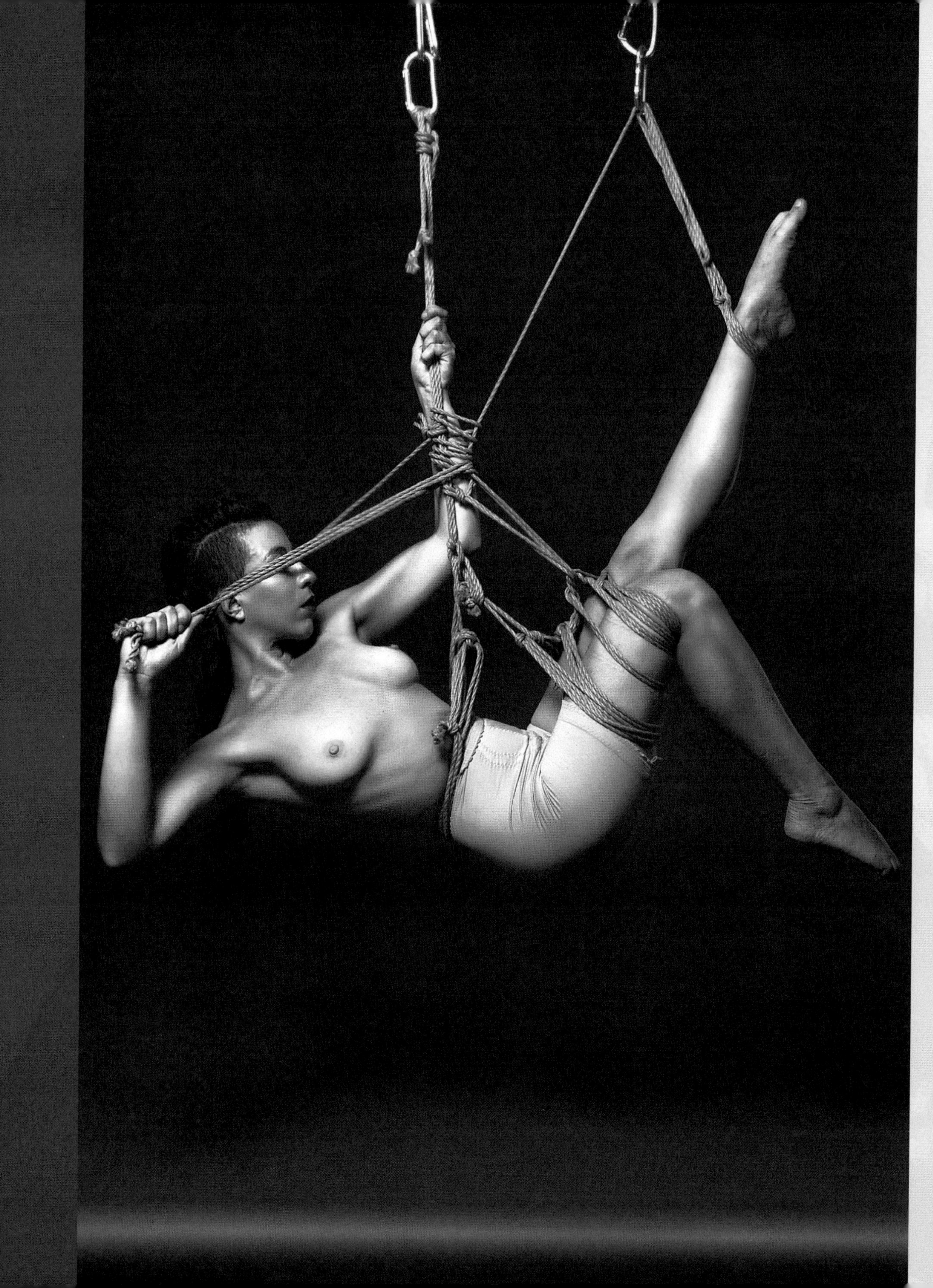

Chapter 11
For Self-Tyers

by Shay Tiziano

Shay Tiziano is an avid and creative self-suspender who has been teaching rope bondage for more than a decade. In addition to presenting and performing internationally, she is the host of BENT (San Francisco's biggest dungeon event), cofounder of RemedialRopes.com, producer of Twisted Windows, and education director for the SF Citadel and Dark Odyssey: Surrender.

"Self-tying is when I get to express myself most with rope. I'm fully independent, and the only constraints are my own limits, as both a top and bottom."
—Abbystract

"I love to fly, I love pushing my body...basically, I self-suspend for the sheer joy of it." —ANakedFlame

The idea that there is a "right way" to do or experience rope is bullshit. Self-tying bucks common thinking about bondage in many ways, and self-bondage practitioners face a number of unique challenges. Some of these challenges are intrinsic in a practical sense (difficulty reaching behind your back to tie knots, for instance), some stem from self-bondage still being a niche activity, and some are a mix of the two.

Self-bondage is very much an emerging practice, but it's been amazing to watch it expand over the past few years. I've been producing events in San Francisco since 2005, and in my first five years of hosting I saw all of two people engaged in self-bondage at my events. At my most recent party, I saw five different people self-suspend! I'm seeing smaller-scale increases in self-bondage as I travel around the country to different kink conferences as well—it's fabulous to see this practice spreading and becoming more accepted in the kink community!

"Wanking Around" in Rope

"I've had people assume that I'm self-tying because I don't have anyone to tie me, which makes far too many incorrect assumptions about me." —Abbystract

"There is a feeling of power and autonomy to satisfying my own needs that makes self-tying a very beautiful and deep experience for me." —Cozima

For many people, self-tying is like rope masturbation. As with masturbation, some people do it because they don't have a partner (or their partner is not available). This is a common approach, but it's important not to conceive of self-tying *only* as a thing people do when there's no one around to tie them. Many of us prefer to self-tie, even when there is the option of partnered tying—just as you might sometimes (or always) prefer masturbation to partnered sex.

Some of the reasons to self-tie include:

- Freedom to set your own pace, explore, and satisfy yourself without feeling the need to please and perform for a partner
- Desiring a very specific type of rope experience
- Wanting a physical challenge or a "rope workout"
- Fitting a "rope fix" into a short window of time
- Practicing ties (rope science or "lab time")
- Learning about rope bottoming

Glü Wür in self-bondage. Photo by Marianana Gallardo Klein

- Challenging yourself or simply adding more variety to the way you experience rope
- Wanting to experience both topping and bottoming

Let It Flow

"Self-bondage takes my anxiety, anger, or sadness and dissolves every single feeling till it's only pain and focus on the knots." —Hyena

"I find it cathartic to be able to 'disappear' in my own world." —Twitch-the-switch

My experience of self-bondage is often about getting into a flow state. The idea of flow originates with Mihaly Csikszentmihalyi, one of the pioneers of the scientific study of happiness.[1] He defines flow as "a state in which people are so involved in an activity that nothing else seems to matter; the experience is so enjoyable that people will continue to do it…for the sheer sake of doing it."[2]

When I'm being tied by someone else, I often have a hard time letting go of my brain chatter and worries: *Is my top thinking that the hip harness makes my legs and butt look funny? Are they enjoying tying me? How are they securing that line?* It just keeps going and going.

It's even worse when I'm tying someone else: *Are they enjoying this? What's the risk of me giving them nerve damage in this tie? Wait, did they say they did or did not like rope dragging across their nipples???* Self-bondage removes all those questions and worries, and allows me to be fully present in the moment, mind and body working harmoniously.

I'm an exhibitionist and often self-suspend at dungeon events. I love having a crowd watching me, yet I'm hardly aware they're there. I become completely focused on my body and the rope, moving and flowing with the knots and my limbs. I feel the energy of people watching me, and it feeds into what I'm doing, but it's also not *for* them, as I'm totally absorbed in bondage, flying, and sensation.

Building Endurance and Body Awareness

"I started self-suspending to get over my fear of suspension in general." —CedoPet

"Self-tying has put me on a quest to be more fit so I will have the energy to do more." —Ebi McKnotty

It often takes time to build up a tolerance to the intense sensations and emotions, including fear, that can be associated with being tied up. As you gain experience, your body learns that you felt all the things and not only survived but actually had fun!

While certainly there are real dangers of bondage, learning to distinguish warning signs of damage from sensations that are intense but not harmful is an essential and crucial rope bottoming skill. For me, self-bondage has been an invaluable tool to learn to make these distinctions, build up my endurance, and feel more confident and calm both with tying myself and being tied by others.

My favorite quote on this subject comes from NASA: "It is a defining characteristic of human sensory and motor systems that they habituate with repeated use."[3] I find it is much easier to habituate with self-bondage, because I'm completely in charge of the experience and have total control of when it stops and how far it goes. The skills I build in this way not only enhance my self-suspension, they also transfer to partnered bondage.

On the Floor vs. in the Air

"I find that the motivations behind self-bondage and self-suspension are the complete opposite. In self-suspension there's pride in one's achievement. In self-bondage I find there´s the desire to feel ashamed, to be degraded (if only by oneself)."
—leaf-in-the-wind

It's fashionable these days to decry the "race to get in the air" and encourage people to spend a lot of time doing floorwork before moving on to suspension. While I see the wisdom there, I also think the ways we measure "experience" are pretty random. If I've been tying up my partner once a month for five years, do I have more experience than someone who dove into the rope community six months ago and has been tying eight hours a week since then? I've seen people with experience in other types of aerial or rope practices (professional theater rigging, trapeze, silks, even sailing) progress very quickly into suspension. We don't all start from the same place, and it's ridiculous to proclaim that we should all follow the same path.

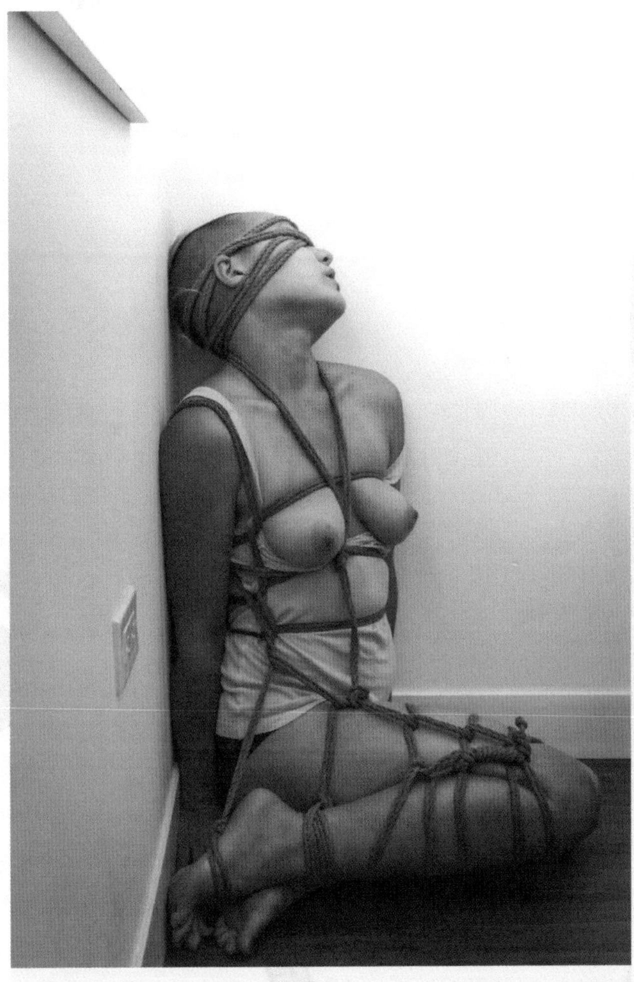

Jagrend in self-bondage. Photo by BoBoChee

It's also quite fashionable to extoll the virtues of floorwork in general, with some declaring it more connective than suspension. While I don't think suspension should be exalted as the ultimate pinnacle of advanced bondage, neither do I think that floorwork is automatically more authentic in some way. Suspension and floorwork are quite different activities and may interest different people, at different times, with different partners—and that is totally OK!

I find the floor/suspension divide is especially apparent in self-bondage. People who are primarily interested in self-suspension (as I am) are often quite a different lot from those focused on self-tying on the ground, which often involves rather extreme immobilization and a humiliation angle. It's been my experience that self-tying on the ground tends to be more explicitly sexual (frequently involving genital bondage or stimulation, or done as part of masturbation), while self-suspension is often more like training or performing on a trapeze, with little to no direct sexual stimulation involved.

This isn't to say suspension types never do floorwork. We do, whether just to practice a new futomomo or as an enjoyable stand-alone activity. But to think of it as a clean progression from floorwork to partial suspension to full suspension is a misconception, even more so to think people should progress through these types in certain periods of time, and this is especially true for self-suspension. While my own perspective is much more focused on self-suspension than on tying on the floor, floorwork-focused self-tying is very popular in its own right, and many self-tyers explore both!

Challenges and Helpful Ideas

Now that we've covered some background, motivations, and misconceptions, let's dive into some specific challenges of self-bondage and ways to address them.

Learning the Ropes

"Not a lot of classes are out there for self-tying or suspension, and a lot of suspension stuff relies way too heavily on the TK [takate-kote], which I obviously cannot tie on myself." —Azura Rose

"I learned from videos online and a lot of trial and error." —scuddle

"Finding resources for more advanced or unusual techniques is really difficult." —AltBronte

Self-bondage has a relatively high bar for entry, combining the requirements of bottoming (body awareness, health, etc.) with the requirements of topping (technical knowledge, possessing the physical supplies, etc.). It demands an extremely high degree of knowledge about your own body and physical limits.

Self-tying is still not widely or publicly practiced, so learning the how-tos is often the first challenge people face. When I started experimenting with self-suspension, I didn't know a single person in my area I could look to as a mentor, and there were zero classes offered...and I live in San Francisco! I'd only seen a handful of people self-suspend, none of whom were located anywhere near me. I couldn't even find videos on the topic (I've since made a few myself, and these days there are some others out there, but there are still surprisingly few online resources for self-bondage). I ended up taking what I knew from years of experience with partnered bondage and applying it to self-tying. This is reasonable but hardly optimal, as the experience doesn't translate 100 percent.

Since many of us who do self-bondage are basically self-taught, we tend to struggle a lot with imposter syndrome ("a feeling of phoniness in people who believe that they are not intelligent, capable or creative despite evidence of high achievement."[4])—this makes it extra challenging to find someone willing to teach self-bondage. I still struggle with this when I teach suspension in general, and self-suspension particularly.

Self-tying is a very creative form of bondage. While I'd encourage you to find a mentor and take classes if you can, sometimes it's simply not possible. There is a lot to be said for the combined wisdom of the community; however, there is *also* much to be said for being creative and independently coming up with what works for *you*. Use established bondage safety wisdom and skills to keep yourself from being harmed, but remember that particular ties are not the "twue" way. People created them...and you can also create your own ties! Self-bondage is an amazing opportunity to workshop and experiment with new and innovative ideas.

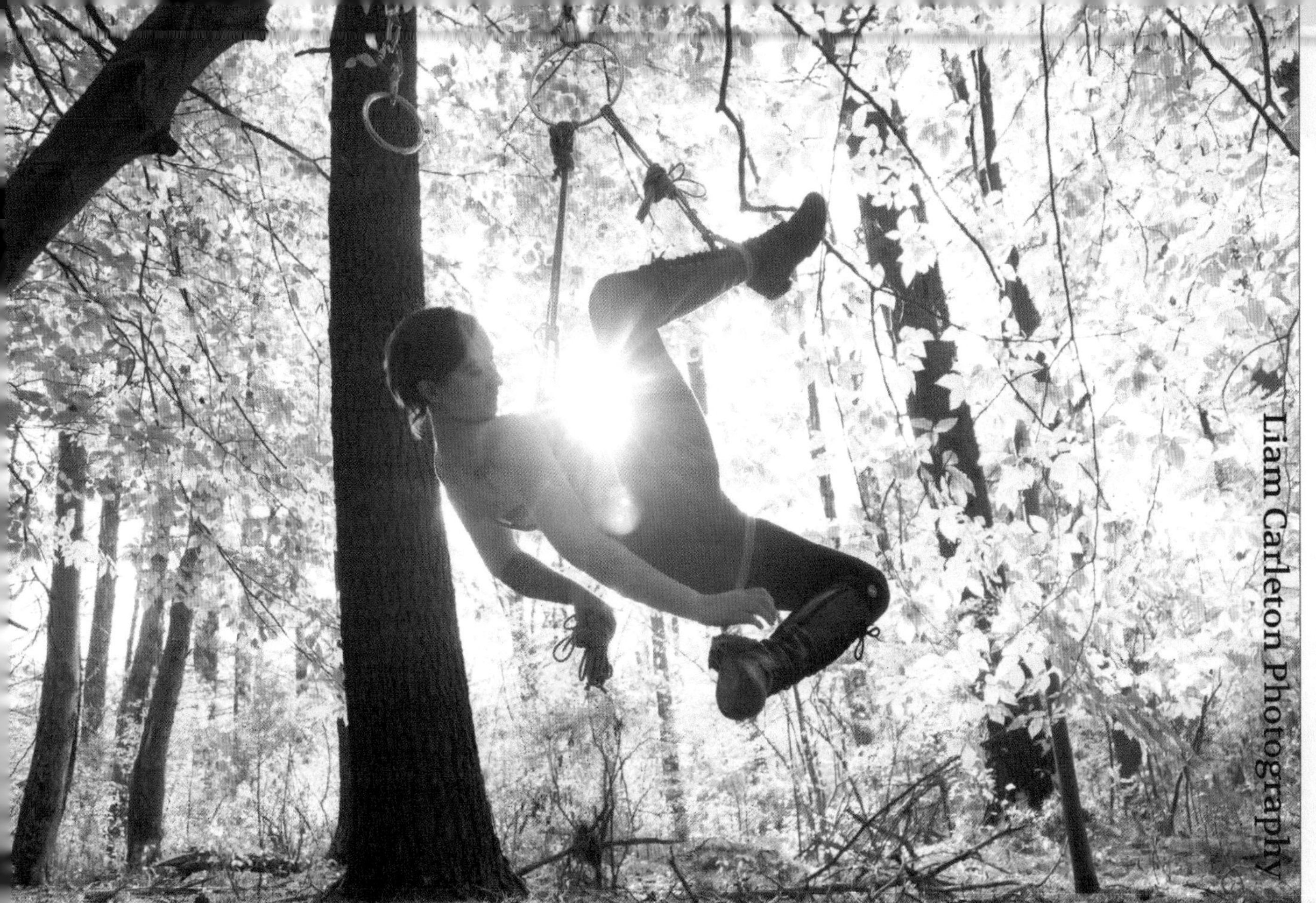

Abbystract in self-bondage.
Photo by Liam Carleton Photography

While I've played around with some extremely intricate rigs over the years, self-suspension doesn't have to be complicated. A pretty common method is to tie a suspension-worthy single column around the waist (tying on top of a high-quality corset makes it significantly more comfortable) and simply suspend from that, or from that and two additional loops that can be swapped between different limbs (this is sometimes called an open-loop suspension). It only needs to be complicated if you like it that way!

> **Important!**
>
> With self-suspension, it's crucial to start getting down before you are overtired—you must have enough body awareness to save some mental and physical reserves to safely get to the ground. When undoing a suspension, generally it gets worse before it gets better; you will usually make the suspension more strenuous just at the point when you're almost done, because undoing lines to come down will make the suspension more intense. If you're experimenting, take all these factors into account, and work with a spotter—more on this in the "Finding a Spotter" section.

Lack of Community Support

"Until recently, I think self-bondage wasn't commonly accepted, so you'd get odd looks, like, 'Why are you doing that by yourself?'" —adrenaline_lust

"I feel that self-bondage is seen as taboo/perverted in others' eyes, even in the BDSM community. That makes

it hard to start publicly learning and makes safety extra challenging." —sincognitoy

Many areas don't have regular self-bondage classes (as we discussed), or a lot of established mentors. In my home community, I've collaborated with other local self-suspenders to build a number of skill-share events, munches, and similar types of gatherings. It has worked out amazingly well—we've built a fantastic little community, and the number of self-suspenders at events has increased exponentially as a result.

You're almost certainly not the only person in your area interested in self-tying or self-suspension. There are even several self-bondage groups on FetLife (type "self-bondage" in the search box at the top). If a local self-tying community doesn't already exist (and odds are it doesn't), create a FetLife group called "Self-Bondage in [Place You Live]" and post about it in some of the local bondage groups, and/or experiment with a meet-up at a local event or a munch. You could also host a mini takeover of an established rope event, skill share, or munch (as long as its leaders are onboard, of course).

Don't worry if your local self-tying community starts out small. Know that it just takes someone to make the first steps, and that person can be you—even if you're just a curious beginner. Building a community takes time. Have awareness of your own internalized imposter syndrome and realize what you have to share and offer.

Finding a Spotter

"Always use a spotter! I have had to use my spotter many times to get me off the ring, especially when I didn't have upline management skills." —OnionSkin

"The proper answer is, 'Yes, I always have a spotter.' The truth is less cut and dried. Sometimes I judge my risks of the tie I am going to practice and proceed on my own. Other times I do the smart thing and wait." —Maralade

"I've never had a spotter. I have a lot of body awareness and previous experience with aerial apparatus, so safety is something that I've always taken upon myself to feel out." —Anna

"Once I began doing transitions, I started to keep two people with me at all times. I broke those rules a few times...and then I had my only truly bad experience, and since then I have never self-tied alone." —Twitch-the-switch

I will definitely go on record recommending that you never self-suspend alone. In terms of self-tying, risk isn't "all or nothing," but rather exists on a gradient, within which you must use your own judgments and make decisions according to your own risk tolerance. Probably most of us have practiced single-column ties on our ankles alone in our living room, and it's hard to think of what could go wrong in that scenario. However, being bound more intensely and alone (either self-tying or being left alone by a top) is highly dangerous, as fatalities can attest to.

Anytime you're attaching yourself to a hard point, I'd strongly recommend having a spotter. This also applies for ties that carry the possibility of asphyxia (when the body is deprived of oxygen), including positional asphyxia (where pressure on the chest impairs breathing, for example in a hogtie) and neck rope. Practicing self-tying a futomomo or a basic chest harness you probably can safely do alone; practicing a new facedown to face-up suspension transition, not so much.

Naturalturn in self-bondage. Photo by anonymous

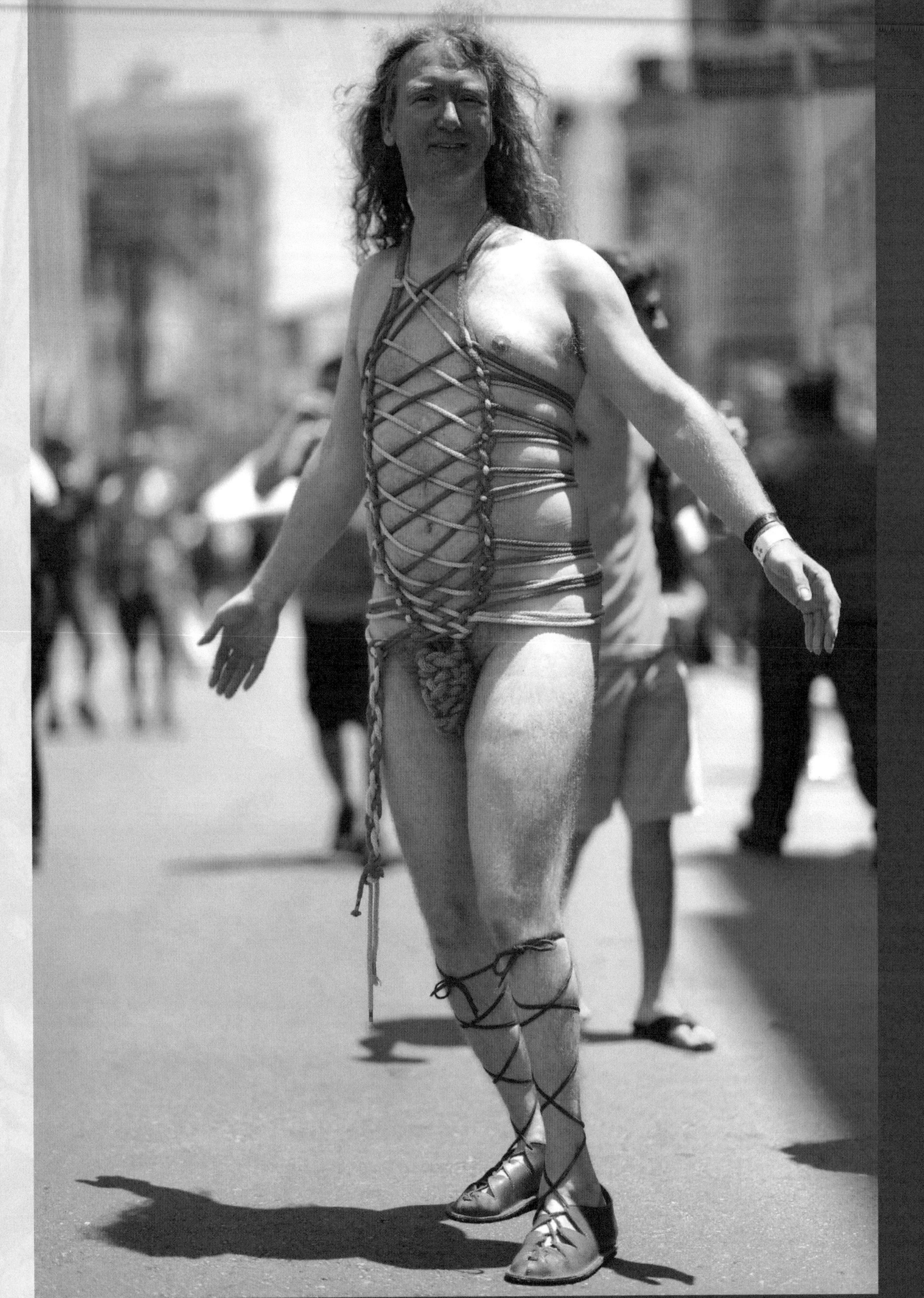

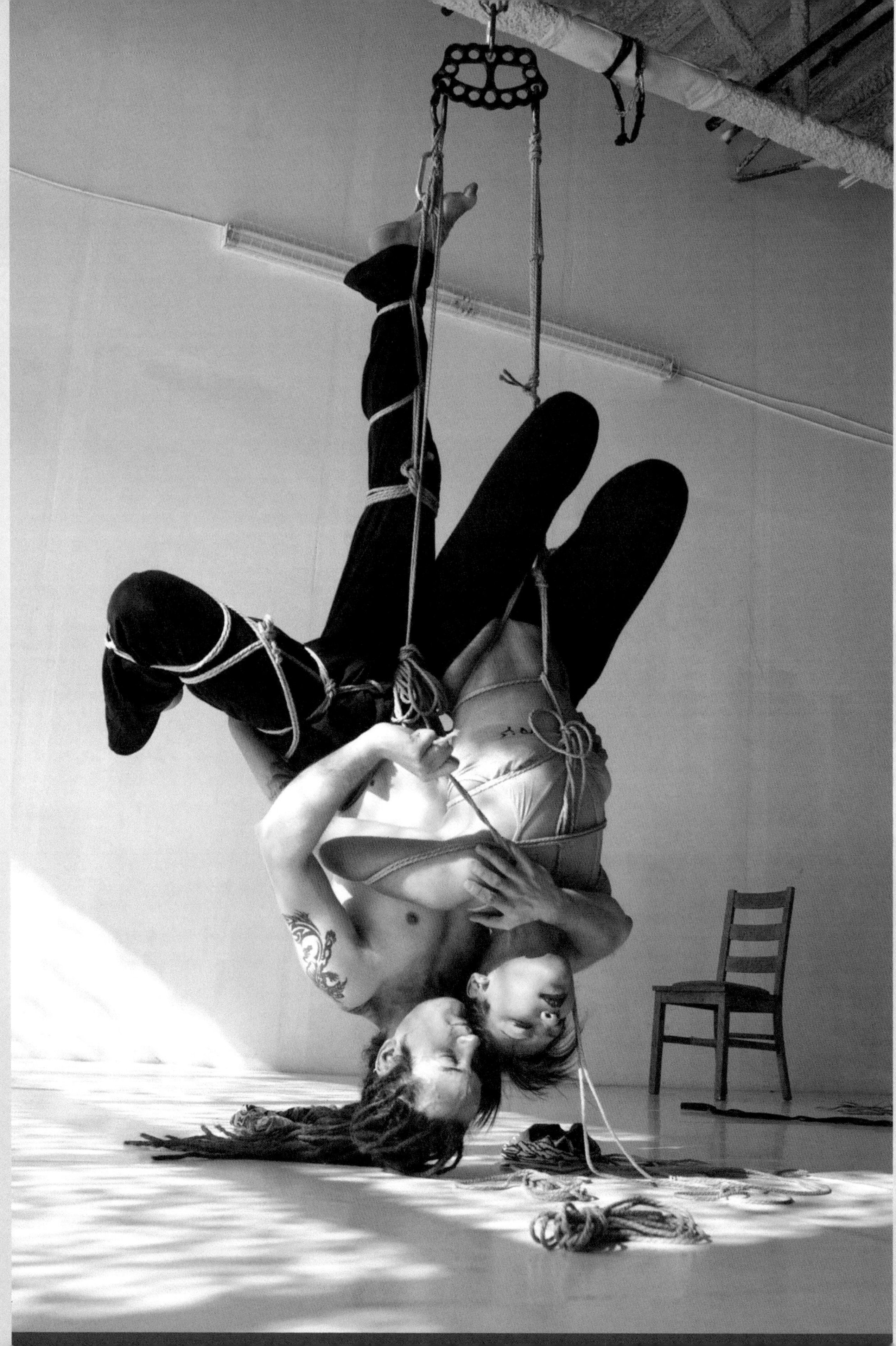

It's important for me to have a spotter even when I'm suspending with lots of people watching, because I have *zero* awareness of what's going on around me. If someone comes into my space when I'm spinning and moving, I won't even notice and they'll probably catch a foot (or high heel) to the head. My spotters need to both keep people out of my space and also be extremely careful how they approach me themselves.

Given that many people get into self-bondage because they don't have a partner to tie them, how can you find a spotter? Some ways are:

- Finding a friend who also self-ties, and taking turns spotting each other
- Finding someone who's interested in learning self-bondage and exchanging mentoring for spotting
- Recruiting housemates
- Practicing at a peer rope workshop or similar gathering where others are available and willing to help if needed
- Asking people assigned to monitor safety at parties and events, often called dungeon monitors (DMs) or playspace monitors. Responses will vary based on the knowledge, comfort level, and duties of the individual DMs, but it's worth making the inquiry!

One of the things to keep in mind is that it's not enough to have a pair of eyes and ears—those eyes and ears needs to be attached to a person who can recognize an emergency and know what to do. What if you pass out? What if you fall? Do they know where your safety scissors or rescue hook is, and how to use it? Do they know what procedure to follow in an emergency? There are entire classes offered on this subject—take one if you can, and if you have a regular spotter, encourage them to go as well. At least talk through some possible scenarios, and make sure your spotter actually knows how to provide assistance.

It's also crucial to discuss with your spotter how they can best help facilitate your solo scene. Some self-tyers like their spotter to provide anticipatory service, such as moving objects out of the way, offering water, helping pick up that piece of rope that's just out of reach, etc. For others, that sort of "help" completely disrupts their scene, and they want to be left totally alone unless they ask for assistance or clearly have an emergency.

Do you want your spotter to watch you intently, because that's what makes you feel safe? Or does someone staring at you seem too intrusive and you'd rather they were there, listening and nearby, but mostly focused on something else? Consider what will make your solo scenes fly, and don't expect your spotter to be a mind reader—clearly communicate what you need from them.

As many self-tyers see spotting as a service someone provides them, it's common for people to give back to their spotters in various ways. This can be as simple as taking turns spotting each other, offering them a massage afterwards, or plying them with baked goods. Consider how to provide an exchange that energetically feeds everyone involved, and you'll get to do happy (and safe) self-bondage with spotters who will be delighted to come back and spot for you again!

Scenus Interruptus

"I've gotten interrupted by ignorant bystanders, as well as asked why I would want to tie myself when there are riggers around who want to tie me." —Kel Bowie

Kim Nova and Miss Avery in dual self-bondage. Photo by RachelKi

Sharing the Journey

Shay Tiziano

I've always been a "rope as a means to an end" (i.e., "tie me up and fuck me") type rather than a "rope as an end in itself" (i.e., "spend two hours putting me in an intricate rope dress and leave me to float in subspace") type. When I first learned bondage, I spent about four years not feeling the need to tie or be tied with anything more complicated than a basic single or double column.

I eventually experimented with suspension bottoming a few times, but ended up feeling like a "bad" bottom when I'd do pickup play, because I couldn't sustain ties for very long and I was mostly interested in exploring how I could move once I was in the air. I kicked a couple of my first riggers in the head—they apparently didn't expect me to toss around the way I did! Not wanting to risk the safety of my community's bondage tops, I set out to learn self-suspension. I never was very interested in upping my self-tying floorwork game—I'm a goal-oriented person, and I wanted to fly!

In 2012, I was put in a mobile (marionette) suspension at a Dark Odyssey event, and I was instantly hooked. I didn't know anyone in my area who did that kind of suspension, so I went home and immediately started trying to reverse-engineer it. Still a "means to an end" type, I was motivated to see how I could use suspension to enhance movement rather than to get in the air only to be immobilized, which was the only type of bondage I'd seen up to that point.

In the bondage community, this category of ties is sometimes (derisively) called "circus bondage," which is a label I actually embrace—I'm an exhibitionist and always wanted to join the circus. Once I'd come up with a reasonable approximation of the marionette rig, I kept working on new variations to challenge myself, make it quicker and easier to self-rig, and explore different types of dynamic suspension. There's always more to learn and try, and I look forward to many more years of experimentation!

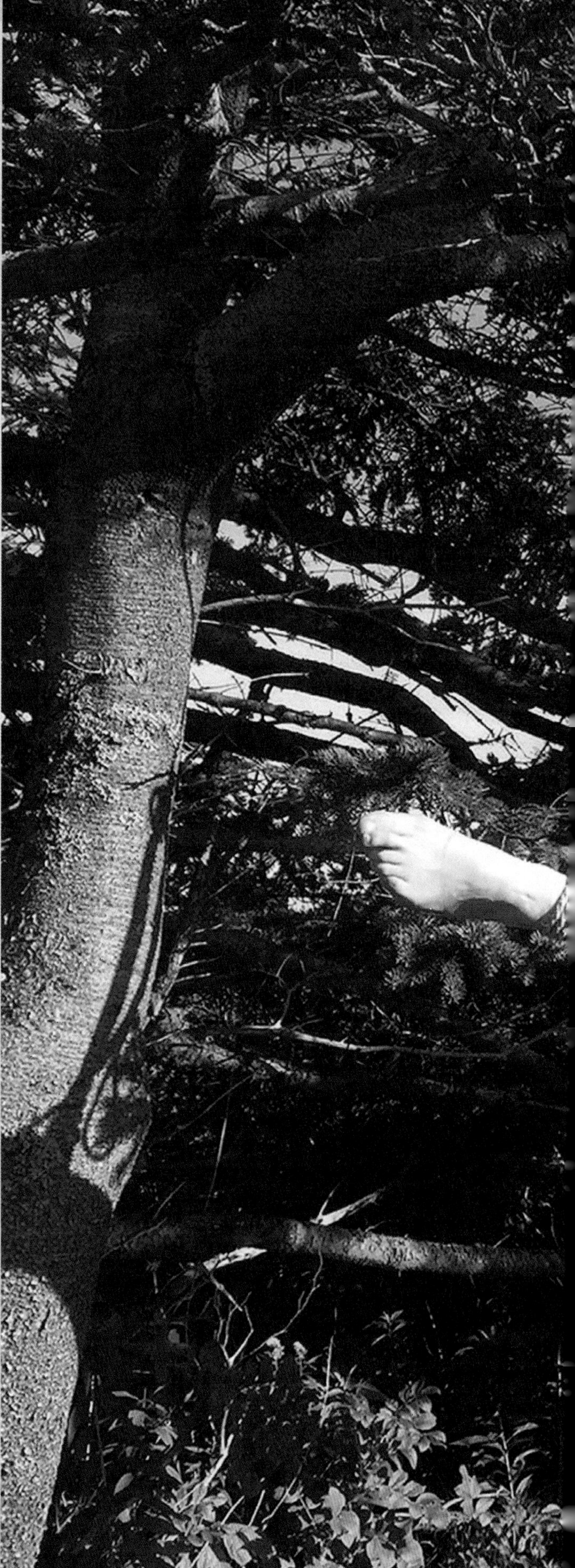

Shay Tiziano in self-bondage. Photo by Gabriel

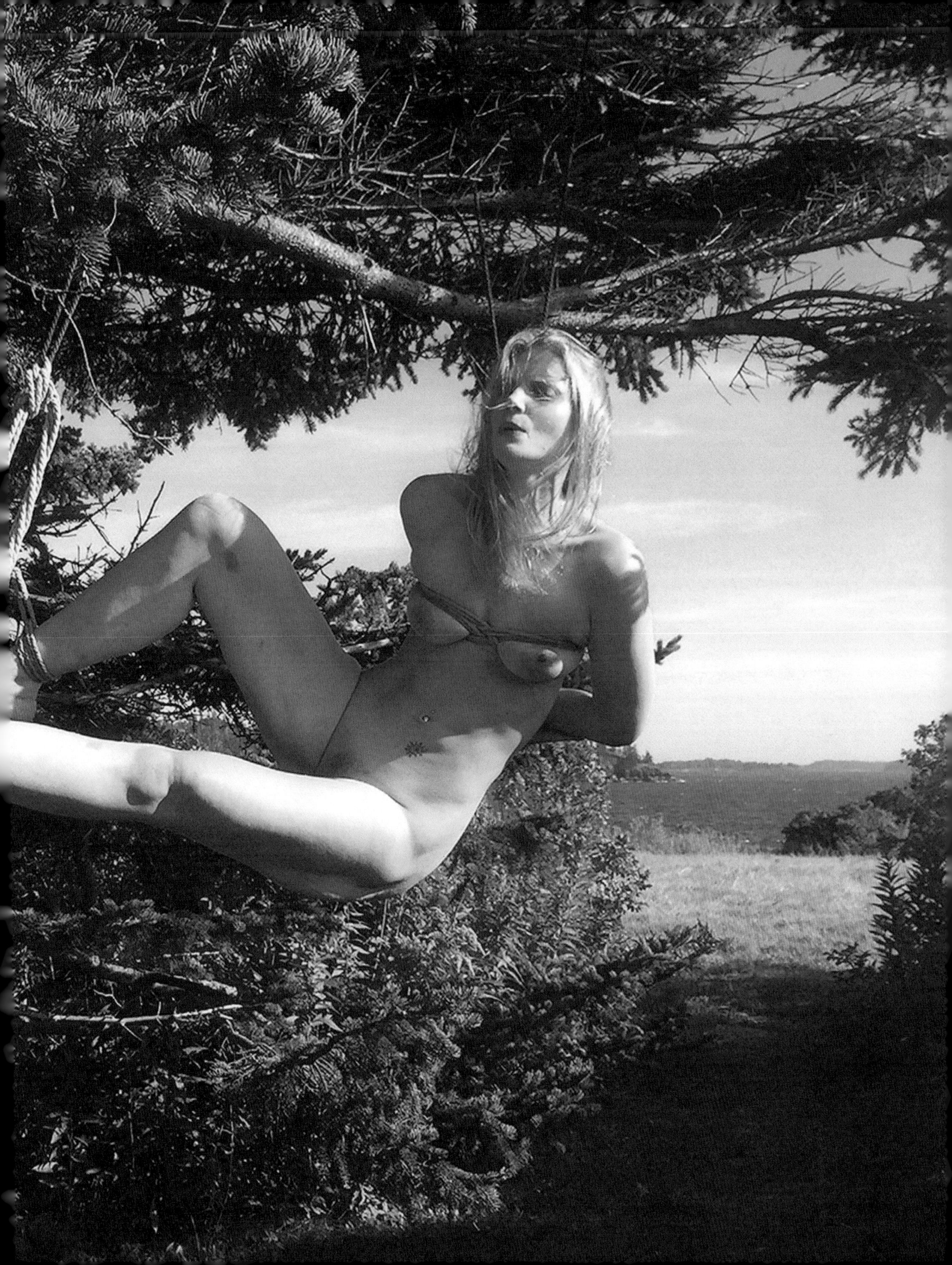

"One problem with doing self-bondage is all the domly doms trying to 'help.'" —volpetta

"A big challenge has been getting my space to be respected as a scene. I have a headspace as much as any D/s [Dominant/submissive] pair do, and being interrupted with 'Do you need help?' from people breaks that headspace." —Azura Rose

Being interrupted while doing self-bondage at a venue or an event where others are present is a common issue. This can take many different forms—clueless observers getting too close, other riggers stepping in to be "helpful," concerned dungeon monitors (DMs) who are unfamiliar with self-bondage asking questions, or even sexual harassment from bystanders. Having a visible spotter helps head off these types of interruptions, and often a spotter can stop someone before they disturb your space.

When you are doing self-bondage in a venue that has DMs, I'd highly recommend talking with them before you start setting up. They may be able to facilitate your scene (advising on best location, sharing any special rules or guidelines you'll need to follow, etc.). It's extremely helpful to tell the DM who your spotter is, or whether you're expecting anyone to enter into your self-bondage scene.

Different venues will have very different guidelines, and many DMs are not very knowledgeable about bondage in general (let alone self-bondage), so taking the initiative and checking in is something I highly recommend.

Injuries

"I've given myself sensory nerve damage. I've accidentally bruised myself and given myself rope burn. I've overstretched muscles, and I think overworked some and underworked others." —Kel Bowie

"I have never had an injury from self-bondage. I tend to put myself into very comfortable ties, and because I am doing it to myself, I know exactly where I'm putting the ropes, how long I plan to stay up, how much tension I want on a rope, etc." —adrenaline_lust

"I've had small injuries. Slight nerve compression causing numbness in a finger for a couple weeks. Pulled a muscle hauling my weight up too quickly once." —Anna

The risk of getting injured in rope isn't unique to self-tyers, of course. But the risks involved in self-tying are a bit different than for partnered tying.

Getting on Your Nerves

Nerve damage is a major concern in the bondage community. The interplay of five basic factors determines whether a bondage nerve injury happens and how severe it is:[5]

- Individual differences in nerve vulnerability
- Anatomical location (where on the body you are tying)
- Duration of compression
- Severity of compression
- Stretch/stress positioning

It is certainly possible to get a nerve injury from floorwork. However, due to the increased loads involved, suspension is generally higher risk than tying on the ground. The risk of nerve damage in self-suspension (as opposed to partnered suspension) is relatively low, as it tends to be dynamic (involving moving around a lot, rather than staying in one position and

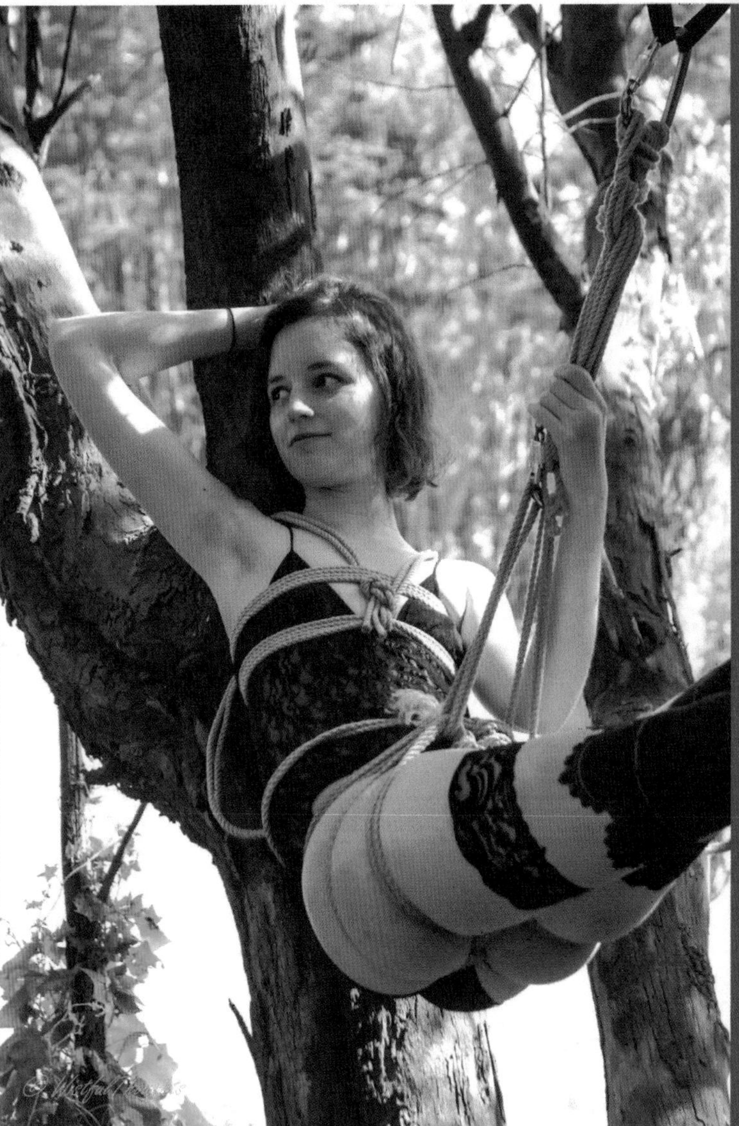

Hyena in self-bondage.
Photo by Wistful Thoughts

putting pressure on any given nerve for an extended period of time) and commonly utilizes lower-risk ties (hip harness vs. TK) with shorter duration. However, your body awareness may be altered as you take on both the top and bottom role, and you may get stuck in a position for longer than intended or strain yourself trying to self-rescue.

It's important to be aware of different kinds of nerve pain—numbness, burning, a sharp or cold feeling, tingling—and do frequent self-checks. Be sure you always have a reliable, safe cutting implement (such as a safety shears) within reach, and know when and how to safely use it.

I have given myself a nerve injury doing self-suspension—I damaged the iliohypogastric nerve, which is vulnerable below the iliac crest. I'd never even heard of the iliohypogastric nerve until I damaged it! As self-tyers do some unique bondage, we may also face some unique risks. It's important to broaden your sense of risk awareness beyond simply checking your arm for radial nerve damage or outer thigh for numbness.

See Chapter 2 for more on anatomy and nerve damage.

Dropping Yourself

"I recently had a near miss...I just managed to catch myself from falling. It would only have been less than a foot, but would've caused some sort of damage." —Angel666Sub

"I had a homemade hoist rigged up that overheated. While trying to get loose (I was about 70 percent into an upside-down self-suspension), I fell backwards and almost broke my elbow when I hit the ground." —David

"An upline attached to a chest harness slipped from my hands and I was inverted very quickly by accident once. It scared the crap out of me, and I'm grateful my hip harness was solid and that the upline was safely attached!" —Sarahblueberry

One of the first self-suspensions I ever saw was a performance at a major rope event in which the performer dropped themself while attempting a tricky transition. There were mats underneath, and

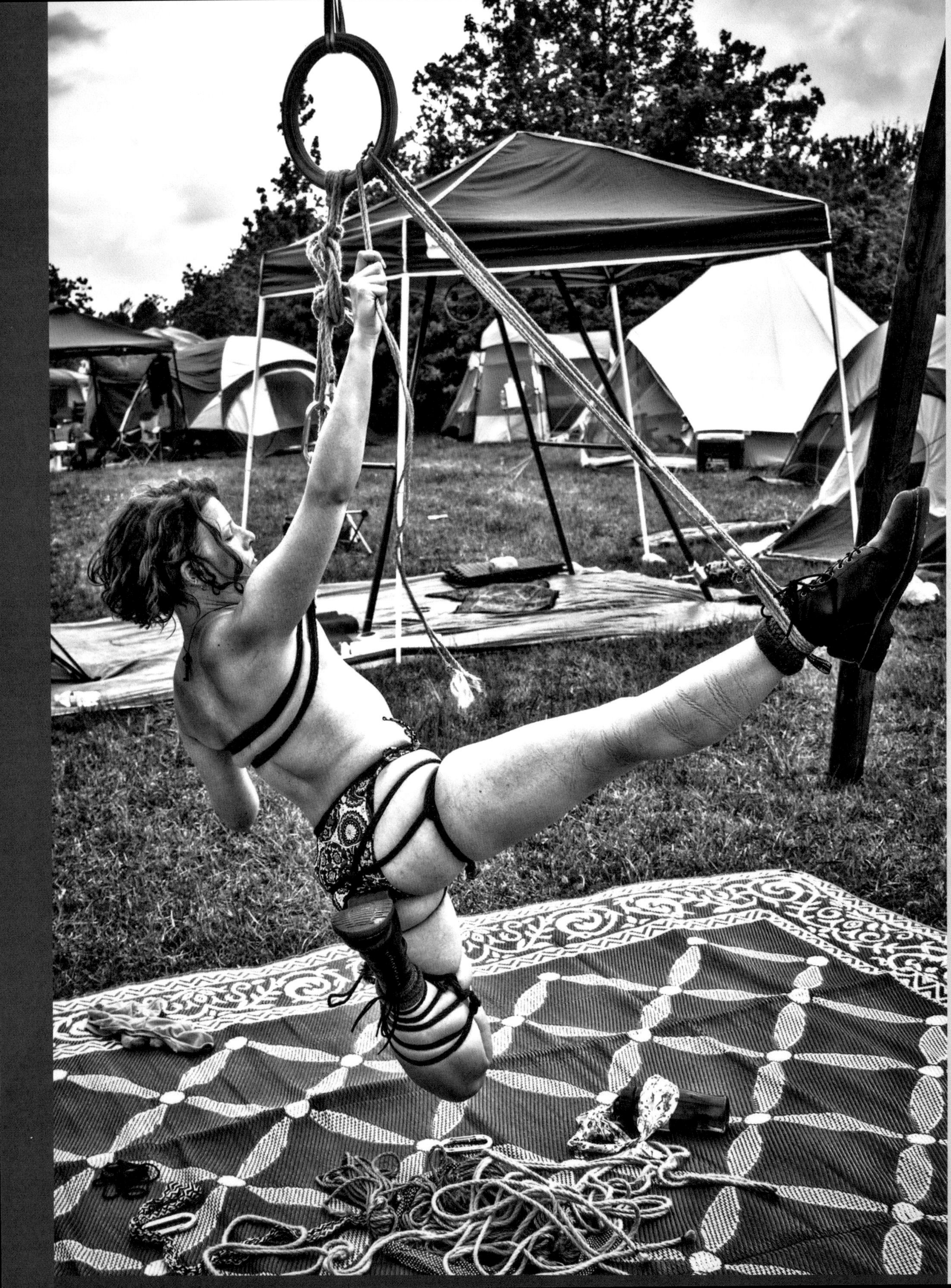

they recovered quickly and with no significant injury (aside, perhaps, from a bruised ego).

Drops from suspension are relatively rare but can have devastating results. Some precautions you can take to decrease the odds of a dangerous self-drop:

- When you're learning (or experimenting with something new), hang your hardpoint very low—being an inch off the ground *totally counts* as a suspension!
- Think about what your critical line is (the line that's keeping your head from hitting the ground) and don't adjust or remove one critical line before completely securing another. For example, securely tie off a chest harness, then raise and securely tie off the hips, *then* disconnect the chest for an inversion...and securely tie off the chest again before lowering the hips. Adjusting critical lines on the fly is a more advanced and risky move, so work your way up to it.
- Use rated rope for your uplines (see the rope kit section on page 162) and properly rated hardware.
- Assess your hardpoint and use your own judgment regarding its safety.
- Use a crash pad, or at least a mat. I have a crash pad of the type that climbers use for bouldering. It was a bit expensive, but I dropped myself onto it once (when I miscalculated my height for a gravity boot-based transition) and can assure you that the investment was totally worthwhile.

Selfless Self-Tying

"I like to experiment and try things out on myself that I then later try on other people when I tie them. Self-tying provides an opportunity to take risks that I may not feel comfortable doing on someone else." —SpecialLibrarian

"I learned more in my first self-suspension than I did in half a dozen previous times suspending my partner." —Pendorbound

"I find self-tying and self-suspending give me an insight into what the person being tied is feeling and experiencing, which I hope will make me a better rigger." —Angel666Sub

Difficulty with finding instruction and mentoring aside, self-bondage is an amazing way to learn how to tie, and I would love to see more people using it as a learning tool. For many other types of BDSM play, we encourage people to start on the bottom, or at least experience play from the bottom's perspective as part of the learning process. While I don't think this is necessary in every case, I do think it's extremely helpful to have the feedback and experience of being in rope.

I also admit to getting a bit judgey when I watch certain rope practices—I'll think to myself, if more riggers had been in rope *ever*, they wouldn't tie the way they do. An experienced bottom with good body awareness and the ability to give clear feedback is invaluable for a beginning rigger, but no bottom can give you the instant, unambiguous input that you get from experiencing *your* ties with *your* body.

Many of the people I've talked to about self-tying mentioned that they self-tie partly so they can practice or experiment without worrying about injuring someone else. An extremely common theme was: "I'd much rather risk an error when my own body is on the line than take a chance with someone else's." This is also one of my personal motivators for self-suspending.

At the same time, don't make the mistake of thinking that your subjective experiences with your own body in rope will translate perfectly when you transition

Kel Bowie in self-bondage. Photo by gaping_lotus

from tying yourself to tying other people. I have found that it's challenging for me when I've been exclusively self-tying for months to remember that another person's experience of my bondage may be completely different from the way I experience the same ties. Your own body will even react differently at different times!

Additionally, the motor skills involved in self-tying differ from those involved in partnered bondage (it's a bit like trying to write with your nondominant hand), so expect to feel awkward or have an adjustment period as you move between the two.

Your Rope Kit

As the joke goes in the rope community, there are two lengths of rope—too long and too short. One advantage of self-tying is that if there is a specific tie you do often, you can have a custom length of rope just for that tie on your body.

Regarding the type of rope you use for floorwork or harnesses against your body, the choice mostly comes down to personal preference—whether you prefer the feel and properties of hemp, jute, nylon, or something else entirely. I use a mix of hemp and nylon—nylon when I anticipate that I'll be moving around a lot and I want to minimize chafing (such as a hip harness in a marionette rig) or maximize comfort (such as with a gravity boot), and hemp when I need to hold frictions and have my rope stay in place completely solidly (such as with futomomos).

Many types of self-suspension involve dynamic, high-friction applications that can impose shock loads. For this reason, I strongly recommend using rated rope for self-suspension uplines. I primarily use 6-millimeter POSH, which is a type of spun polyester that has a breaking strength of 1,200 pounds. Reinforced jute is also becoming more common. For static uplines I won't be adjusting (pulling myself up, etc.) or particularly high-friction rigs like mobile suspensions, I use ⅛-inch AmSteel, which is a synthetic rope often used for sailing that has a breaking strength of 2,300 pounds.

Tying It Up

"I consider self-tying and self suspension to be my favorite form of self-love. I am giving myself something I truly love." —Sarahblueberry

"Rope helped me to love myself. To look at the beautiful women suspended in pictures with appreciation, not shame or envy. Kink is about finding what works for you, not becoming what you think you should be." —Phyllis

"Self-tying is about reclaiming my body and space. I'm a disabled woman, so most of my life I'm given the message that my body is not mine to enjoy. Self-tying allows me to be in complete embodiment of myself, and to feel my body working with me.... It's my art, my meditation, and my self-care." —Azura Rose

Self-bondage has motivated me to become a better version of myself. It has become the reason to take care of my body, the means to quiet my mind, a healthy outlet for my exhibitionism, and a constantly shifting challenge. Self-tying can be an amazing way to explore movement through rope, get into a flow state, enhance your mind-body connection, build skills as a rope top and rope bottom...or just a fun way to spend a quiet afternoon! Stay safe, enjoy your explorations, and savor this unique rope experience.

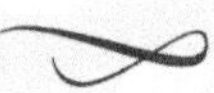

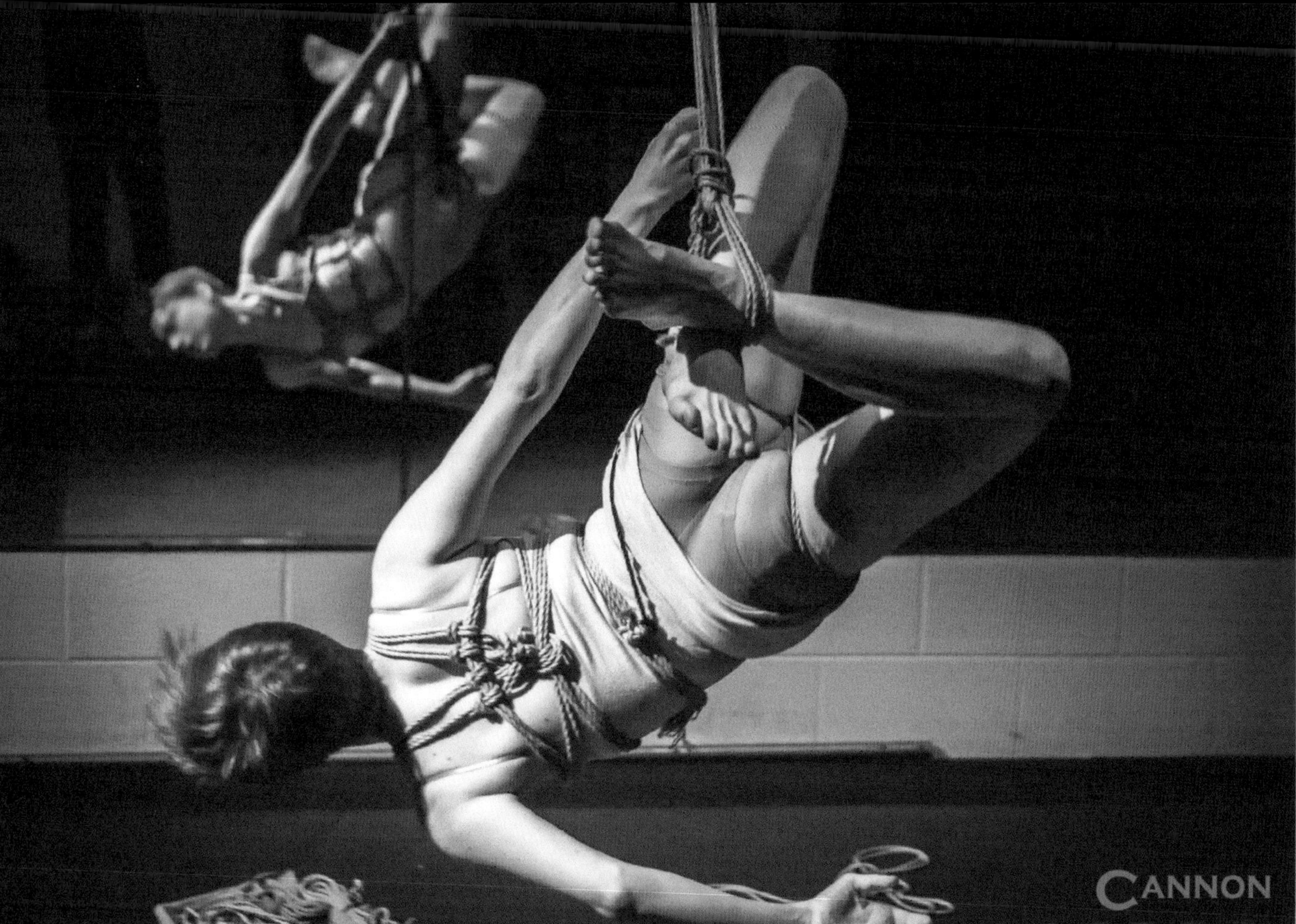

Parker RopeBoi in self-bondage; www.ropeboi.com; @ropeboi on Twitter. Photo by Cannon; www.riggercannon.com

Notes

1. Csikszentmihalyi, Mihaly, and Csikzsentmihalyi, Isabella Selega, eds. *Optimal Experience: Psychological Studies of Flow in Consciousness.* Cambridge: Cambridge University Press, 1988.

2. Csikszentmihalyi, Mihaly. *Flow: The Psychology of Optimal Experience.* New York: Harper & Row, 1990.

3. "Adapting to Artificial Gravity at High Rotational Speeds," NASA Astrophysics Data System

4. Harrin, Elizabrth. *Overcoming Imposter Syndrome.* The Otobos Group, 2011.

5. Stewart, John. *Focal Peripheral Neuropathies*, 4th ed.

Chapter 12

Ties for Limited Range of Motion

Photo credits

Model: Terri F.

Bondage by Demonsix and Zetsu Nawa

Photos by Retrotie

Hair and makeup by Anastasia Panagiotidis

It's no secret that different bodies have different ranges of motion in the joints—those areas where the ends of two bones come together, like the shoulders and elbows. Injuries, diseases, disorders, inflammation, infection, and more can prevent a joint from moving through its normal range of motion.

"Normal"—ugh. I hate that word here, because "not normal" has negative connotations, and because I've never met a rope bottom without some kind of physical limitation. Let me repeat that: *Never.* So really, limitations are actually the norm.

But to determine whether a range of motion is limited, there needs to be a standard to measure against, so for lack of a better word, we'll stick with the medical profession's use of "normal." If you're curious about what the normal ranges (in degrees) are for flexion, extension, rotation, and so on of the various joints, check out www.verywell.com.[1]

For bondage purposes, we're going to consider it limited range of motion if you can't *comfortably* move the joints into positions as required by standard ties, like the takate-kote. "Comfortably" is the key word here, because having your joints forcibly moved past that point isn't just painful; it can potentially aggravate your condition.

The good news is, you don't need to do any specific tie to have an awesome experience in rope! Really. If anyone tells you that they can't tie you because you can't be in certain ties, they are actually telling you that *their* knowledge base and skill set are limited. And if they tell you this in any way that makes you feel bad about yourself, consider yourself lucky that you didn't end up tying with such an insensitive jerk.

Remember too that "lab time"—when you tie for the

The Instructors Behind the Ties

Demonsix and Zetsu Nawa, the rope bondage teachers who came up with these ties, don't just have well over two decades of rope experience combined; they have a passion for rope that has nothing to do with seeking fame or fortune. They both generously gave their time and effort for this project—as did our effervescent model, Terri F., our awesome photographer, Retrotie, and our fabulous hair and makeup artist, Anastasia Panagiotidis.

Demonsix is one of the founders of the Devil Mask Society in Los Angeles, which offers classes by local and international bondage instructors. And Zetsu Nawa, a student of Yukimura Haruki since 2011, is a licensed instructor of Yukimura ryū and the owner of L.A. Rope studio, which offers classes and private lessons. He also created KinbakuToday.com and is a purveyor of kinbaku and shibari books via www.ainawa.com—check 'em out!

sake of learning and exploration rather than pure fun—is for bottoms as well as tops. You can use it to figure out ways of tying that work for the range of motion that is available to you.

Normal vs. Limited: Examples

Because the TK is so popular, and because many bottoms have trouble with it even outside of suspension, we'll focus here on limited range of motion in the shoulders and elbows.

This is within the normal range of motion:

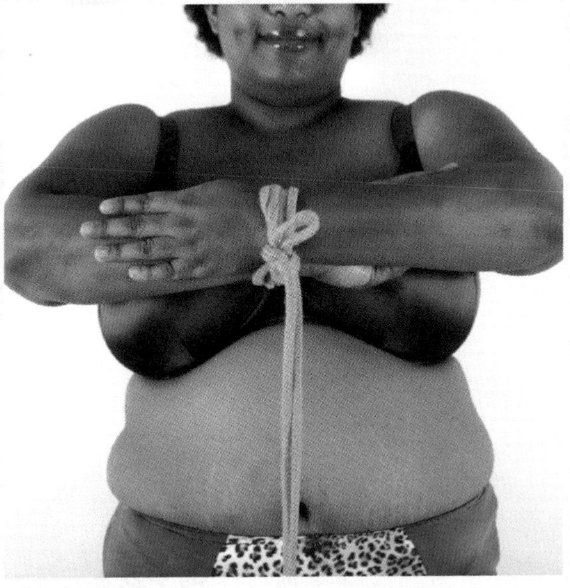

You can see in the photo above that the rope can safely be tied above the wrist joints on both arms without the elbows being forced together. (Tying on the wrist joint increases the risk of nerve compression.) So even though the fingertips don't reach the elbows, forming that perfect box shape, it's not limited range of motion.

This is limited range of motion:

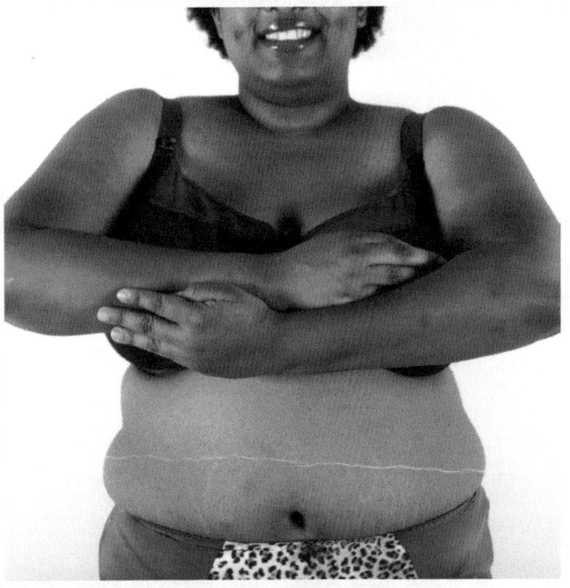

You can see in the photo above that there's no way to tie the arms together above the wrist joints on both arms. You could get rope above the joint on one arm, but then it would have to go around the hand on the other arm. So if this, or with the elbows further apart, is the range of motion you're working with, a standard TK is not the ideal tie for you.

The Shibari Show

We're showing all Japanese-style ties because, you know, Japanese style is the best, most authentic, most historically accurate form of tying, and you should never do anything else or you are not doing true bondage.

Ha! Kidding, of course. Whatever makes you happy is the best style of bondage for you. These ties are Japanese-style because the two highly esteemed rope instructors who came up with them have trained in the Japanese style—plus, the Japanese have been tying people up and thinking about ways to improve ties longer than Westerners have. But the concepts are easily transferrable to Western-style tying, so feel free to riff on them to your heart's content!

These ties are *not for suspension*. There's no way we could impart all the instruction needed for safe, suspension-worthy ties in just a few photos. Think of them as modular floor ties: They can be a piece that is added to, for a tie that includes the lower body, feet, hair, and so on. Or they can make for a fabulous scene all by themselves.

You can learn about suspension-worthy non-TK ties in other places; check out, for example, Topologist's video tutorial for a hands-free chest harness at http://crash-restraint.com/ties/130.

Show Me the Ties!

I know, you want to get right to the tying—don't we all. But bear with me. It behooves you to know first that:

• Size has absolutely nothing to do with range of motion or flexibility. Our model, Terri, has beautful curves and had to dial back her range of motion for this shoot, for instance.

• Cotton rope has more "give" than hemp or jute. That extra bit of rope flexibility can help you be more comfortable in a tie if you have limited range of motion. We used cotton rope for this shoot.

• Honest communication with your rope top about limitations is essential. If you try to hide them, you'll increase your chances of getting hurt, and if your partner finds out later, you'll have earned some mistrust. Plus, worrying about getting hurt can distract you from enjoying the scene fully.

• The ties described in this chapter, while not as risky as something like a TK in a suspension, still do carry the risk of motor and sensory nerve damage. So pay attention to how your fingers, hands, and arms feel and report any numbness, tingling, etc. to your top. (See Chapter 2 for more on nerve damage.)

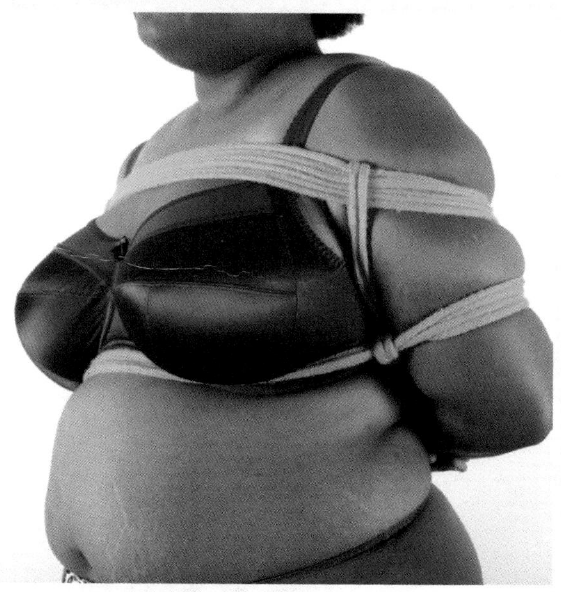

A word on kannukis: Notice in the photo above how the top rope is coming over and down instead of under and up. This type of cinch pulls those top wraps down, away from the brachial plexus (the network of nerves that sends signals from the spine to the shoulder, arm, and hand), so it carries a lower risk of nerve damage than one that pulls the rope up toward it.

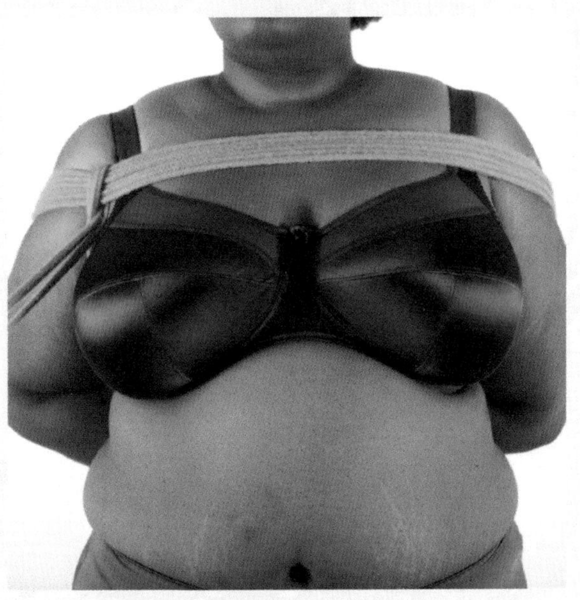

Here you can see the effect of pulling the rope when the cinch is tied over and down instead of under and up—it moves those top wraps down and away from the danger zone.

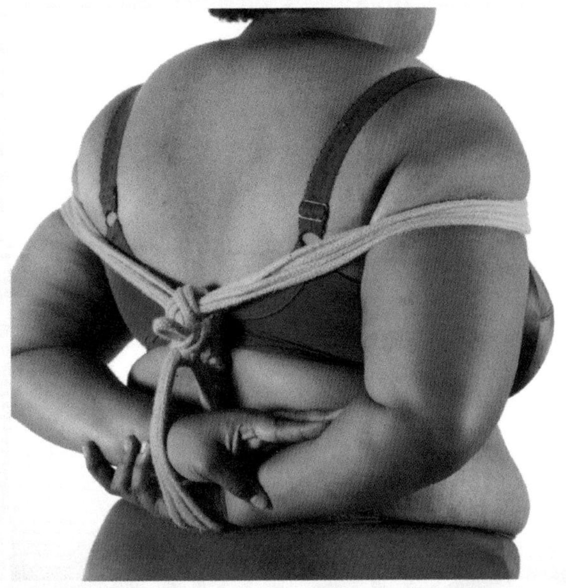

Lastly before we get to the ties, know that the wrists don't need to be tied tightly for a chest harness (TK or other) to be effective. Tying the wrists tightly is a rookie mistake that increases the risk of nerve damage and (unproductive) discomfort for the person being tied. Look how loosely the wrists are tied in the photo above, allowing Terri to switch which arm is on top as needed and to keep the elbows a comfortable distance apart. The wraps around the arms, including the lower ones when added, are what makes the tie secure. And with such loose tying around the wrists in a standing position like this, you don't need to be concerned if the wraps slip up past the wrist joint, because there's no compression.

5 Nonsuspension Ties for Limited Range of Motion

Here we go! These ties don't require anything fancy—someone with basic bondage knowledge should be able to figure them out by looking at the photos. If not, get creative! They don't have to be exact to be effective. And remember to think of them as modular pieces. If you were lying facedown on the floor, for example, your partner could put each leg separately in a futomomo, bind your legs together to look like a mermaid's tail, tie your ankles to your hair, or come up with something else. Have fun experimenting.

You can probably guess that the names are not Japanese, by the way...I made 'em all up.

1. Wrap and Cuff 'Em

From the front, this doesn't look like much, does it?

But in the back, it's a different story. Having the wrists tied behind the back can create a vulnerable feeling—because for one thing, you wouldn't be able to break a face-plant with your arms. And having the shoulders pulled back even a little opens the chest and energetically makes the heart feel exposed. The wrap around the upper arms makes this tie feel more binding than the cuffs alone would.

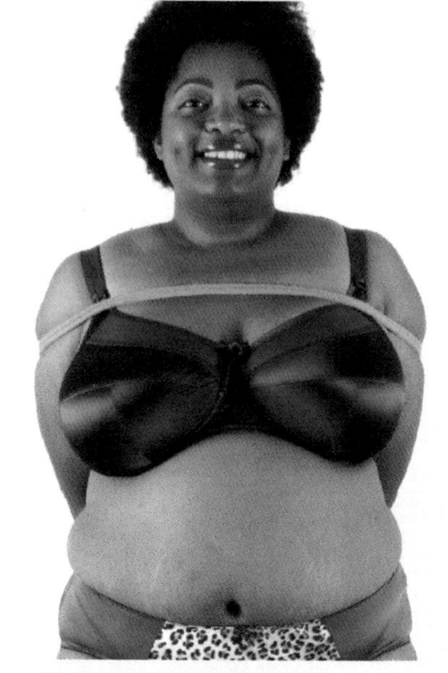

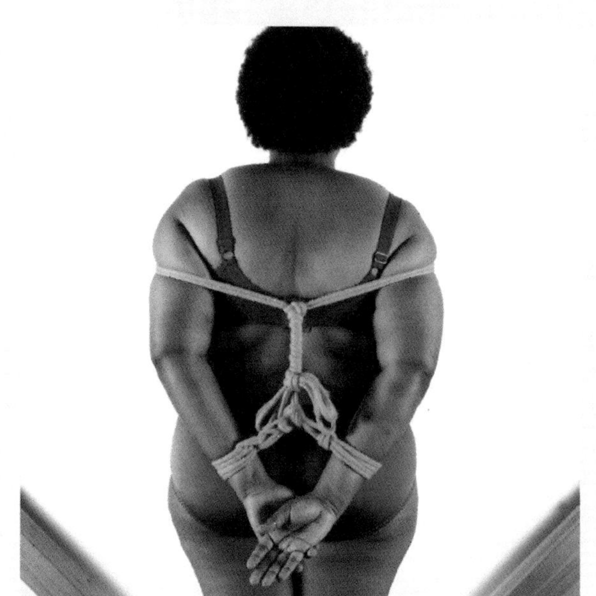

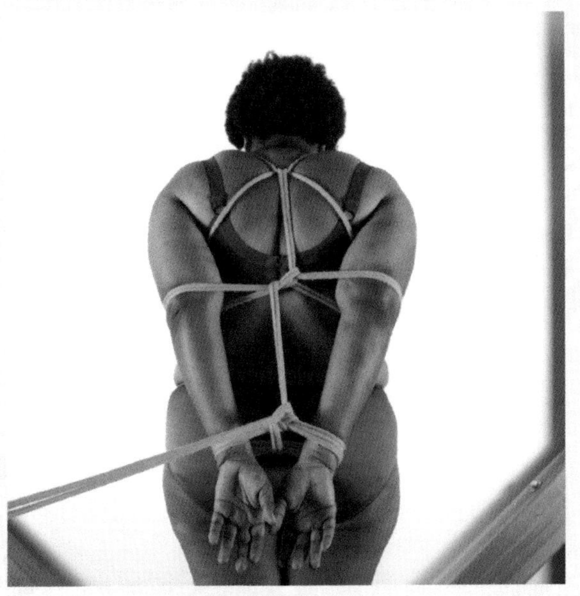

2. Self-Adjusting Strappado

This beauty of this tie is that it works whether the elbows are an inch or a foot apart, and whether your partner pulls your arms up (putting pressure on the shoulders) only a teeny amount or a lot more. You could even just use it as a regular armbinder and not pull the arms up into a strappado at all.

Safety notes: Notice how the rope at the neck and under the arms avoids the brachial plexus. Also, avoid tying directly over the elbows, because there's a higher risk of nerve compression, the area tends to move around a lot, and overall it's just more delicate than other parts of the arm.

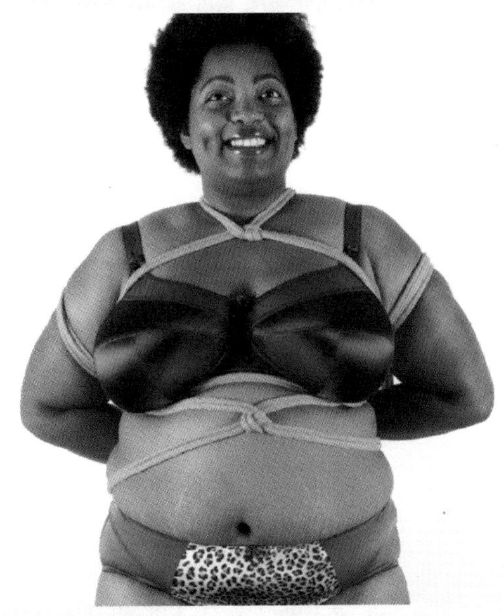

3. Knot Below the Neck

This tie is pretty simple but has some deceptively complex benefits. See that little knot just below the clavicle? It pushes in just the right spot to add lovely pressure and the feeling of being at someone's mercy, but without any worry about being strangled.

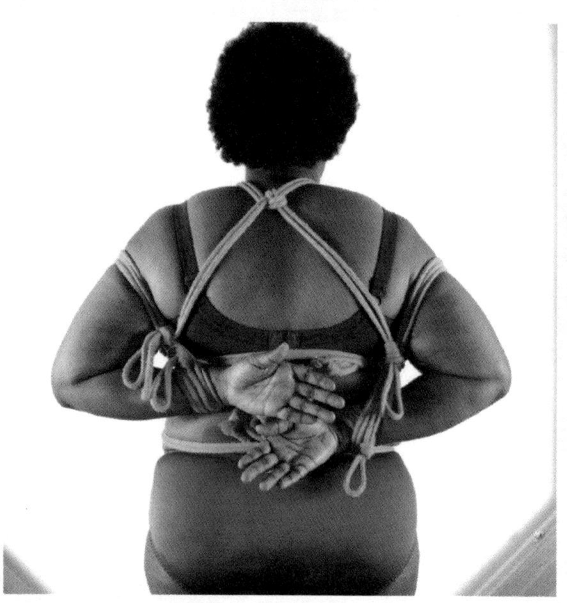

And check out the back: The placement of the arms and hands, along with the wide wrist cuffs, means you won't have to work to hold your arms and hands in a certain position, the way you do in most TKs. And, as in tie #1, the shoulders are being pulled back to open the chest and energetically expose the heart, increasing the feeling of vulnerability.

Also notice that the rope is binding in multiple ways, wrapping the upper and lower chest, arms, wrists, and abdomen. That coverage makes you feel more tied up than it may look. And some bottoms find symmetrical ties like this one soothing, because you're not doing all that extra mental and physical processing that asymmetrical ties require.

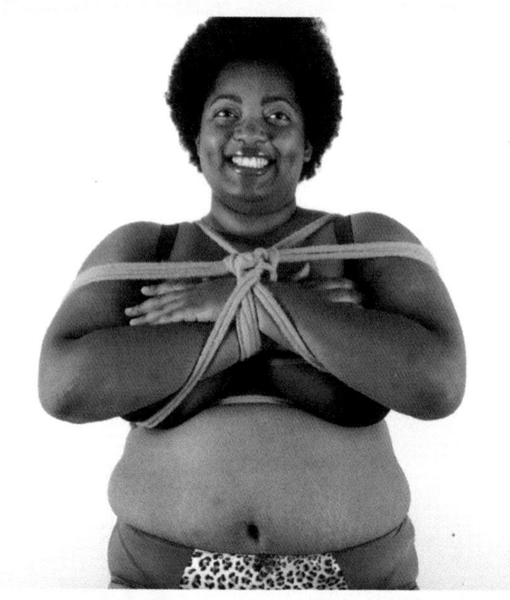

4. Hand to Heart

Crossing the hands over the chest creates a different feel: You're less exposed and are in a sense "protecting" your heart. This tie can feel more comforting, more nurturing, more inward-gazing than the others—which may or may not be your cup of tea. But in any case, you're still nicely bound. And it might not feel as comforting if, say, your partner then lays you on your back, spread-eagled, and ties each ankle to a hook in the ceiling. Just sayin'.

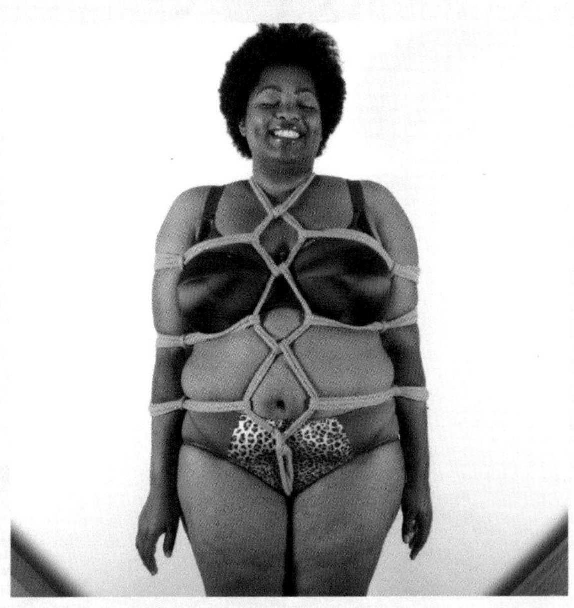

5. Diamonds and Pearls

Decorative *and* satisfyingly snug! Your hands can move a bit in this one, but your arms won't be going anywhere. Plus, it looks cool. And you've got that sweet "pearl" pressing right below the clavicle. (If you were thinking the pearl part of the tie's name had anything to do with those innocent rope strands meandering down below the belly button, you have a dirty, dirty mind, and I hope we meet someday.)

• • •

So now you have five fun ties to play around with. And who knows? Maybe this will inspire some bondage instructors to come up with others—and maybe even teach more classes on ties for bottoms with a limited range of motion (hint, hint).

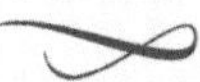

Notes

1. https://www.verywell.com/what-is-limited-range-of-motion-189733

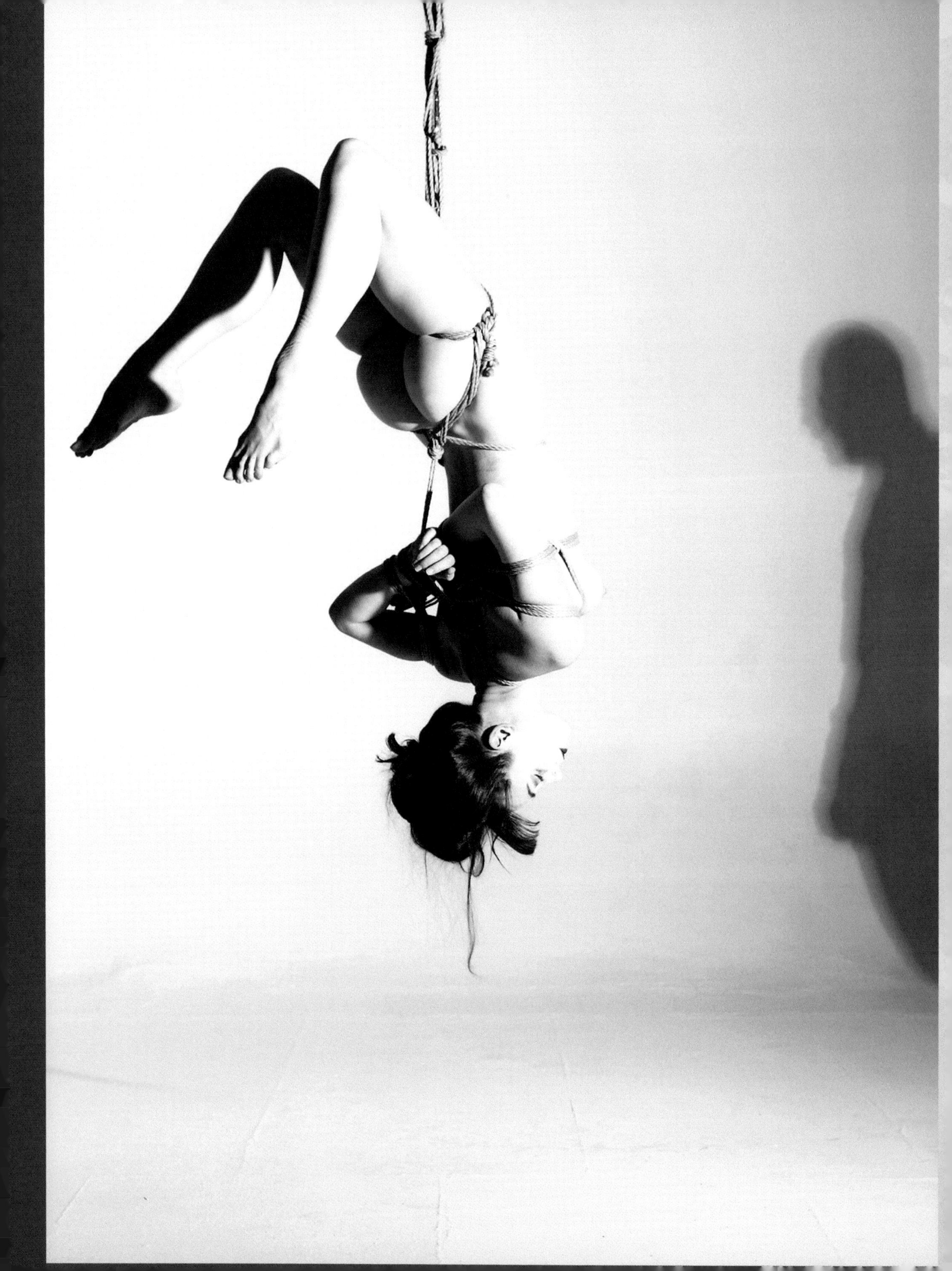

Chapter 13

Rope Bottoming Beyond Play

There are plenty of reasons for getting tied up besides the pure pleasure of being in rope. And with more and more people showing interest in bondage, the opportunities for bottoming beyond just play are greater than ever.

Even if you do bottom only for play, maybe sometimes you like to be tied at a club or dungeon. Or maybe you like to be tied somewhere else that's semipublic or even fully public. Anytime people are watching or the environment is unfamiliar, it can change your experience of the rope and your partner, and can affect your decision-making. It's good to be aware of those possible effects beforehand, both to minimize safety risks and to get the experience you're hoping for.

Later on we'll look at some specific considerations for different types of bottoming beyond play, including modeling, performing, and guerrilla bondage (aka rope bombing). And of course there can be an element of play in all of the types—maybe you get off on being photographed while dangling naked from a tree in the deep, dark woods, for example. But in most of them, the elements commonly considered part of playing/scening (intimacy, connection, ropespace/subspace) are not the primary goals.

First let's look at some overall considerations.

5 Basic Questions

These are good to ask yourself anytime play is not the primary goal. And hopefully, you'll be working with a partner/photographer/client you already know or have researched and deemed trustworthy.

1. Why do I want to do this? To be tied on something unusual, like a public statue, or in a special location? To make money? To get an amazing photo? To feel more social? To get attention? To be entertaining/contribute to other people's good time?

These are just a few possible motivations, and identifying your motivation can help you create the experience you desire. If you crave attention and have a crowd-pleaser scene planned, for instance, but you go to a dungeon on a night when everyone's at the party across town, it might not feel so fulfilling. Ditto if you're hoping for a stunning photo but your partner just wants the thrill of tying on that secret beach.

Be honest about your motivations. The term "attention whore" carries a whiff of judgment, but if attention makes you happy, who cares? Some ropesters consider performance bondage inauthentic. Again, who cares? It's your rope experience, and the only person you are ultimately accountable to is *you*.

If you do consider performance bondage inauthentic, by the way, True Blue's essay in this chapter might change your mind.

2. What is an acceptable level of risk for me? Am I OK with possible nerve damage or other injuries because I don't want to interrupt the show, cut things short, appear like a failure or "unprofessional," disappoint the photographer/director/client? If sexual contact has been negotiated, am I OK with the possibility of getting an STI? If photos are involved, am I OK with the possibility that they may end up in places I didn't intend?

Gestalta; www.gestalta.co.uk. Bondage by Pedro. Photo by Murhaaya; www.murhaaya.com

True Blue

True Blue is a rope switch, performer, and teacher as part of the duo Bondage Erotique. Find her at voxbody.com and on Instagram as miss_true_blue.

I am hanging in a double ankle inversion, and Kanso is about to attach a main line to my hip harness. I know that within minutes, I will be lifted more than 30 feet above a crowd of hundreds by that hip harness line alone, in a very strenuous backbending, face-up suspension. So, I am acutely present with the rope as Kanso ties off the line. It is surreal how hyper-aware of that rope I am! I feel the vibration as the jute runs back through the Y-hanger. I know exactly where his hand is as he locks off the line. I am sensing all these details as if the rope is a part of my body. I am upside down, and coursing with endorphins from the already challenging sequence he has taken me through. I trust the line and he who has tied it.

And while I am so clearly aware of these subtle, vital details, I also hold a scope of the bigger picture: the brisk evening air, the music, the pace we are keeping, and how I imagine it feels for the audience. We are at Symbiosis Gathering in California.

This is how it can be for me, performing in rope: There is a micro and a macro. It is an internal process, and an intimate one to share with my partner, yet has a broader scope and an awareness from the perspective of the viewer, all at once. How do those two spaces—the personal and the public—get bridged?

The first time I saw Akira Naka and Iroha Shizuki perform, he shared an idea with the audience before the performance began: He wanted us to imagine that we were peering through a keyhole at two partners engaged in an intimate moment. My memory of that evening's performance is as if none of us watching dared breathe, so as to not be caught looking in on something so personal. I have channeled that notion as best I can ever since, every time I perform in rope.

For me, rope is intimate. No matter how fancy or technically advanced the ties, the true beauty lies in what transpires between the two partners engaged, and in the personal journey the bottom takes in the ropes, facilitated by the rigger. Whether it be semenawa, circus bondage, slow and sensual, rough and edgy, it is at its essence about the energy shared between the partners, and how they both lock in on the experience they are having and let the rest of the world drop away. And so, this is my starting point. This is what I seek to share when I find myself performing in rope. I want to find a genuine way to convey outwardly what I am feeling inwardly.

I am also an ex-burlesque dancer who ran away with a vaudeville circus once upon a time, so I do understand the importance of story and color and line and arc in performance. We do have an audience to engage, after all.

Performance is an opportunity to communicate what is happening inside of us, whether that be through a specific choice of costuming or song, or the way we turn our head or curl our toes. We are storytelling. From the moment we walk onto the stage, before the rope is even picked up, we are setting a tone.

"My role in society, or any artist's or poet's role, is to try and express what we all feel. Not to tell people how to feel. Not as a preacher, not as a leader, but as a reflection of us all." —John Lennon

When Kanso and I have a performance to prepare for, we rehearse three times. I have found over and over again that it is in the third time running through a specific piece that we will discover the story we need to tell with it and unfold the deeper meaning of this particular sequence. Maybe it concerns something personal happening in our lives we want to share, maybe it is a certain mood it makes us feel, maybe it is that one moment of the sequence holds a very potent, charged, challenging, connective, or symbolic weight to it, and then we draw all our colors, props, and music from there. That is to say: First we examine what the rope means to us, and then we envision how to share that.

Back to the performance 30 feet above a crowd of hundreds. We had gone to the stage that afternoon to check the pulley system and run through the lift with the stage riggers. I was nervous. If anything were to go wrong, I would be doomed. I would have a headpiece on with a footlong deer antler attached to it, and in the backbend, my mouth would be tied off to my ankle. Full commitment to that moment. The story was something of the deer, the vulnerable,

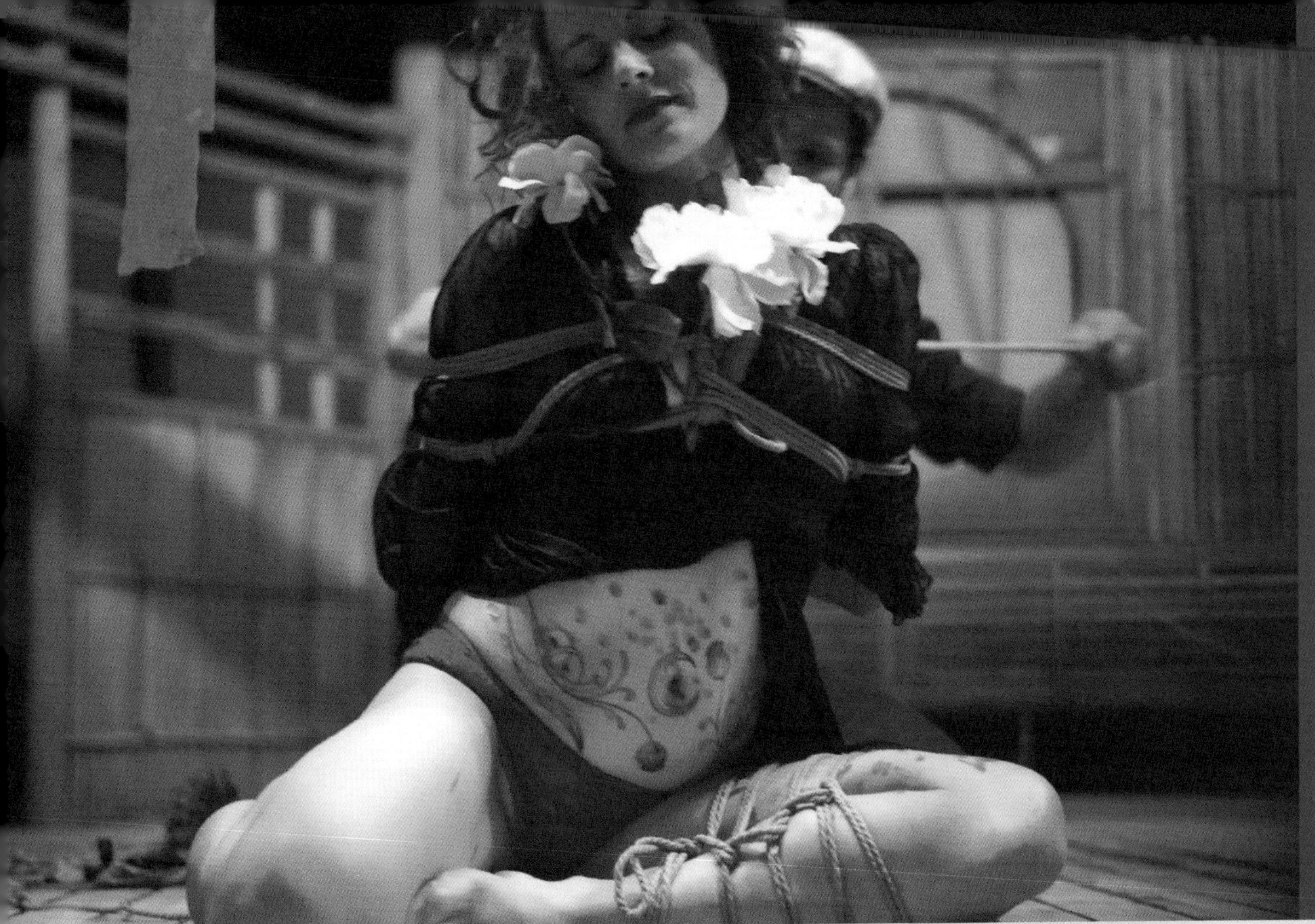

True Blue and Kanso. Bondage by Kanso. Photo by D.L. Frazer

the hunter and the hunted, a love story of sorts. As much as the antler on my headpiece added to the risks involved should I slip or fall, I felt it also to be a talisman of power. The power of the trust and surrender I was offering, of myself, to the piece, to Kanso, to the audience.

I later received a message from someone who had been in the audience that night:

"I know little of erotic bondage. My kinks express themselves with less deliberation. What I saw that night was easily one of the most arresting performances of the weekend. You opened my eyes to a side of intimacy that I had never been exposed to, and I am so grateful for it. Never in my life have I seen such a romantic, communicative, trusting display of intimacy in public.... I was spellbound by the story you told." —Max

I had had what I would consider a healthy amount of anxiety during the run-through that day. But that evening: lakeside, starry skies, moody warm lighting, an amped-up and, frankly, stunned crowd, and the opportunity to walk onto the stage with Kanso and share this rope that we both so deeply love, I was calm. The line was locked off, Kanso carefully stuffed some arrows into the ropes surrounding me, his catch, and up I went. Serene and surreal. Grateful to be able to share such an internal, challenging moment in such an absurd and visual way. I spun slowly as I rose up. I closed my eyes sometimes, and felt the stage lights bright against my eyelids. I opened my eyes sometimes, and looked down, upside down, on a crowd of uplifted faces. I felt their energy as they felt ours. The moment, as they seem to do, slowed down. I believe my calm was the result of a balance I had struck between my innermost thoughts on this sequence, and how it was being conveyed. I do see performance as an opportunity to make an offering of oneself, and cherish this moment in particular as an example of that, of offering my surrender, my physical self, my love, in a way I can only do through rope.

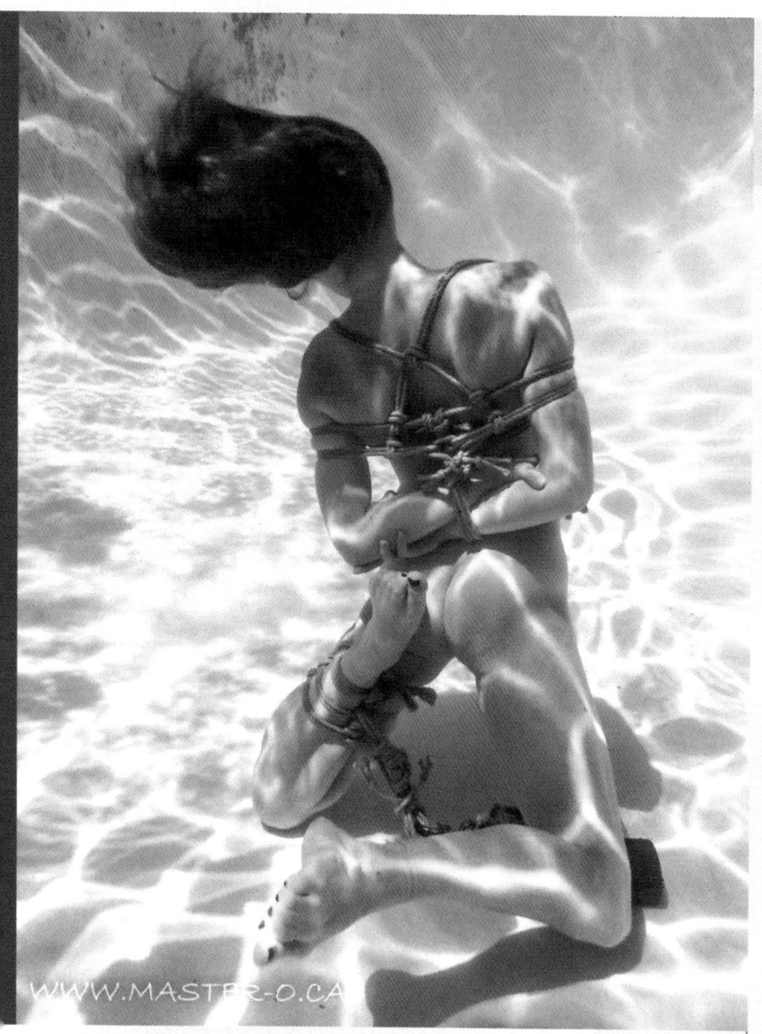

Saffron Tresses. Bondage by LaughingDragon. Photo by Master_O. Please see all the safety precautions taken for this photo in the column below

Tying in front of other people can increase the pressure—whether it exists only in your mind or whether people have paid money to see you—to appear "perfect." Communicating about needing an adjustment or to come down entirely can be hard for a lot of rope bottoms even when they're alone with their partner; add all those extra eyes or a camera lens and you may communicate even less or not at all, putting yourself at greater risk of injury. Being realistic about your likely behavior and what is acceptable risk—and sharing that info with the person tying you—can reduce unexpected outcomes.

A rope bottom who is also a circus performer once told me she wasn't particularly worried about nerve damage, and in fact in some places it actually helps her circus act, because her routine would be quite painful otherwise. I was pretty shocked at the time, but acceptable risk is entirely personal. I recommend, however, if you are similarly not worried, that you clearly inform your partner, because it may not be an acceptable risk to *them.* And if you won't be communicating to your partner about signs of impending injury during a scene, clearly let your partner know that beforehand as well.

As for its being "unprofessional" to ask for adjustments or even to ask to come down during a performance, I would argue that in fact you would be setting the better example by demonstrating respect for your personal safety.

And speaking of risk, the photo at left is a great example of a situation that only *looks* super risky. What you don't see are all the safety precautions: 1. The model is an experienced scuba diver. 2. Just outside the frame, a certified scuba instructor monitored her and frequently gave her a regulator with air. 3. The weights weren't so heavy that she couldn't be pulled out of the water in seconds. 4. There were three other people in the pool at all times to help her.

So while amazing photos like this can be inspiring, please don't be inspired to re-create them without seriously considering how to stay safe.

3. Have I negotiated for sexual touch? Many people unfamiliar with kink assume that bondage and sex go hand in hand. Not necessarily! Sexual contact, whether it's a playful nipple tweak or a triple penetration, is something to negotiate.

Even if you've performed/acted/shot with a partner in the past without any issue, it can be helpful to go over every time what's acceptable and what isn't. People forget; they have multiple partners and get confused; they feel they know you well enough to know what you want even if you haven't asked for it. And sadly, some rope tops, as in the rest of the world, are unethical asshats who simply take advantage of people, especially when there are gray areas.

Of course, it's a good idea to negotiate for all the other usual things too, but it's easy to assume that everyone is on the same page about whether sexual touch is or isn't on the table. If you're new to negotiation, you can search for checklists online. Tifereth, a well-known ropester, performer, and educator, recommends that performers discuss two things at the minimum in addition to sexual touch: health conditions/injuries and rope placement/preferences—a great idea for everyone!

4. What will aftercare look like? In many nonplay situations, you're responsible for handling your own aftercare. You may get it from a performance partner, especially someone you regularly work with, but it's highly unlikely that a photographer or director is going to snuggle you or whatnot afterward, even if they put you through the ringer.

Nonplay scenes can be just as intense, if not more so, than play scenes, and you can experience sub drop and everything else that goes along with play. So it's a good idea to have an aftercare plan, whether you call on a friend or your teddy bear.

5. What's my backup plan? In a play scene, if you're having an off day or something unplanned happens, it's usually not too hard to switch things up or even throw in the towel. In a performance with a hundred eyes on you, a photo shoot that took hours to set up, a film with a crew of people depending on you, and so on...not so much.

So, in addition to taking the gig seriously and preparing well—showing up rested and hydrated, warming up, having eaten enough, and the like—it's good to have a backup plan. While obviously you can't plan thoroughly for the unknown, you can consider things that logically might go wrong and have a plan for if they do.

A partner and I once did a performance in a multiperson show that involved a mock abduction and hard-core resistance play. Of course I was planning not to get (too) hurt; I knew him well and trusted him completely, and we had practiced a bit too. Still, before we went on, we discussed possible concussion, sprains, and bone breaks. "I'm just gonna say, 'Broken,' and you can drag me off by what's not broken so we don't ruin the rest of the show for everyone," I told him. It was less glib than it sounds.

What would you do if a photographer you don't know well changes the location at the last minute to a place you're not familiar with? Or if you're supposed to be a supporting actor but get asked to fill in for the star who called in sick? What if you're doing guerrilla bondage and someone walks up? For every kind of scenario, you can probably think of at least a few things that could go wrong, and having a backup plan can mean the difference between feeling like the gig was "ruined" and eagerly looking forward to the next one.

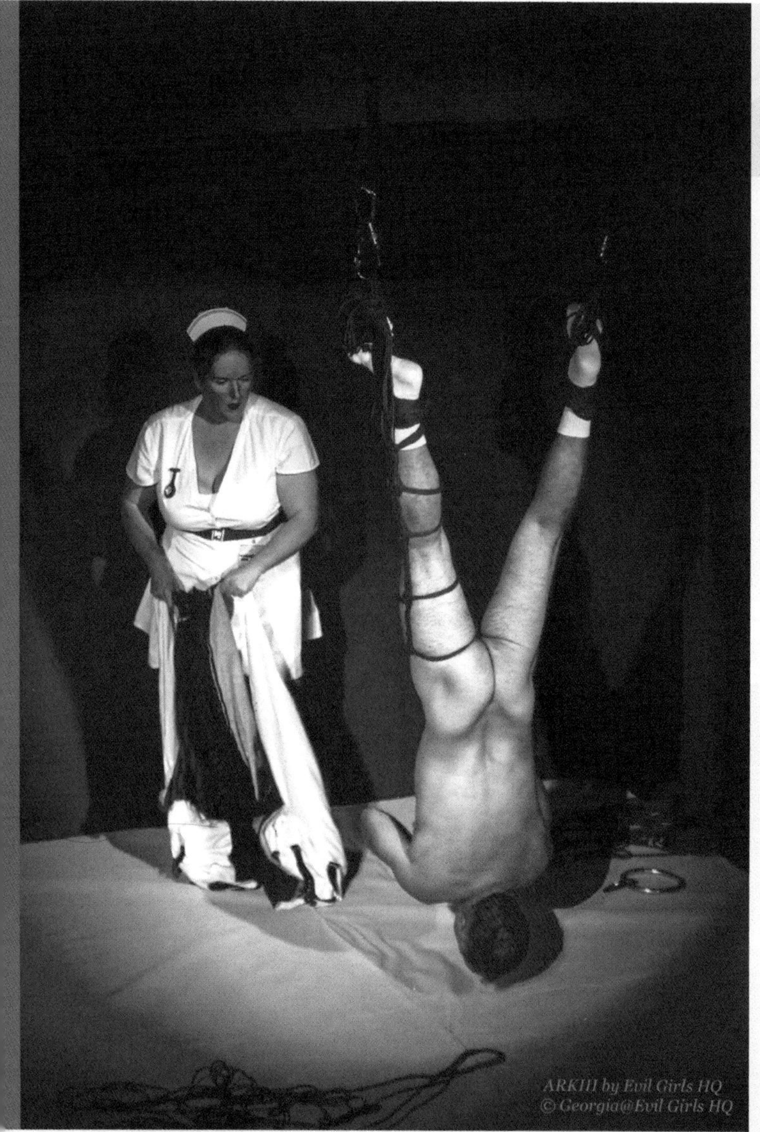

Submissive_Lion and -DeepDarkDesire-.
Bondage by -DeepDarkDesire-.
Photo by Georgia from Evil Girls HQ

Specific Considerations

Bondage Performers

Doing a bondage performance in front of an audience can mean anything from rocking out on amateur night at the local club to taking the stage for a paid gig in front of hundreds of people. Some people rehearse extensively, get costumes and props, and choose special music; some just come up with something on the fly or do their usual play style, in which case it's sometimes called a "playformance." Bondage performances often involve suspension.

When I started in rope, bondage performing was pretty rare—and at first I didn't get it. To me, bondage is personal, intimate, connective; why on earth would anyone want to turn it into a dog-and-pony show? Now it seems like it's become the entertainment du jour at certain kinds of parties and other events, and not only do I get it, but I do it! There's the joy of sharing what I love with others, the possibility of helping someone discover a new passion, the satisfaction of providing good entertainment, the thrill of shocking any "vanillas," and, of course, all the attention and feeling special. It seems obvious now, but bondage can be whatever you want it to be—personal, showy, playful, serious, even crowd-interactive.

It can also be pressurizing, given the audience and that mentality of "the show must go on." So it's especially important to discuss ahead of time things like:

- How will you communicate? Vocally? Through hand or other bodily signals?
- Will the rigger check in on you periodically as well? If there's loud music and dim lighting, you might not readily be heard or seen.
- How will you both handle it if you need to come down?
- If you're winging it, do you have at least some idea of the format? Predicament bondage, multiple transitions, rough body play with rope on the floor, etc.?

All of these considerations may also apply when you're not technically performing but people are watching anyway, like in a club or dungeon.

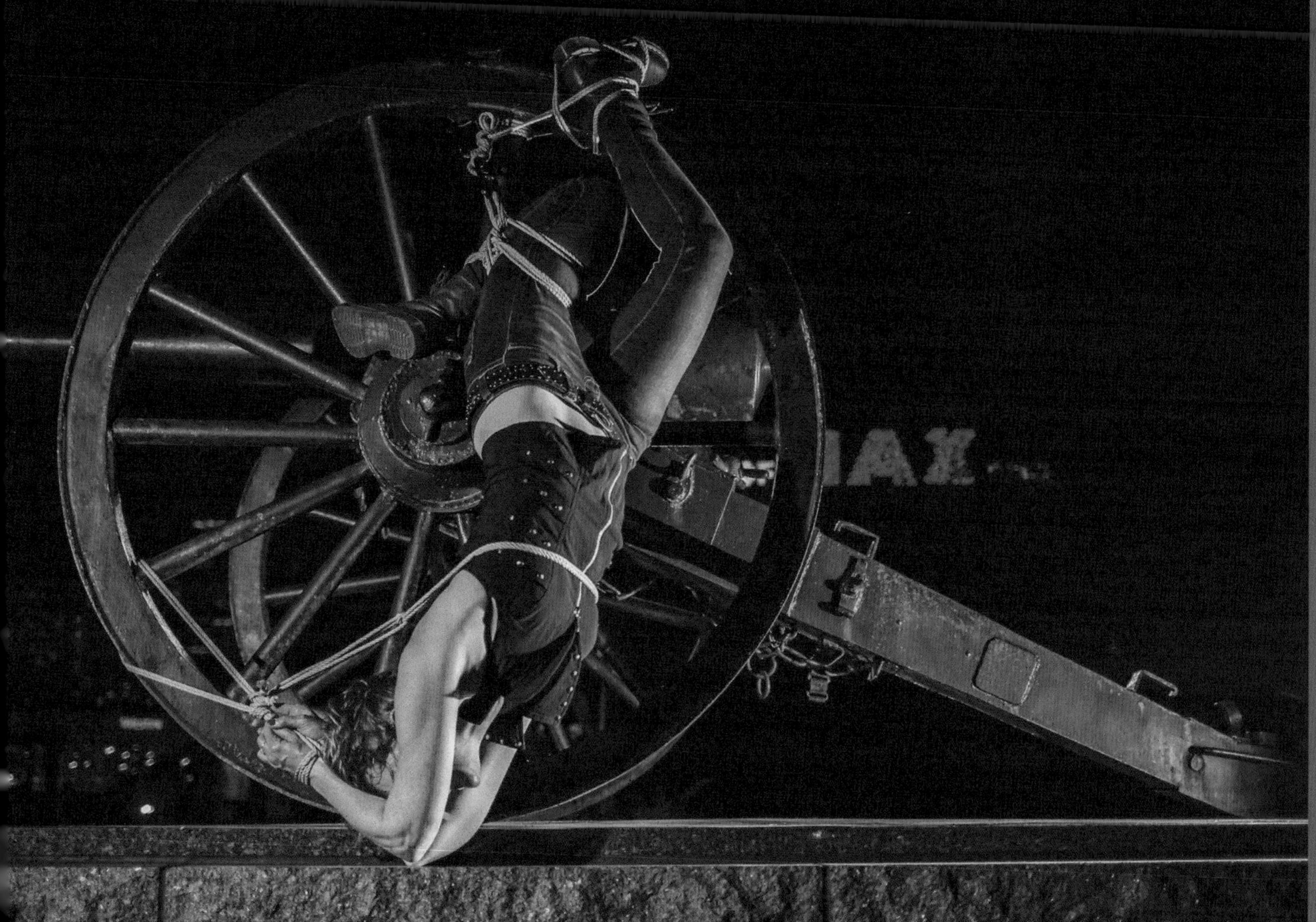

Curious-one. Bondage and photo by BDSLR

Models

Some bottoms get tied up in the name of art. Often the art is photography, but it can include things like walking around at an event for "ambience," posing as a kind of art installation, and holding a pose so people can sketch it. Some ropesters also call anyone who gets tied up a model, even if it's in a play scenario, but that seems odd to me because in a play scene you're not modeling the same way you would model for art.

Sometimes models have no prior bondage experience, which can be dangerous. And sometimes a "photographer" is really just a creeper with a camera. If you're considering bondage modeling, I would first recommend getting to know your body in rope well before you add the camera. And read "A Guide for Rope Bottoms and Bondage Models" by Clover, which you can download for free at KinkyClover.com. The better you know your body, the more you can lower your risk of getting injured. Bonus: You'll probably look better in the photos too, because you'll have a better understanding of how your body responds in rope.

Second, learn how to keep yourself safe in terms of not being preyed upon. The general Fetish Models & Photographers group on FetLife has almost 15,000 members, and it seems like a great place to ask questions. It also has indexes of models and photographers in the sticky section. You can find local modeling groups for many regions as well. Get to know other models; get references for photographers ahead of time in addition to checking out their work; listen to your instinct; consider having a friend accompany you to the shoot if you have any doubts. (But also be aware that a boyfriend or girlfriend staring daggers at the photographer the whole time might not get you the best photos.)

Some other considerations:

- Will the photographer be doing the bondage, or someone else? Of course, check out the quality of the tyer's work beforehand.
- Are you comfortable communicating and advocating for your needs, especially if the shoot involves extreme positioning, an unusual setting, or anything else unfamiliar to you? If not, can you bring someone along who can advocate on your behalf?
- Have you negotiated regarding nudity or lack of it?
- Will you have rights to the photos, and if so, for what type(s) of use? For instance, a photographer may let you post the photos on Facebook but not let you sell them. Will you be required to sign a model release?
- Are you comfortable with the fact that your photos may up on websites or other places you didn't intend, and that once they're out there, they're pretty impossible to take back?
- If the shoot involves other models, how will you be interacting with them? If the shoot involves multiple models and you'll have some downtime, by the way, you might want to bring a robe or nice big blanket to stay warm and comfy when it's not your turn.

Film/Video Actors

Rope bondage in porn videos and even in more mainstream films has been around for quite a while (raise your hand if you've at least considered recreating that tied-to-the-railroad-tracks scene in *The Perils of Pauline* from 1914). Now it's even in music videos, and there are so many live-cam sites, it would be hard to keep track of them all.

Videos and clips can get lifted and distributed on sites other than the ones you signed up for, so you can't assume that you'll stay under the radar. And they may affect your job prospects—so if you're thinking of running for office, say, doing filmed bondage might not be the best career move.

Bondage videos don't have to include sex, but many do. Not every company is perfectly conscientious about requiring documented STI test results, and condom use is not the norm as of this writing. So decide acceptible risk ahead of time and stick with it. Also decide what your limits are in terms of bondage, other BDSM activities, and sex, so you can clearly communicate them. For instance, maybe you're OK with bondage and having dildos rammed up your ass, but you draw the line at having your face slapped.

You'll want to research the production company, the director, the tyer, and anyone else you'll be interacting with. Doing a video shoot can mean anything from someone filming you with a handheld in their bedroom to a full crew and a catered set, and the person(s) can be anything from sleazy to super professional. In one recent highly publicized case, a kinky porn actor was accused by other actors of sexual assault, including rape. Do your research and talk with people who've worked with the people you're

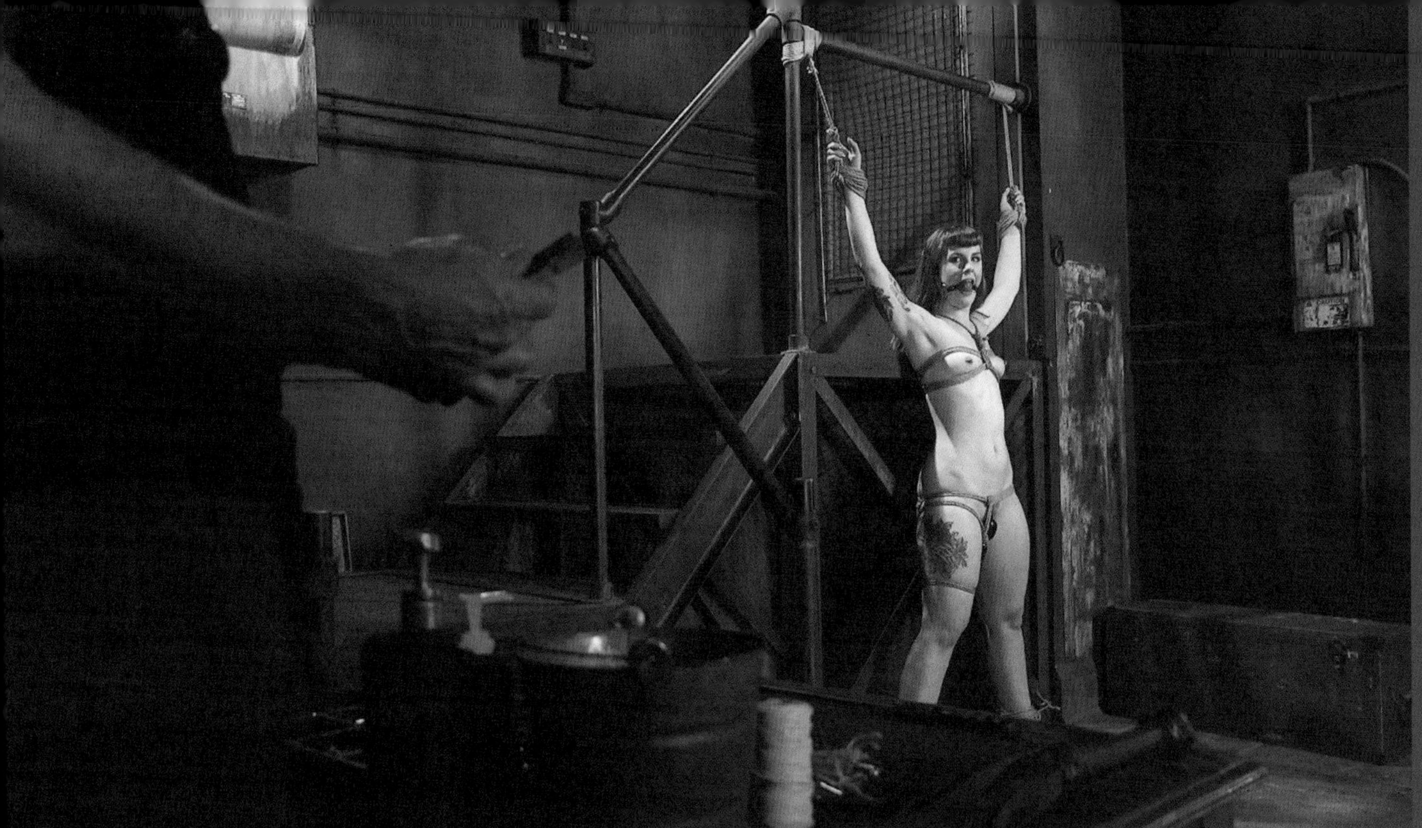

Barbary Rose on the set of The Training of O.
Bondage by James Mogul.
Photo courtesy of Kink.com

considering working with. And consider checking out the International Entertainment Adult Union (http://www.entertainmentadultunion.com/).

Some folks bypass production companies entirely and make amateur videos or set up their own live-cam (webcam) sites.

I've gotten tied up often as a guest on The Upper Floor, a Kink.com channel, but I've never done paid bondage in films or videos. So here to help is model, actor, and performer Barbary Rose. Her Twitter handle is XOBarbary, and you can learn more about her at www.BarbaryRose.com.

"I have an equal love for exhibitionism and bondage," Barbary says, "and I was so excited to be able to get paid to do what I love." It probably won't surprise you, however, to learn that bondage on camera and bondage for play aren't the same thing. Although both can be challenging and require good communication, "on camera it is less about my connection between the person who put me in bondage, since sometimes that person isn't the one topping you or isn't featured in the photos or video at all," Barbary says. "In play I prefer to have a connection and a whole experience with the bondage top."

What's it like doing bondage on camera? "It depends on the experience," Barbary says. "Certain sites that I've shot for—for example, DeviceBondage.com and HardTied.com—really focus on predicament bondage and impact play, whereas other sites and most of the photo shoots I've done are more about artistically displaying the rope, or the bondage is part of a plot line." In some scenarios, "you might be asked to act like you love or hate the bondage, which can feel silly doing."

What advice would she give a newbie looking to get into this line of work?

- "Try to do some experimenting with bondage in your personal life or with someone before trying it on camera. This will allow you time to figure out what you do and don't like, as well as how to tune into what your body is telling you during bondage scenes.
- If you are shooting with a new director or photographer, don't be afraid to check references from other models. Don't be afraid of speaking up during a shoot if something doesn't feel good, and don't ever feel like you need to do something you're uncomfortable with for money.
- Bring a friend or someone else experienced to any shoot for your safety; plus it never hurts to have extra hands on set if needed.
- Signing release forms is a great practice to ensure legality and that both parties are consenting to whatever has been negotiated."

Barbary says she's never had a bad experience in the industry, by the way. I'd like to just reiterate, as mentioned elsewhere, that sexual pleasure can lower your pain perception, increasing the risk of injury. And even if you're fully confident in your negotiating skills in play, being paid can make you feel pressured to do something you're not fully comfortable with, so bringing along someone who can advocate for you might be a good idea.

Demo Bottoms and Practice Partners

Wherever a bondage instructor is teaching or a ropester is learning—classes, workshops, private lessons, peer skill shares, in front of YouTube in the living room—you'll usually find a demo bottom or practice partner. Tying their own legs, a mannequin, a pillow, or the back of a chair only gets someone so far, after all.

Demo bottoming for instructors is a great way to experience a range of tying styles, and being tied by highly skilled people can be very enlightening—not to mention just plain awesome! I'm usually the first one volunteering when someone travels to San Francisco to teach. Still, there are some considerations:

- Just because someone teaches bondage doesn't mean they are actually *qualified* to teach bondage. It also doesn't guarantee that they're ethical. I've had only good experiences demo bottoming, but anytime someone is in a position of power, there's the opportunity to abuse it. So it behooves you to do your homework and talk with other bottoms they've tied, rather than putting the teacher on a pedestal based on assumptions.
- Demo bottoming is work as well as fun. In a day-long workshop, you could be in a TK for a few hours or more! You may have to do unfamiliar or strenuous ties. You may have to stand, kneel, or sit on the floor without back support for longer than you're used to. Being well-rested, fed, hydrated, and warmed up go a long way here. So does knowing ahead of time what the class will cover.
- As with performing, people will be watching, which adds pressure. If you feel like you might be less comfortable communicating about adjustments, consider having a mini session with the instructor beforehand, so you can work out the best placement of the wraps and so on.
- My take on demo bottoming in general is that I'm there for the instructor—to be focused on them, make them look good, and facilitate learning. If I want to share bottoming thoughts with the class, I ask first if it's OK. Otherwise, I try to speak only when spoken to. Teaching takes a lot

of focus and energy, and detracting from that doesn't help anyone. If you're easily distracted, are very chatty, or care more about your own experience than the class's, demo bottoming may not be a good fit. Ditto if you slip easily into nonverbal ropespace, for obvious reasons.

Being a practice partner for someone who's learning is less "glamorous" than demo bottoming, but there are still lots of reasons to do it. In addition to your helping deepen the knowledge pool among tyers, which benefits all bottoms, it tends to be a less risky way to meet new tops. As with demo bottoming, you can experience a wide range of styles, and you might discover new things you like. You might also do it as a trade—for bottoming "lab time," dinner, time practicing your own tying, a foot rub...whatever you two agree on.

The biggest consideration in this scenario is that someone who's learning may make dangerous mistakes. If you think you can't get dropped out of a suspension in a class because an instructor is supposed to be overseeing everything, or you can't get nerve damage or otherwise get injured, go look at FetLife's Rope Incident Reports group. I always insist that the instructor come over and double check everything about my class partner's work—the tie, the rig, the support lines—before going up into a suspension. Yes, the person might feel a bit bad because I'm doubting their ability, but it's my body literally on the line!

In a more private practice session, you have to be even more careful. Don't be afraid to ask questions: How many times have you done this tie before? How confident are you that you can do it safely? Have you ever injured anyone? And listen to your instinct—if something doesn't feel right, say so, even if you can't put your finger on exactly what it is.

Lest you think bottoming in a class or other practice session is totally boring, by the way, I can tell you that I've gotten *quite* rope high on more than one occasion, and a few times it seemed like the least likely setting!

Professional Submissives

The first time I heard that people get paid to be tied up, flogged, whipped, and whatnot, my first thought was, "Where do I sign up?" Pro subs earn money doing BDSM scenes with clients, usually through a company or group (like Fantasy Makers in the San Francisco Bay Area). While sex work may include kinky play, pro subs are *not necessarily* sex workers—in fact, you may be required by law to carefully document everything you do to show that no sex was involved.

Let's get the scoop from Cupcake SinClair, a lifestyle and professional submissive who also teaches classes on BDSM, polyamory, sex work, and more. Her Twitter handle is subbie_cupcake.

Cupcake was already in the BDSM lifestyle before she started working as a pro sub out of Sanctuary, a dungeon in Los Angeles. "Rope bondage is a popular request and by far one of my favorites," she says, but she also caters "to a wide variety of fetish and kink interests—within my limits!" Yes, just as in performing, modeling, acting, and demo bottoming, you get to have limits; getting paid doesn't change that. In fact, Cupcake doesn't do rope suspensions with clients. "Rope suspensions are a form of edge play that I only feel comfortable doing with trusted partners I have played with for a while," she says.

So what exactly does getting tied up as a professional entail? "A rope scene can vary drastically," she says. Sometimes clients just need someone to practice ties on in a class. Others are into role playing, "where perhaps I am the helpless damsel and they enjoy the energy of a squirming, helpless partner as they feel the rope quickly sliding across my skin and beneath their fingers." (Did that turn you on, or is it just me?) The possibilities are limited only by the imagination and what both parties consent to. "The variety of interests that are presented by rope bondage constantly keep me enthralled," Cupcake says.

If you're interested in this line of work, here's her professional advice:

- "Always, always take time to negotiate a scene ahead of time to ensure that you and your client are on the same page about how the scene will go—particularly in a rope bondage scene! Limits and triggers are important to be aware of, along with making your safeword known before the scene starts.
- Always start off small with a rope scene with clients, and if they desire so and you feel comfortable, expand to a larger scene. There are so many ways that nerve and general body damage can happen from improper ties, and your comfort is always a priority, so seeing how they do basic ties is important before allowing more intricate ones.
- If you are new to rope, consider taking rope classes so that you know what proper ties look like and you can experience the ties for yourself in a no-pressure environment.
- Lastly, don't be afraid to turn down rope sessions if you don't feel confident—after all, a professional submissive's or bottom's main goal is to ensure their client is having a great experience, and that depends on you knowing yourself well enough to have a great experience to offer!"

You may also be wondering how to protect yourself while playing with someone you just met. Who's to say they'll even honor your safeword?

At Sanctuary, "there's an intercom system in all of the rooms," Cupcake says. "The receptionist keeps the time for ongoing sessions and will buzz in to give 10-minute warnings. The girl sessioning—not the client—must verbally respond. If there is a lack of response after a few minutes, someone will physically come to check in on the scene to ensure everyone is OK."

Also, none of the playroom doors lock. "That way if anyone feels uncomfortable at any time, they are free to leave." And most of the rooms "have mirrors so both parties can watch the other to see what is occurring even if their back is turned."

Even with these precautions in place, "we encourage submissives on our staff to never have all three of their senses hindered—for example, being tied up and blindfolded are OK, but then do not allow yourself to be gagged," Cupcake says. She says she has never had a bad experience as a pro sub, but as with modeling and acting, I recommend researching the company and listening to your instinct about it as well as about potential clients.

Guerrilla Bondage

Lastly, for those of you wanting to take your tying out of the bedroom or dungeon and into the great outdoors, check out the considerations on the next pages from a master, and have fun exploring all the possibilities for rope bottoming beyond play!

Cupcake SinClair. Photo by Ashes Wednesday

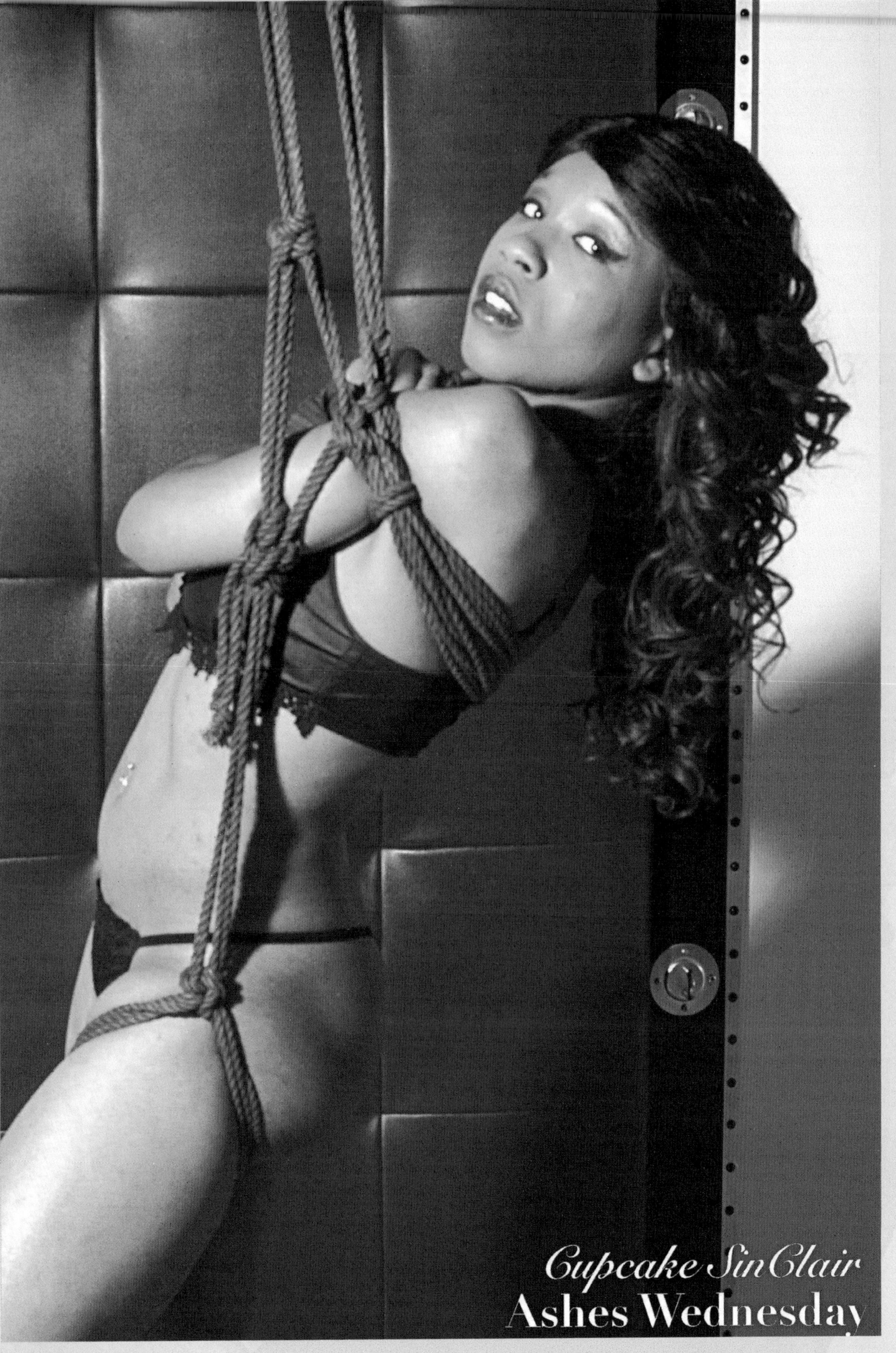
Cupcake SinClair
Ashes Wednesday

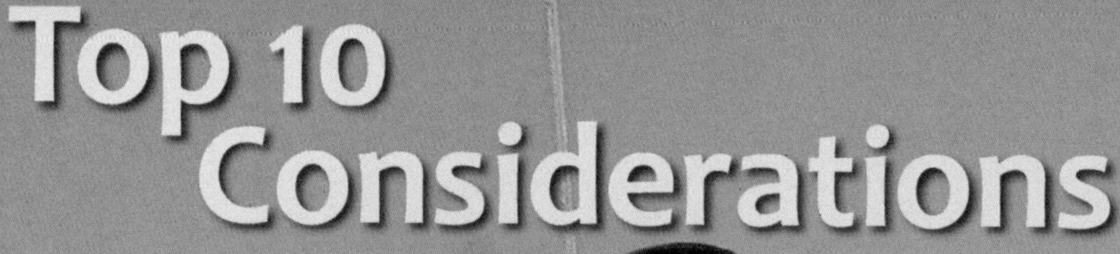

Top 10 Considerations *for Successful Guerrilla Bondage*

by Dallas Kink

Dallas Kink has been doing guerrilla bondage for eight years. He is the founder of Bondage Expo Dallas and Bondage Expo Denver and, with Cat Nawashi, makes and sells high-quality jute bondage rope through the My Nawashi store on Etsy. For more info, check out PinkRopes.com and www.etsy.com/shop/MyNawashi.

More people than ever are taking bondage to the streets—and to trees, monuments, and other outdoor structures. And there are extra considerations when doing bondage in a public space, whether for a great photo or just for fun. These are my top 10 for both tops and bottoms.

1. Risk

Identify your personal risk profile. How much risk are you willing to take in terms of physical safety and potential legal consequences? What is the reward for taking that risk? A good photograph may not be worth a trumped-up "inciting a riot" charge or a mass of splinters from that tree bark. A legendary photo? Priceless.

Bondage and photo by Dallas Kink

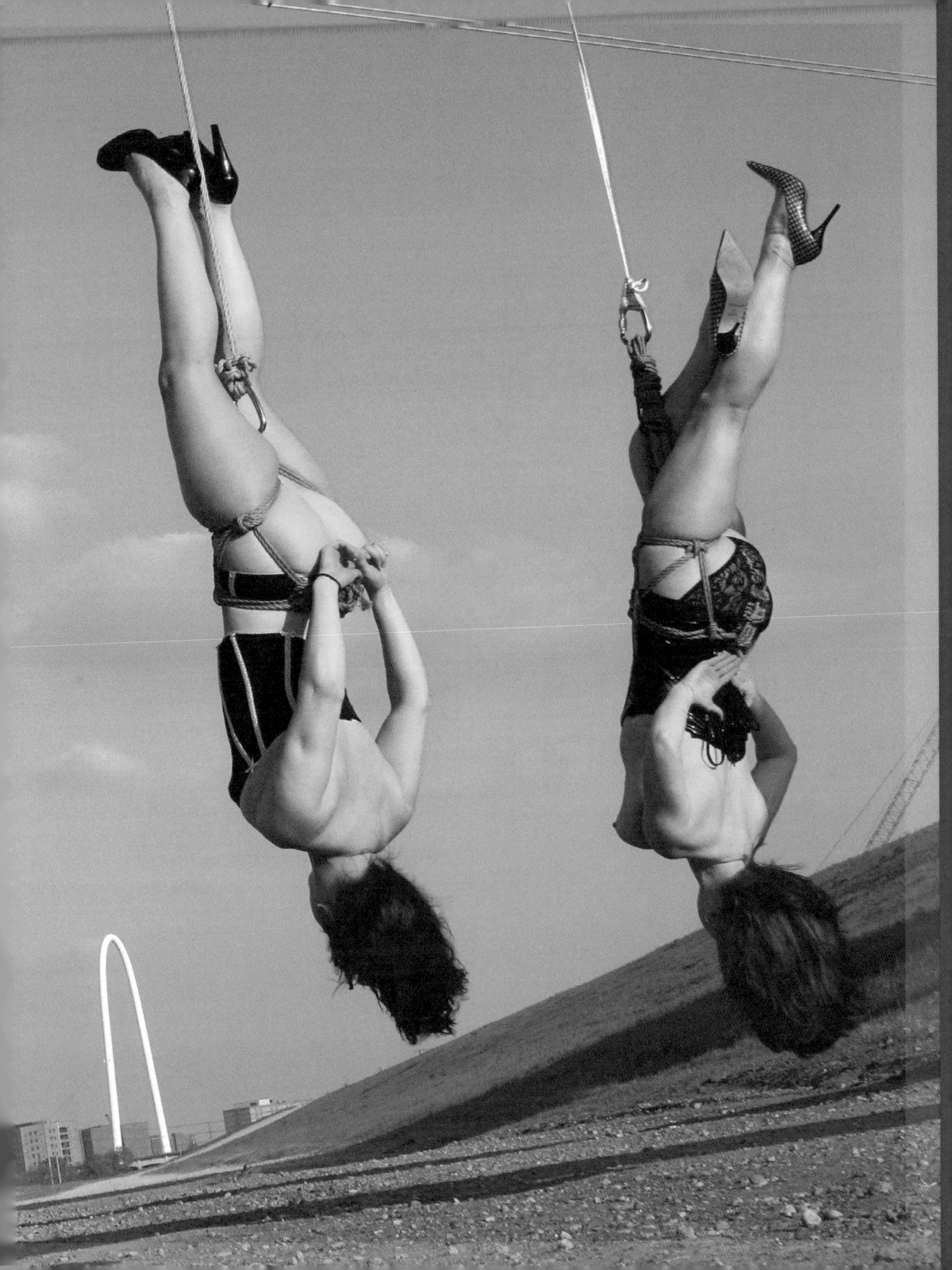

2. Attention

Avoid drawing attention to yourself and your situation. You may want to shoot photos without a flash or dress casually until the last minute. Unbundling rope, tying people, climbing ladders, using a bright flash, etc. all attract attention. Consider doing as much prep away from your target location as possible—you could even tie your TK in advance and hide it under clothing. Most important, both of you should move with confidence. (If you are carrying a load of bondage gear through a hotel lobby, for example, be discreet, know where you are going, and act like you are almost late and don't have time for pleasantries.) More than likely, if you look and act like you are supposed to be there, you won't get questioned. Wearing a black leather vest in the summer stands out. Looking at the front-desk staffer with an "Are you looking at me? Do you see what I'm doing?" face is a red flag.

3. Equipment

Lugging a tripod, lights, rigs, triggers, umbrellas, etc. along with rope even short distances can quickly become cumbersome. Be efficient but don't forget necessities. Bottoms may also want to bring something they can cover themselves quickly and easily with, like a big jacket—and keep in mind that you may be colder after you come down than when you went up, especially if you're shooting outdoors, so that big jacket or a blanket may come in handy for more than one reason.

4. Permission

Will you ask permission ahead of time or possibly have to beg forgiveness later? Public or semipublic bondage requires you to examine yourself. How will you feel if you expose a minor to rope bondage? A religious grandmother? What if someone wrecks their car while watching you? How do you feel about art vs. consent (exposing people to something they may consider indecent without their explicit consent)? What are your odds of being denied permission vs. your desire for the shot or the experience?

5. Behavior

Understand local, county, and state/province views on nudity, trespassing, permissible related behaviors, etc. Federal laws may indicate it's OK to do something, but a city ordinance or municipal code may indicate otherwise. The phrase "art project" tends to diffuse a situation quickly, especially if you're not naked or seminaked; however, security officers on private property will typically respond differently than law enforcement officers. Find municipal codes for your city and state at https://www.municode.com/library/.

6. Communication

Verbal and nonverbal communication is key to any successful scene but is especially important when the setting is unfamiliar and the bondage may be "quick and dirty." Walking each other through what you will do beforehand, and communicating while it is happening and how you are feeling in a play-by-play kind of way, will help you both stay on the same page and know what to expect when adrenaline is pumping through you in the moment. And remember that you may have to climb to a location or otherwise exert yourself physically in addition to doing any tying or being in rope, so communicate whether that affects your stamina or strength.

7. Location

It's a good idea to evaluate where you intend to tie beforehand. If you are suspending from something, what is it? How can you assess its structural integrity for suspension? It's a good idea for bottoms to learn how to do this instead of just trusting the top—it's your body on the line. For help on evaluating a hardpoint, see http://crash-restraint .com/ties/124. You might also note traffic patterns at the site as well—maybe you'll discover a regular 5 a.m. jogger or midnight patrol person, for example. Studying the site lowers the chance that you'll get a surprise visitor during your tying time.

8. Motivation

Why do you want to do this? Is there a location you want to capture, or a bondage vision burning a hole in your brain? Is a site being demolished? Is it a new build? Do you just get a thrill from tying in a public or semipublic place? If you're a bottom, are you doing it just because your top wants to, or are you equally excited about it?

9. Capturing

Are you trying to get video footage or a photograph? Often the more spectacular the shot, the more difficult it can be to capture. Can you rig and then just whip out your smartphone to get the shot? Or do you need a fish-eye lens or someone on the rooftop of an adjacent building? Would a quadcopter or drone with a cam be the best way to capture what you want?

10. Engaging

What will you do if someone shows up to your scene? Are you prepared to deal with a nosy drunk? An angry landowner or upset security officer? A park ranger or sheriff? Can you diffuse the situation? Can you patiently outwait prying eyes? This is not the time to be defensive or argumentative, even if you're 100 percent sure you're not doing anything illegal.

I once had a rope hanging from a tree within reach, by the art building at Southern Methodist University, and a girl in a chest harness covered with a sweater standing next to me when approached by police. I just pulled out my camera and started shooting random stuff until he started asking questions.

Him: *What are you doing?*

Me: *Taking photos.*

Him: *What is the rope for?*

Me: *Art project.*

Him: *What kind of art project?*

Me: *Just an urban photography thing.*

Him: *What is the rope for?*

Me: *It's part of the project.*

Him: *You're not going to hang her, are you?*

Me: *Is that even possible? No. This isn't a lynching situation. It's just an art project.*

Him: *OK. Well, I'm gonna come back and check on you two.*

Me: *OK, thanks for checking in on us. We'll be done pretty quick.*

At that point in a scenario like this, take more random shots. Some of the rope, some of the person who will be tied. None of the police officer. Just keep waiting. When they're finally gone, you'll have a small window in which to work. Diffuse the situation. Your patience may pay off. Get to work, get the shot, and go. We were walking to the car as the officer was returning.

Guerrilla bondage can be thrilling, can produce amazing photos, and can create incredibly memorable experiences. Doing your homework before you head out can make it more likely that you'll remember it for all the right reasons.

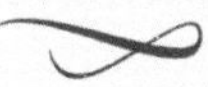

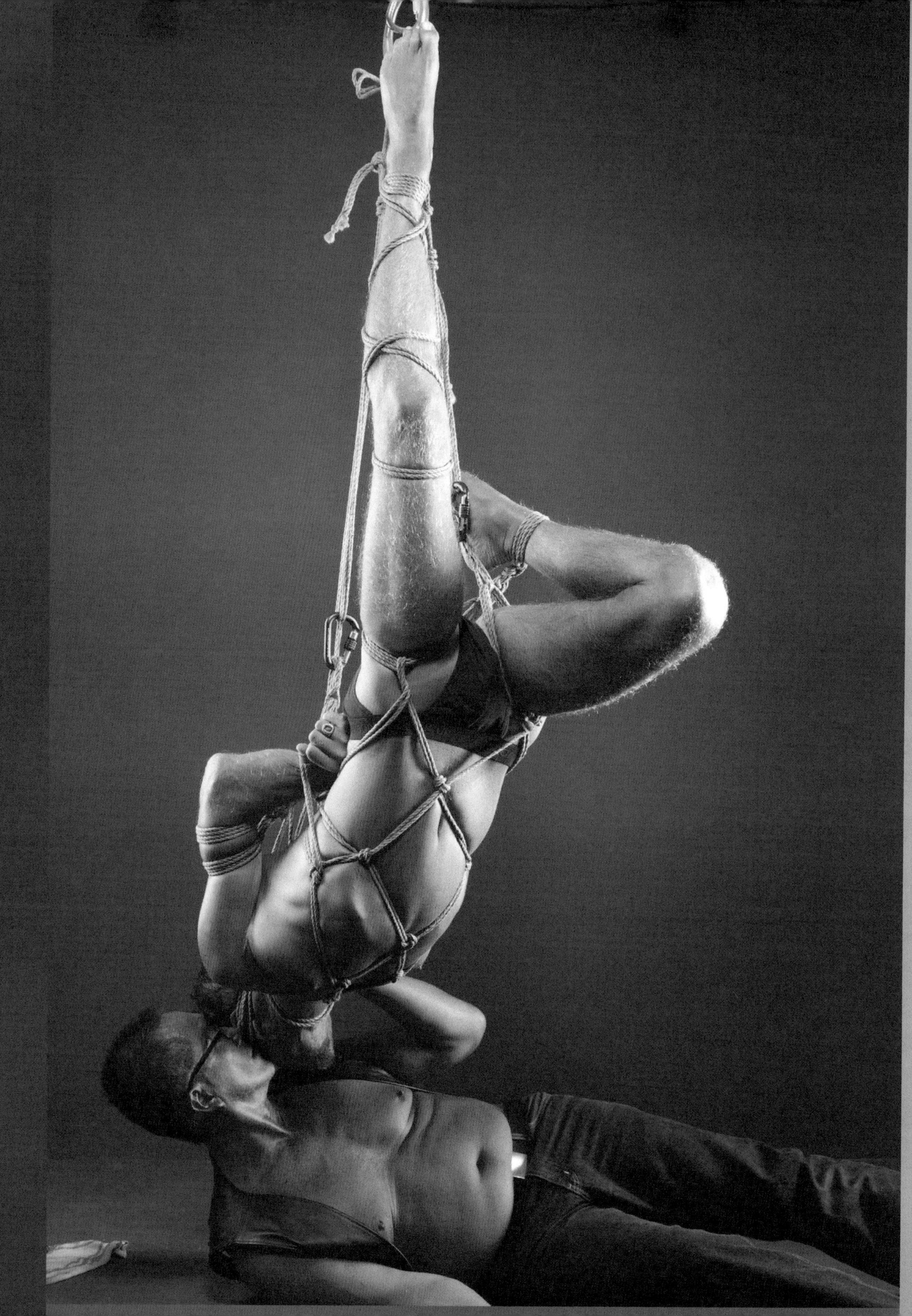

Chapter 14

A Quick and Dirty Guide to Rope Relationships

by Eri Kardos

Eri Kardos is an International Communications and Connection Coach, a speaker, and the best-selling author of the book Relationship Agreements: A Simple and Effective Guide to Strengthening Communication, Reducing Conflict, and Increasing Intimacy to Design Your Ideal Relationship. *She specializes in empowering people to choose their own adventure in relationships, career, and life. She provides private video and phone coaching sessions to clients around the globe. Visit www.EriKardos.com for more info.*

Relationships, as you probably already know, are complicated. As an International Communications and Connection Coach, I work with people around the globe to help them navigate their relationships and explore new ways of creating meaningful intimacy. People come to me because they are tired of trying to fit the mold of "find your Disney prince/princess and ride off into the sunset for happily ever after." Whether you are single, partnered, monogamous, polyamorous, confused, or curious, there is so much to explore. One of the greatest tools I have found for building intimacy and opening space for vulnerability is rope play. Yet a relationship that involves rope can be just as complicated and complex as any other meaningful relationship.

It is easy to apply your own life perspective and judgment when you are brand new to the rope world. A common theme involves projecting mainstream romantic and play partner relationship "rules" onto rope relationships. It's easy to fall prey to the idea that a rope relationship has the same structure and involves the same assumptions as one that began on a vanilla matchmaking site. But the truth is so much juicier...

Types of Rope Relationships

- *Just Me and My Rope*
- *Pickup Play*
- *Monogamous Rope and Sexual Partner (Same Person)*
- *Monogamous Rope Partner + Monogamous Sexual Partner (Different People)*
- *Monogamous Rope Partner + Polysexual (Sex With Multiple Partners)*
- *Monogamous Rope Partner + Monogamous D/s (Dominant/submissive) Partner*
- *Triads*
- *Monogamous Sexual Partner + Multiple Rope Partners*
- *Monogamous D/s Partner + Multiple Rope Partners*
- *Polyamorous With Rope*
- *Swingers With Rope*
- *Relationship Anarchy and Rope*
- *Professional Rope Bottoms + Partner, Artist, Client, and/or Employer*

Rope itself can be a form of sex—incredibly intimate, raw, powerful—even without any sexual touching. This can be a hard concept to grasp when you're first starting out, but many soon discover that rope play can be transformative and empowering for everyone involved. I've also watched many new people come out of this deep experience feeling lost, confused, and hurt. Most of these latter experiences could have

NJWaterDog and BoundToFly. Bondage by BoundToFly. Photo © 2016 Studio NoMad NYC

been better navigated had those involved had an understanding of the power of rope and the many different paths it can take, whether mentally, emotionally, or experientially. If the experience also involves additional complexity, such as multiple partners, alternative dating structures, or poor communicators, the risk for suffering is even greater.

There are some common themes throughout all the possible structures, including navigating jealousy and practicing good communication, as you'll see in the 9 Tips for Fulfilling Ropemances at the end of this chapter. But the particular flavors of rope relationships can vary. Let's break it down.

Just Me and My Rope

As a bottom, the more time I spent around rope, the more I felt drawn to it. I loved its smell, its texture, and the way it moved across my body. I didn't need to have someone else put it on me to get lost in the sensation. So I bought my own rope and found ways to engage with it alone. Sometimes it rested heavily across my eyelids while I masturbated. Other times I would wrap it around my shoulders like a scarf and wear nothing but the rope as I danced around the house, feeling sexy and empowered. Later I learned how to tie knots and rig so that I could do self-suspensions and get lost in the power of just me and my rope.

Just as being partnered with someone is not the path for everyone, so too may be your love relationship with rope. Keep your love affair private or flaunt it in the company of others through your own one-person rope scenes! There's no need to feel incomplete because you choose to have a solo relationship with rope; it's as valid as any other relationship choice. And see Chapter 11 for more on self-bondage.

Pickup Play

You've probably felt this: when you meet a stranger and discover a yummy spark between you, one that maybe then ignites into a night of passion. This same concept can be true in the rope scene. Perhaps you are out at a local party or bondage club and you feel a pull to connect with a rope top. Maybe it's the way the rope seems to dance through their hands, or the way they take command of the room. Whatever it is, you both make space for the spark to turn into a flame. This may involve getting tied up right at the event. Or it may mean finding a more private place to play. Whatever the situation, be safe and do your homework.

One way to do this is to find out how this person is connected to the community and what their experience level is before engaging—*especially* if you are playing somewhere without a dungeon monitor. Pickup play with rope, especially for suspensions, seems to be less common than for other kinds of kinky play. This may be due to the complexity involved in having a good connection, a safe space, the right equipment, and both people choosing to arrive at a playspace or an event without a play partner or previous plans.

Doing rope play on the fly can make you more cavalier about negotiating, especially when it comes to aftercare that may be needed in the days following. (Are you with me, con attendees?) I recommend that even as the spark swirling between you is threatening to drag you off to the bondage area *this instant*, try to slow down, take a deep breath, and negotiate your scene just as you would with someone you've been getting to know over weeks. This includes discussing sexual touch (or not), injuries, and aftercare, including in the days following. It's also a good idea to get

Vivi Marie and Sal Marquez. Bondage and photo by Naturalturn

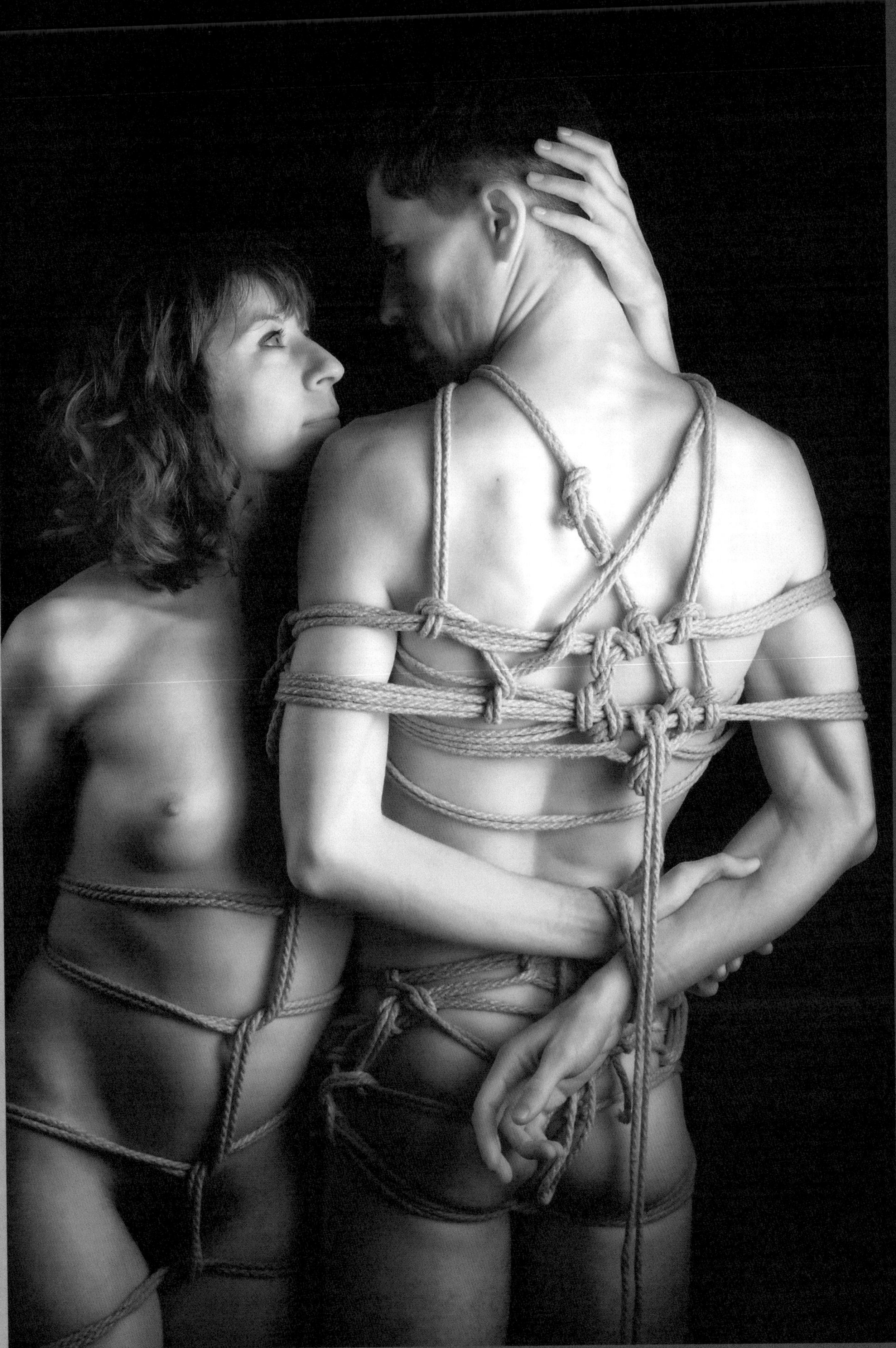

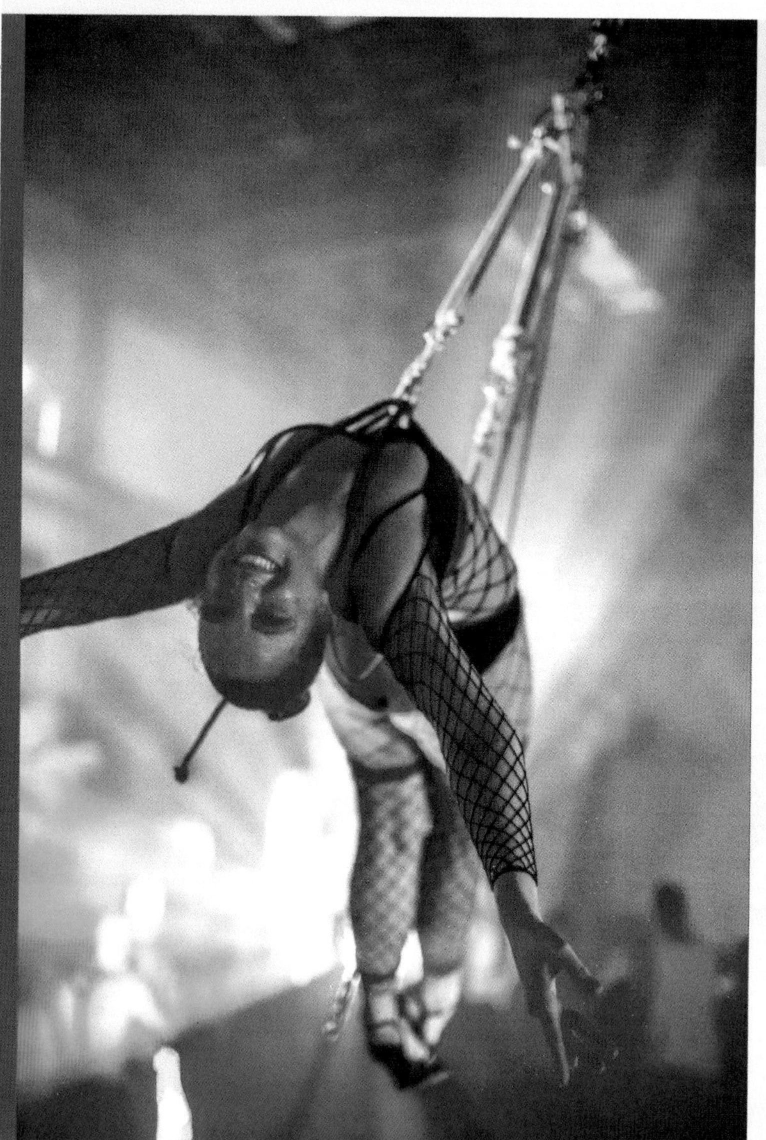

Eri Kardos. Bondage by Geo. Photo by IRDeep

your potential partner's contact info in addition to asking about training and experience.

See RemedialRopes.com for an article on negotiation basics for bondage pick-up play.[1] For general BDSM negotiation ideas, check out Jay Wiseman's long and short forms at www.evilmonk.com.[2]

Monogamous Rope and Sexual Partner (Same Person)

When the person you are partnered with is both your lover and your rope top, it can be surprisingly simple and complex all at once! Having one person for both roles certainly makes it easy to figure out who you will play with. However, it can also add complexity depending on how you both connect in these potentially different ways.

Key questions to ponder in this structure include:

How might our usual communication style need to change for rope play?

Do we both enjoy the same style of rope connection? For example, some people have a very strong D/s (Dominant/submissive) component to their rope play, while others don't. How will your rope connection work to satisfy both of you?

What is my own experience level with rope? My partner's experience level? As with any activity, becoming a skilled rope bottom or rope top takes time, patience, and practice. If one of you is more experienced than the other, it is important to clearly communicate about it and discuss how any imbalance might affect your love relationship. You could also arrange "lab time" for practicing in a purely cognitive and not sexual way. This creates a safe space for the less experienced person to get lost in the puzzle solving, self-knowledge building, and skill mastering required with little pressure from the other person to turn them on or be "perfect."

Be aware too that just as jealousy may surface in a monogamous love relationship, so too can it rear its head in the context of rope. Even if you've been with your partner for years, you may feel hurt if you see them practicing rope on someone else, even if there's no sexual or romantic intent whatsoever, or if you

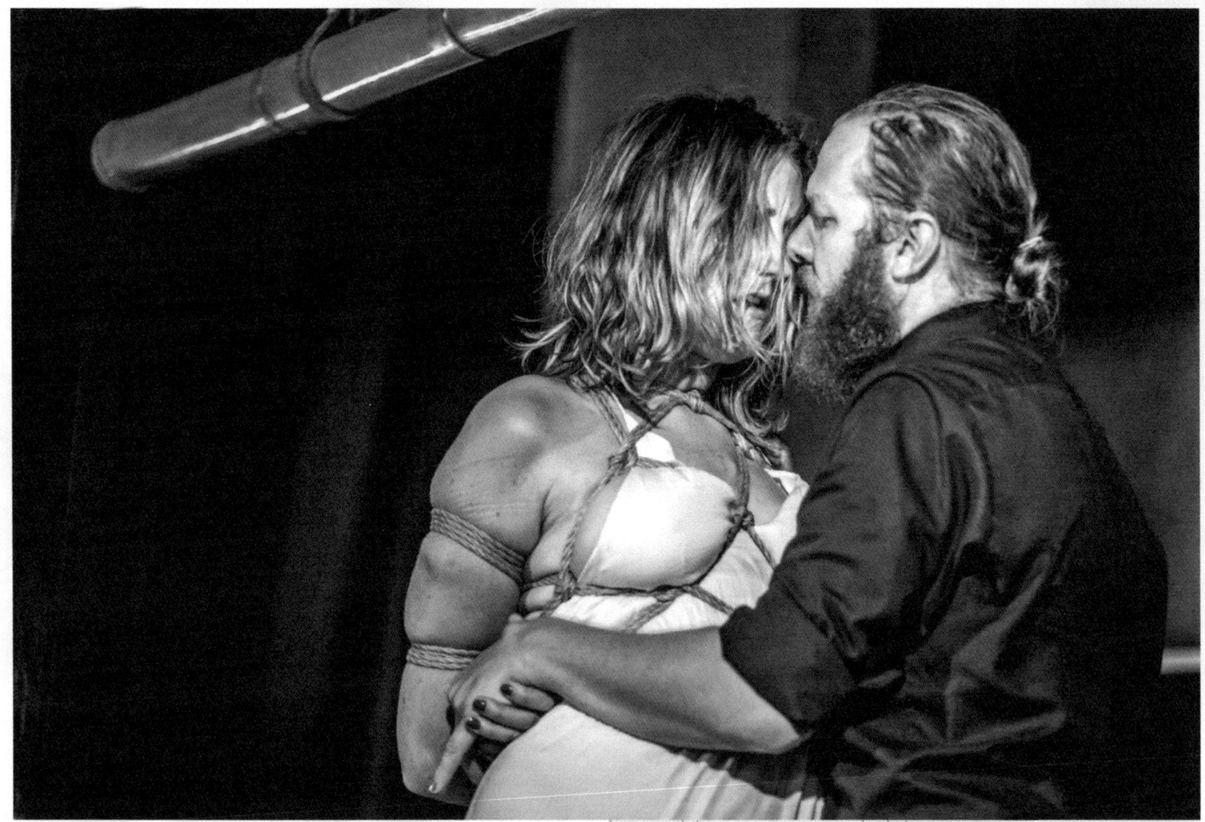

Addie and Barkas. Bondage by Barkas.
Photo by DomWithLens

see someone else in the rope world flirting with your partner or trying to tie with them. So it's important to practice open and honest communication regarding your feelings and expectations around rope, just as you would around romance and sex.

Monogamous Rope Partner + Monogamous Sexual Partner (Different People)

In this relationship structure, you engage in rope play with just one person and are sexually monogamous with a different person. This can be a wonderful, powerful dynamic for all three people. As rope can also be a form of sex without actual sexual touching, each person in this dynamic needs to feel confident in their choice of boundaries and connection styles. What are everyone's physical and emotional boundaries? How is time allocated so that everyone involved feels cared for? How will you handle conflict if/when it arises? Is the bottom responsible for navigating all dialogue between partners? How often will you all check in with one another?

Also, in this type of structure, either your sexual partner or your rope partner may already be in place when the other person comes into your life (for example, you've been in a monogamous marriage for a few years and are just beginning to explore rope, which your life partner isn't interested in). It's good to be aware that the newer partner may need extra support and encouragement to relax into the idea of coming into an established relationship. And the established partner may need extra reassurance that they aren't lower in your estimation for not being able to fulfill all of your needs or join you on all aspects of this phase of your journey.

Monogamous Rope Partner + Polysexual (Sex With Multiple Partners)

Here the rope partnership is reserved for only one person, whereas other forms of connection through play and sexuality can be shared with multiple people. Want this to have a greater chance of success? Be really clear about your dynamic with rope and how you keep it sacred with one person *before* you engage with anyone else (especially other kinksters). How will you make your partner feel special when you are drawing a line that excludes certain possibilities? How will you feel fulfilled in your rope relationship without sex, and how will you feel fulfilled in your sexual encounters without rope?

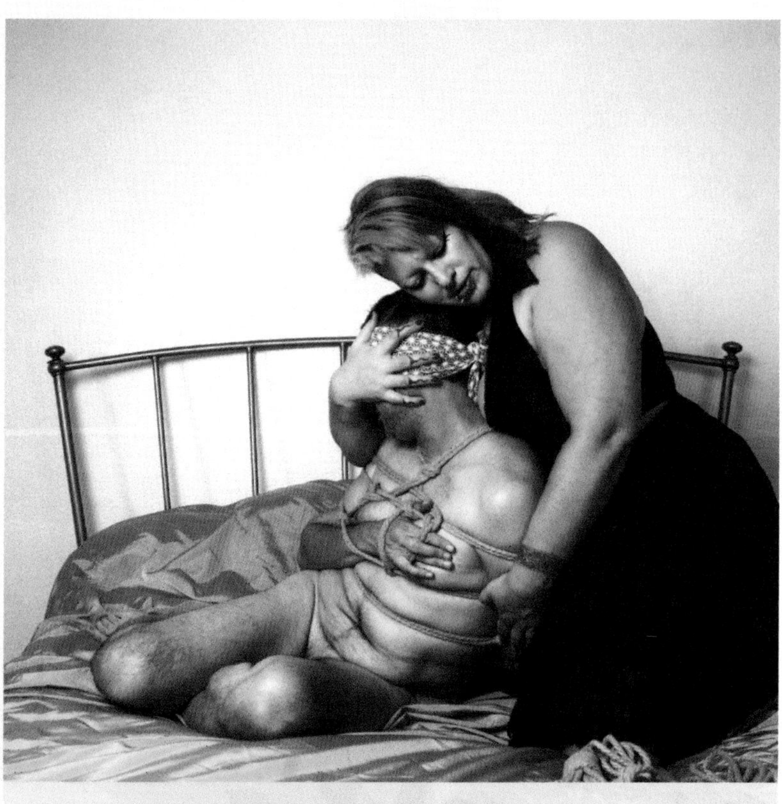

Strngrinthealps and MzFur. Bondage by MzFur. Photo by Strngrinthealps

A monogamous rope relationship when there are multiple sexual partners is rare, in my experience—people open to multiple sexual play partners are often open to multiple rope play partners. More common would be multiple rope partners but only one sexual partner, due to the perception that rope is a lower-risk activity in terms of being exposed to infections and developing long-term emotional attachments. But if you're in a monogamous rope relationship, remember that rope actually *can* create a deep emotional attachment, and that you are trusting your partner to keep your physical and emotional well-being in mind. So treat this relationship structure with the same care as you would one based on a monogamous sexual relationship with multiple rope partners.

Monogamous Rope Partner + Monogamous D/s (Dominant/submissive) Partner

Having only one rope partner and a completely separate D/s relationship tends to work best when the D/s partner is not passionate about rope play. The beauty of having multiple relationships like this is that everyone can have their needs met and passions fulfilled. However, it involves additional considerations, such as:

- A ropester wanting to tie with someone who's a submissive in a D/s relationship may have to negotiate through the dominant. The dominant may even want to be present during the scene.
- If you're the submissive, does your dominant's power extend to your rope relationship, or is it completely separate?
- If you're dominant, does your submissive have any say in who you tie with? What will you do if your submissive is jealous or otherwise doesn't want you to tie with a particular person?

Things can become tricky if either partner decides they want to explore the "other" world of rope or D/s and add it to the relationship. Having agreements (especially written) in place before such a curveball is thrown can be helpful.

Triads

Three people who are all seeing each other—usually all romantically and sexually involved and often exclusive to one another in those areas, although perhaps not exclusive regarding rope or other nonsexual kinky play—are considered a triad. Toss in some rope and you have a yummy and potentially confusing concoction! Now to decide: Who is/are the top(s)? Bottom(s)? Switch(es)? Is the role each person takes sexually the same they play when rope is added? For example, perhaps you like to bottom to rope, but you are a top within the triad. You can tell your relationship bottom(s) exactly how to put rope on you for your pleasure.

Before you engage in this dynamic, I encourage you and your other two partners to talk about how to keep a flow so that no one feels like a third wheel. And of course, if anyone has rope partners outside the triad, discuss your dynamic openly with the rope partner(s) and make sure your triad partners know about your rope partner.

Sexy tip: Create your own secret codes or signals! You can apply them to any great connection, and this works expecially well in threesomes and group sexual activities. Create two code words or signals: one for "I love you!" (or a similar sentiment you share) and one for "Something is not OK—please help." Maybe you have a certain squeeze on a limb or a strange phrase that can be uttered/moaned/shouted. Having these pre-established codes can increase the feeling of connection and safety amongst partners.

Monogamous Sexual Partner + Multiple Rope Partners

Here the central person is in a sexually and/or romantically exclusive relationship with one partner, and has the freedom to connect through rope or other kinky play with multiple other people. It's important to pre-establish boundaries with everyone involved to keep certain aspects of the heart and body sacred to the monogamous relationship, while still leaving space for fun, exploration, and connection with others. For example, you may reserve PIV (penis-in-vagina) sex for your monogamous partner, and share meaningful rope and oral sex connection with others. Or you may have no sexual contact whatsoever with partners outside of your monogamous romantic partner. This is a fairly common dynamic.

Monogamous D/s Partner + Multiple Rope Partners

In this dynamic there is only one dominant or submissive, but there is the opportunity for kinky and sexual connections with multiple others, even including a topping or bottoming role but sans the D/s power dynamic. For many years I had a Sir while I engaged in kinky, fun, and romantic play with many others in our community. Clear communication about desires and boundaries up front and whenever new connections arose helped make this dynamic easier to navigate. Other tools such as physical symbols of the D/s dynamic (for instance, collars, rings, or branding) and noting relationship statuses on FetLife can also help keep the boundaries clear.

Polyamorous With Rope

In polyamory, people maintain or are open to multiple sexual and/or romantic relationships at the same time. "Ethical" polyamory involves open knowledge and consent from everyone involved, but it's not a given—some partners in open relationships may have a "Don't ask, don't tell" policy. So be clear about what level of communication you need and what your own boundaries and practices are.

In a similar vein, a rope connection can be shared within these multiple relationships, and it's a good idea to talk about this dynamic with all parties involved. Open relationships, and especially polyamory, are still mostly uncharted waters for mainstream society. Make use of the wonderful resources available in the form of books, podcasts, websites, coaches, and therapists to help you choose your own adventure and create meaningful relationships and rope dynamics for everyone involved. (See the Resources section at the end of the chapter too.)

Swingers With Rope

There's a small contingency of people who swing with the added juiciness of rope. Swingers are people who are often coupled and have multiple sexual partners—often casual ones, like people they just met at a party—in addition to their existing romantic relationship(s). Unlike in polyamory, these relationships tend to focus on sexual connection over romantic or emotional connection. Rope usually appears for these folks during swinging parties when a partner swap happens or a new connection is made and a rope dynamic is established among the players.

If you are playing with a new partner, make sure you are honest with yourself and your partner(s) about your current state (playing with rope under the influence of drugs or alcohol isn't advised) and are able to negotiate play well. Practice negotiating *before* you meet someone you want to connect with. This will lead to smoother, faster talks so that you can get to the juicy, sexy stuff faster.

See resources for negotiating in the Pickup Play section above, and see more info in the "Safer sex and STIs" section at the end of the chapter.

Relationship Anarchy and Rope

Sometimes when multiple play partners and multiple sexual/romantic partners are involved, everyone involved engages in any relationship they see fit—without restriction, duty, or obligation. Talk about freedom and responsibility for self! This dynamic is *far* from mainstream ideas and education. It relies heavily on every person involved doing a lot of self-work and having exceptional communication skills. If/when something happens that could potentially affect anyone in their relationship network, a

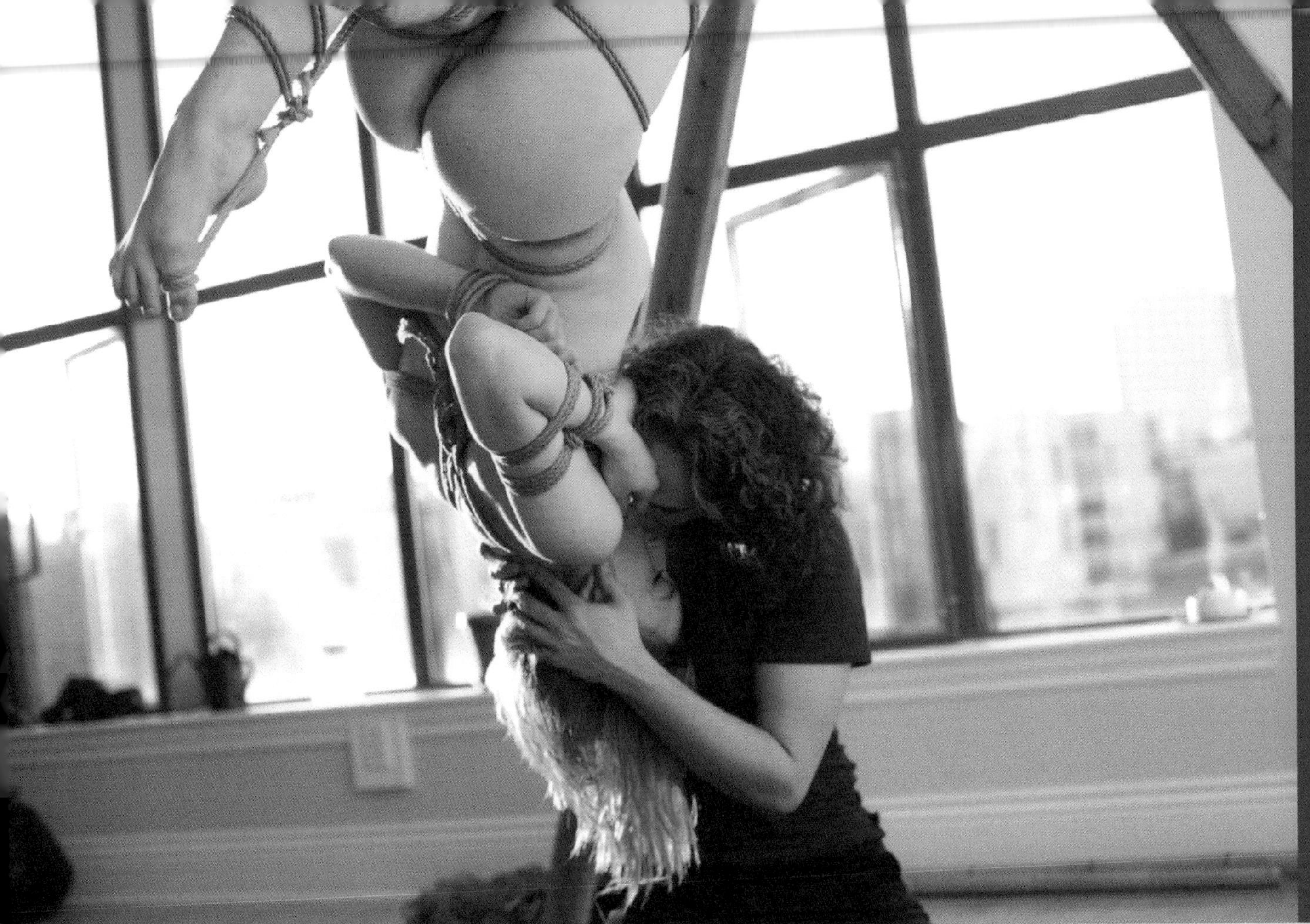

RachelKi and Topologist. Bondage by Topologist. Photo by June St. Paul

person can clearly, quickly, and honestly disseminate the news. How does rope factor in? Any way the individuals choose! It's all about the connection shared by the people involved in that moment.

Professional Rope Bottoms + Partner, Artist, Client, and/or Employer

Sometimes a rope bottom is paid, and sometimes they bottom for reasons other than pure play enjoyment or financial compenstion—the compensation might take the form of attention or a great photo, for instance. Examples in the "professional" category include performers, models, film and video actors, demo bottoms for classes and private lessons, and hired submissives and sex workers who include getting tied up as a service. It's important to understand that the motivations behind professional rope bottoming are often different than for regular play, and that the relationships created may be temporary—even if the intensity level is high. Aftercare is included less often in these scenarios, so it's good to prepare for self-care or alternate aftercare in advance. See Chapter 13 for a detailed discussion of bottoming for reasons other than pure play.

Please know also that sexual touch is something to negotiate in any kind of BDSM scenario, professional or not, and is neither a given nor a requirement whether you're getting paid or not.

Now that we've delved into specific types of rope relationships, let's look at some ideas that can be applied more generally to ropemances—and really, to any type of relationship.

9 Tips for Fulfilling Ropemances

1. Know yourself. Before you engage in any rope relationship, take some time to reflect on what you want from the experience, both as an individual and as a relationship partner. What is your intention for the connection? What boundaries do you have? What do you need for self-care before and after you engage? Ultimately, you are the only one responsible for your own pleasure, safety, and growth.

2. Communicate clearly. Once you've taken inventory of the desires and boundaries of your heart, mind, body, and soul, it is time to share them with your partner. If you are not feeling confident in your ability to voice them, try journaling and sharing via e-mail or in a letter to be opened together.

Discuss the hopes and desires of all parties involved to reduce surprises and set you up for fulfillment. What are each of your hopes and fears for this relationship? Walk through hypothetical situations and allow yourselves to talk about the scary topics; it may prevent harmful experiences from happening in the future. Take inventory of your relationship. Are there any unresolved issues you haven't brought up with your partner? Is something bothering you that has not been addressed yet? The idea that your partner can read your mind in or out of rope might sound sexy, but this is highly unlikely and can set you up for unmet expectations. In the end it is sexier and easier to navigate when everyone is on exactly the same page through clear communication.

3. Let go of assumptions and expectations. Even as you're contemplating your desires and intentions for a relationship, having specific expectations for individual rope scenes can lead to feeling unfulfilled. Instead, consider thinking of each scene as a journey that you're traveling together—you may have a destination in mind, but you may also miss something delightful along the way if you rigidly stick to a predetermined path. Similarly, if you make assumptions about your partner in or out of rope, you may be missing wonderful things they can offer you that you never even considered.

4. Set boundaries and make agreements. Before you head off on a grand new relationship adventure, take some time to talk about language use. How will you describe your relationship and boundaries to others? Do these labels mean the same thing to you both, or are there nuances you might need to clarify before you go? There is power in language—use it carefully. What agreements and boundaries might you need for this event/relationship? Sexual boundaries? Emotional boundaries? Spiritual boundaries? Think through your individual needs and consider making requests of one another. Deciding on a plan ahead of time and staying open to the idea of renegotiation allows for more comfort and ease in the dynamic. I strongly suggest creating a relationship agreement, with the understanding that it may change as you and your relationship evolve. For more in-depth information, I invite you to check out my book on the subject. You can also find many examples online; just search for "relationship agreement examples."

5. Explore how to deal with jealousy. Jealousy can be successfully navigated with a few learned skills. Kathy Labriola, author of *The Jealousy Workbook*, likens jealousy to a smoke alarm. It can be a helpful tool for alerting you to potential danger, informing you that it's time to check whether your relationship is actually on fire, or whether it is just a false alarm.

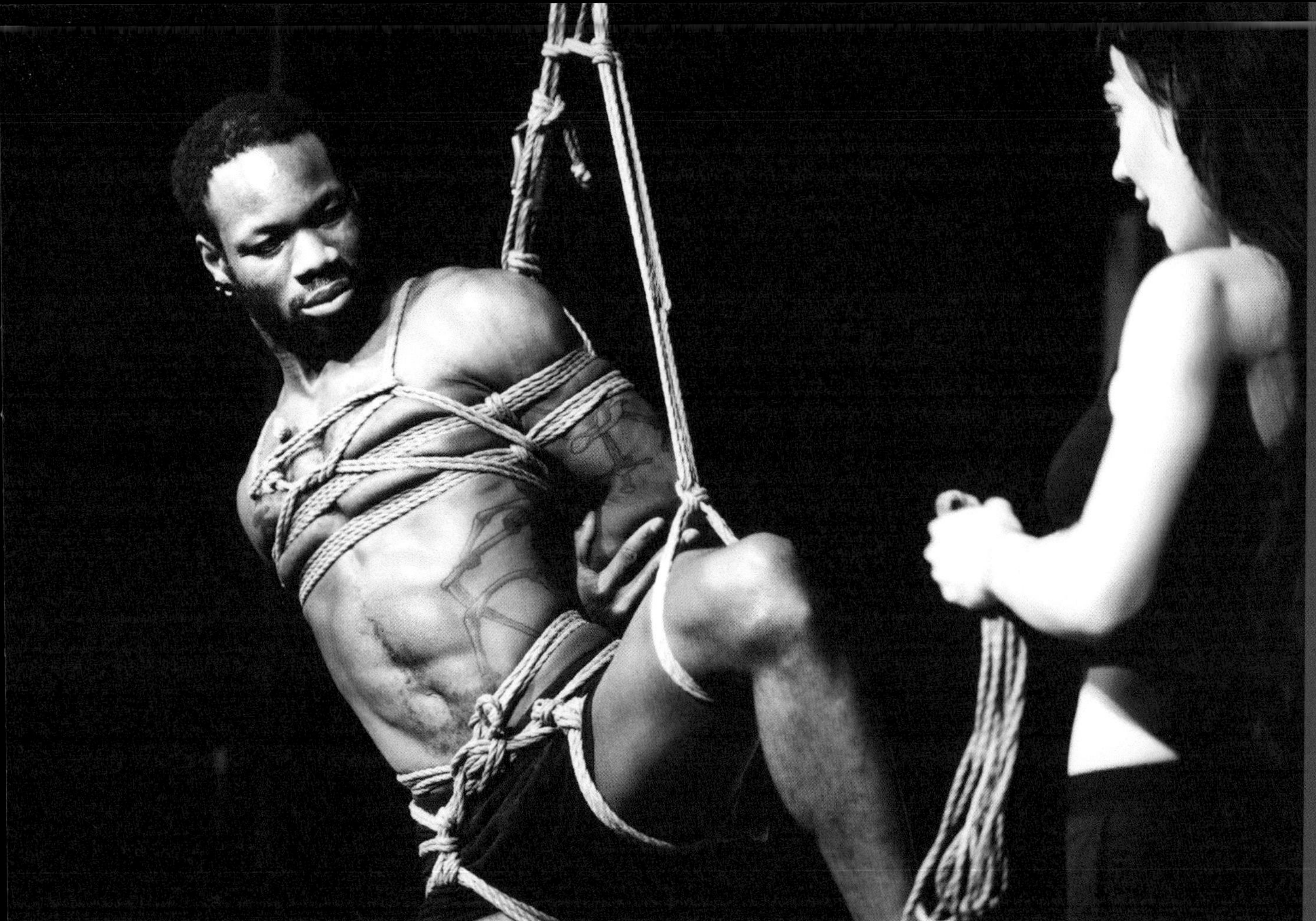

Bishop Black and Gestalta.
Bondage by Gestalta; www.gestalta.co.uk.
Photo by Amaury Grisel

It's a tool you can calibrate with practice to make sure that it doesn't go off every time you metaphorically burn a slice of toast, but does when there is an actual fire. Sadly, most of us don't use it like a tool. We assume that when the alarm goes off, there is always danger, whereas underlying fears of abandonment or being replaced are usually at play. When your partner has time and space to listen to your emotions, reactions, and fears, be sure to share them. Action is not always needed—just being heard often quiets the frightened inner voices of jealousy.

6. Care for yourself. One of the best ways you can take care of a relationship is by taking care of yourself. Rope relationships are often filled with intense experiences and highs and lows—how will you process them? Journaling, drawing, meditating, dancing, and doing yoga may all be helpful, and talking with others in similar situations may help as well. Make sure to create space and support for yourself so you can process and refresh.

7. Care for your partner. Once you have taken care of yourself, turn your attention to your partner. Do they need anything specific to feel secure and fulfilled in the relationship, whether it's words, a massage, or something else? Check in with them regularly about their desires and energy levels. Consider learning about the five love languages so that you can care for partners in a way that will resonate with them.

8. Use your calendar. We've already noted that relationships are complicated, and this can apply to

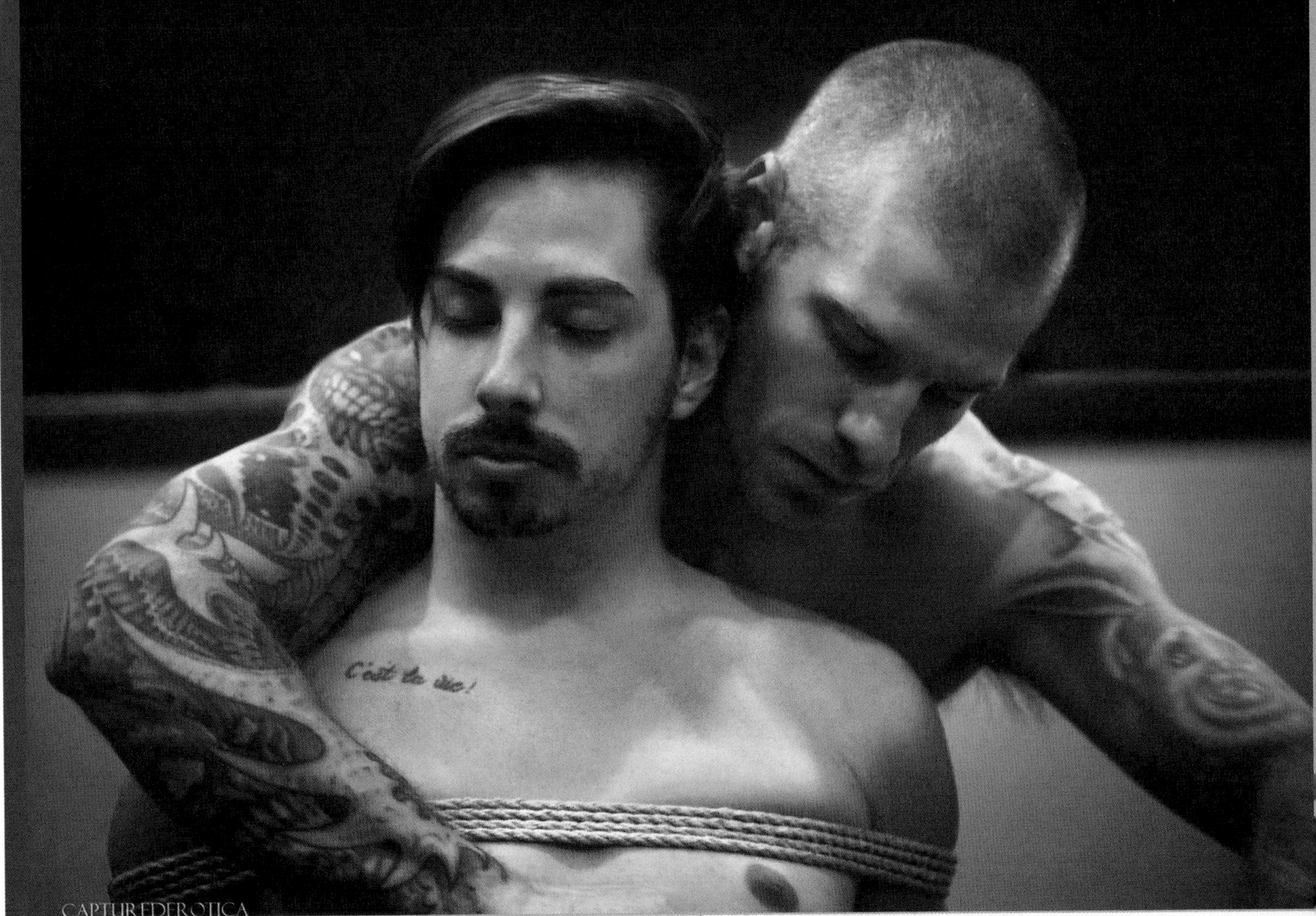

justanotherknot and FredRx.
Bondage by FredRx.
Photo by Captured Erotica; CapturedErotica.com

scheduling too. Use your calendar and spend time intentionally making space for everyone involved. Remember that rope is rarely just a matter of bodily sensations—it usually involves the hearts of people who deserve time, compassion, and respect.

9. Educate yourself. With so many wonderful resources out there on rope, kink/BDSM, open relationships, safer sex, conflict resolution, jealousy, and alternative relationship styles, you can easily find information from a variety of sources and in a way that appeals to your specific learning style.

Resources. You could schedule time with a professional coach; check out your local dungeon or sex store for classes; pick up books that address relationships, like *More Than Two* and *The Ethical Slut*; reach out to the community via FetLife and other social networking sites as well as groups like the Society of Janus and TES; and check out the plethora of online resources including podcasts, websites, videos, and forums. KinbakuToday.com and RemedialRopes.com are two great online resources for ropesters.

Safer Sex and STIs. Whether you are monogamous (or -ish), single, or in an open relationship, make sure to brush up on safer-sex education before you connect with more than one sexual partner or switch to a new monogamous partner. Get tested for STIs (sexually transmitted infections), understand your results, and

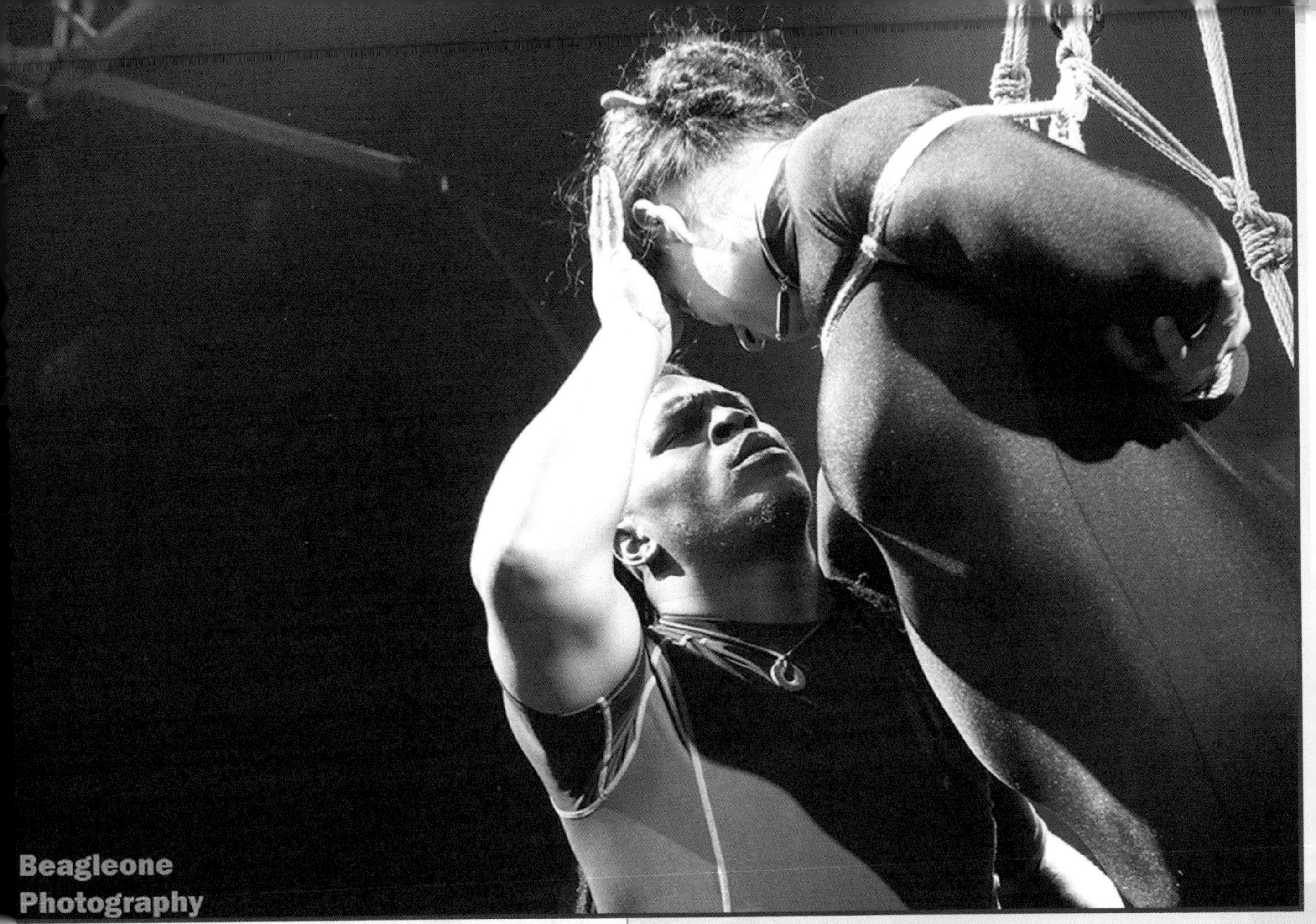

Beagleone Photography

share them honestly with your partners. If having "the talk" is difficult for you, search online for Reid Mihalko's Safer Sex Elevator Speech (it's even in video form) and practice until it becomes easy. Learn how different STIs are transmitted, think about what impact they might have on your life, and decide on your comfort level with sexual risk. STIs are often accompanied by social shaming, and it is time that we respond with compassion and educated questions instead of fear and shunning.

Wondering whether STIs can be transmitted via rope? Check out the sticky section of FetLife's Riggers & Rope Sluts group and do your own research. Many pathogens, including bacteria and viruses, can indeed live on inanimate surfaces from hours to days. Some rope bottoms keep their own rope to use on their juicy bits.

Murphy Blue and Diamond Blue.
Bondage by Murphy Blue; MurphyBlue.net.
Photo by Tony Morales/Beagleone Photography

• • •

Editor's note: I hope everything everything discussed here, and in all the other chapters, will help you enjoy your rope relationships and scenes even more. Happy and safe tying! —*Evie*

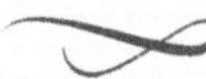

Notes

1. http://www.remedialropes.com/bondage-safety-articles/bondage-pick-up-play-real-talk-aka-bondage-negotiation-basics/
2. http://www.evilmonk.org/a/wiseman10.cfm
3. Kramer, A., Schwebke, I., and Kampf, G. "How long do nosocomial pathogens persist on inanimate surfaces? A systematic review." *BMC Infectious Diseases* 2006 6:130.

Acknowledgments and Resources

I am deeply grateful to everyone who made this book the celebration of community that it is. First and foremost, thank you to MrKiltYou for always being there and being a voice of reason in my crazy moments, as well as for being such an awesome performance partner, and to True Blue for being an eternal inspiration and a truly beautiful soul with such a deep heart. Thank you to MJ Maxam for realizing early on that this book was as much about the photos as about the words, and for all the encouragement along with the amazing book design. Thank you to David Delp not just for designing a stellar cover (again) but for keeping my string lit when so many bulbs were out.

Many thanks to The Silence. You may be quiet, but your talent, passion, and dedication to creating beautiful memories speak volumes.

Thank you to Neuromancer28, Shay Tiziano, fuoco, MissDoctor, and Eri Kardos for contributing entire chapters and for being so good-natured about the editing process—I'm honored to have collaborated with you! The same goes for Lee Harrington, Clover, Peter Acworth, Hedwig, Morgana Muses, Naiia, Lady_Hunny_Bunny, Dallas Kink, Erin Houdini, Barbary Rose, and Cupcake SinClair, who dealt with the back-and-forth with such grace and good humor. Special shout-outs to Shay for the extra reviewing help, for being a cornerstone of kink education, and for creating opportunities like Twisted Windows for kinksters to share their stuff; and to Peter for always being supportive and for furthering the acceptance of kink on a grand scale.

Thank you to each and every survey respondent, photographer, model, and tyer throughout. You've put a piece of your heart out there, and your contributions have brought the soul to this book. Special thanks to Terri F. and SatineAngelic for the enthusiasm and energy they brought as models to the longer shoots; to iambic9, BoBoChee, Naturalturn, Marcuslikesit, and Marshall Bradford, who all responded kindly to "Can I please have just one more photo?"; to Zetsu Nawa, Demonsix, Retrotie, and Anastasia Panagiotidis for giving up a weekend day to make our L.A. shoot rock; to Ian Snow for the insightful teachings; to Bri Burning for the helpful commentary; to Glü Wür for being a visionary artist; and to Topologist for letting us shoot in his studio on the fly without batting an eye.

Thank you to Ebi McKnotty and Goodmosttimes, and to Anna Bones of Anatomie Studio, for the helpful leads and for all of their educational efforts.

Thank you to Yuki Sakurai for all of her hard work translating the previous book into Japanese and patiently answering all of my questions. And to Sin, both for orchestrating the translation and for helping market it in Japan. Thank you to Daniel S. for all the marketing help and for being a good friend to boot.

Thank you to Stefanos for being an integral part of the S.F. kink scene as an unflaggingly enthusiastic leader. Thank you to _impysh_ for letting us shoot the cover in her beautiful backyard, and to WickedlyKinky and nano_bites for the proofreading help.

Thank you to all the rope bottoms in our local meetups and other discussion groups, and to those who have shared their bottoming wisdom through writing. Your gems of insight have been so valuable.

Thank you to S.H., J.B., and Caroline Carrington for all the personal and emotional support, and to C.V. for keeping my secrets and loving me through thick and thin.

And thank you of course to L.H., light of my life and joy of my heart. I love you more than all the stars.

Select Resources

For clickable versions, visit my EvieVane profile on FetLife. Also, this is by no means a complete list.

FetLife Groups

Ask a Rope Bottom, Rope Bottom's Roundtable, Riggers & Rope Sluts, Rope Incident Reports

Also on FetLife

TwistTies's extensive list of resources for rope bottoms, including many personal essays: https://fetlife.com/users/9434/posts/2622521

Guilty's "Bondage Safety for Bottoms": https://fetlife.com/users/3765943

Tifereth's Makeup for Rope Bondage Commandments: https://fetlife.com/users/1140442/posts/1392399

Videos

"Anatomy for Rope Bondage" by IPCookieMonster and co.: https://youtu.be/u9-VzX9_pzg

Evie Vane channel on YouTube

"Bombproof Bottoming: Suspension from Sub's Side with Tifereth and Cannon": https://www.kink.com/shoot/36252

"Neural Glides for Ulnar, Median, and Radial Nerves" by Doctor Jo: https://youtu.be/yZJ1MfKqByY

"Femoral Nerve Guide Floss 1" by Rehab My Patient: https://youtu.be/OjbDUpypE7E

Websites

RemedialRopes.com—Devoted to risk-awareness-based education for bottoms and tops

Crash-restraint.com—Includes info on nerves and self-check-ins, a downloadable list of do's and don'ts for bottoms and tops, and how to evaluate a hardpoint for suspension

KinbakuToday.com—Articles by bottoms and tops (news, opinion, and history) plus photo galleries

Fit & Bendy (http://www.fitandbendy.com/)—Flexibility and contortion training

Writings and More

"A Guide for Rope Bottoms and Bondage Models" by Clover: http://kinkyclover.com/resources/rope-bottom-guide/

"Negotation and Negotiation Forms" by Jay Wiseman: http://www.evilmonk.org/a/wiseman10.cfm

"Mobilization of the Plexus Brachialis Nerve Branch by Sin: http://www.kinbakutoday.com/mobilization-of-the-plexus-brachialis-nerve-branch/

Frozen Meursault's downloadable Nerve Injury Reference Card: http://www.frozenmeursault.com/nerve-injury-reference-card/

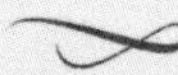

Dylan Cabral Stevens. Bondage and photo by Marc Taylor

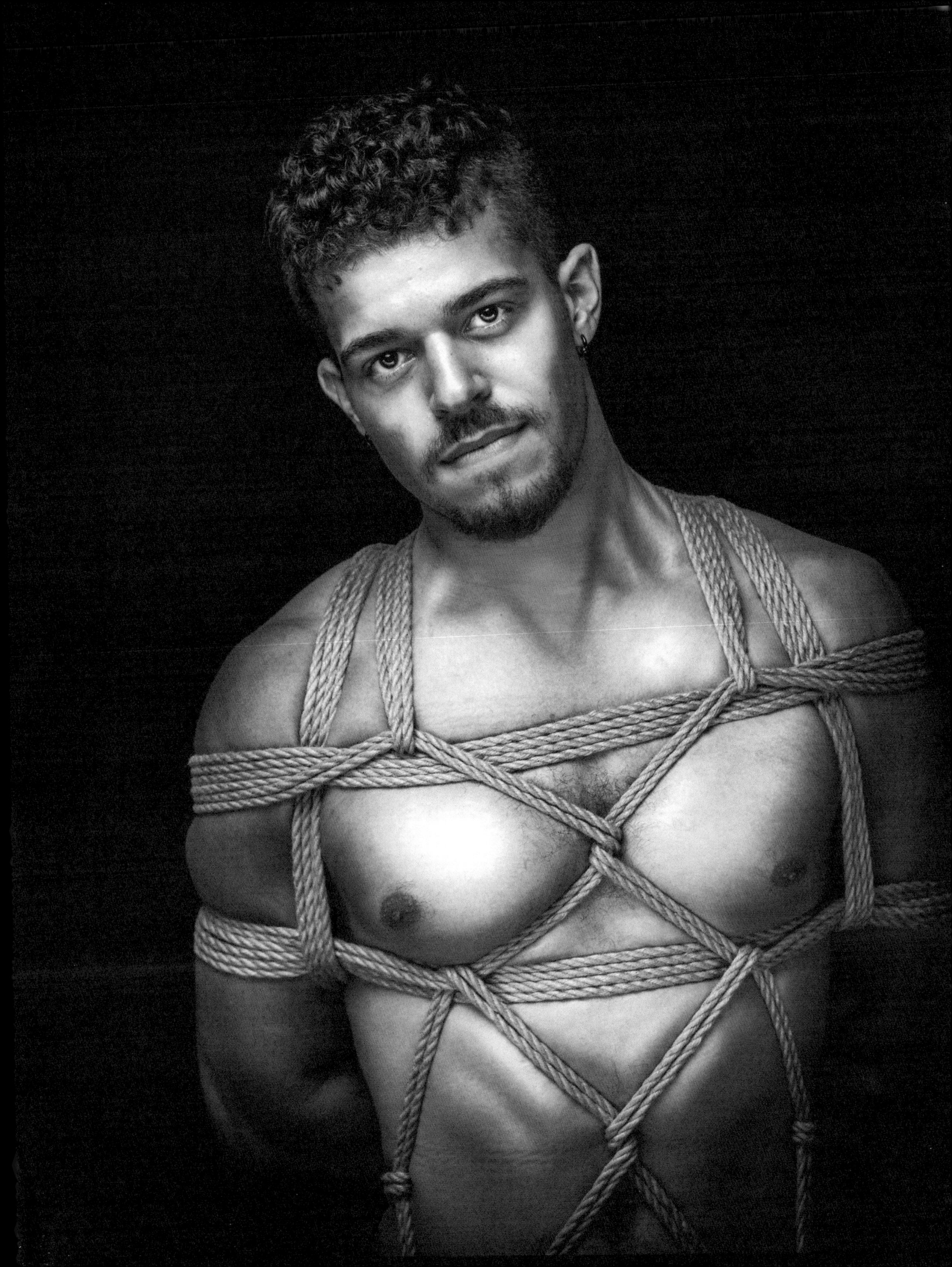

Printed in Great Britain
by Amazon

58190036R00113